Weight Management

State of the Science and Opportunities for Military Programs

Subcommittee on Military Weight Management
Committee on Military Nutrition Research
Food and Nutrition Board

INSTITUTE OF MEDICINE
OF THE NATIONAL ACADEMIES

THE NATIONAL ACADEMIES PRESS
Washington, D.C.
www.nap.edu

THE NATIONAL ACADEMIES PRESS 500 Fifth Street, N.W. Washington, DC 20001

NOTICE: The project that is the subject of this report was approved by the Governing Board of the National Research Council, whose members are drawn from the councils of the National Academy of Sciences, the National Academy of Engineering, and the Institute of Medicine. The members of the committee responsible for the report were chosen for their special competences and with regard for appropriate balance.

Support for this project was provided by U.S. Army Medical Research and Materiel Command through contract no. DAMD17-99-1-9478. The U.S. Army Medical Research Acquisition Activity, 820 Chandler Street, Fort Detrick, MD 21702-5014, is the awarding and administering acquisition office. The views presented in this report are those of the Subcommittee on Military Weight Management and are not necessarily those of the funding agency.

International Standard Book Number 0-309-08996-4 (Pbk)
International Standard Book Number 0-309-52681-7 (PDF)
Library of Congress Control Number: 2003111596

Additional copies of this report are available from the National Academies Press, 500 Fifth Street, N.W., Lockbox 285, Washington, DC 20055; (800) 624-6242 or (202) 334-3313 (in the Washington metropolitan area); Internet, http://www.nap.edu.

For more information about the Institute of Medicine, visit the IOM home page at: **www.iom.edu.**

Printed in the United States of America.

The serpent has been a symbol of long life, healing, and knowledge among almost all cultures and religions since the beginning of recorded history. The serpent adopted as a logotype by the Institute of Medicine is a relief carving from ancient Greece, now held by the Staatliche Museen in Berlin.

"Knowing is not enough; we must apply.
Willing is not enough; we must do."
—Goethe

INSTITUTE OF MEDICINE
OF THE NATIONAL ACADEMIES

Shaping the Future for Health

THE NATIONAL ACADEMIES

Advisers to the Nation on Science, Engineering, and Medicine

The **National Academy of Sciences** is a private, nonprofit, self-perpetuating society of distinguished scholars engaged in scientific and engineering research, dedicated to the furtherance of science and technology and to their use for the general welfare. Upon the authority of the charter granted to it by the Congress in 1863, the Academy has a mandate that requires it to advise the federal government on scientific and technical matters. Dr. Bruce M. Alberts is president of the National Academy of Sciences.

The **National Academy of Engineering** was established in 1964, under the charter of the National Academy of Sciences, as a parallel organization of outstanding engineers. It is autonomous in its administration and in the selection of its members, sharing with the National Academy of Sciences the responsibility for advising the federal government. The National Academy of Engineering also sponsors engineering programs aimed at meeting national needs, encourages education and research, and recognizes the superior achievements of engineers. Dr. Wm. A. Wulf is president of the National Academy of Engineering.

The **Institute of Medicine** was established in 1970 by the National Academy of Sciences to secure the services of eminent members of appropriate professions in the examination of policy matters pertaining to the health of the public. The Institute acts under the responsibility given to the National Academy of Sciences by its congressional charter to be an adviser to the federal government and, upon its own initiative, to identify issues of medical care, research, and education. Dr. Harvey V. Fineberg is president of the Institute of Medicine.

The **National Research Council** was organized by the National Academy of Sciences in 1916 to associate the broad community of science and technology with the Academy's purposes of furthering knowledge and advising the federal government. Functioning in accordance with general policies determined by the Academy, the Council has become the principal operating agency of both the National Academy of Sciences and the National Academy of Engineering in providing services to the government, the public, and the scientific and engineering communities. The Council is administered jointly by both Academies and the Institute of Medicine. Dr. Bruce M. Alberts and Dr. Wm. A. Wulf are chair and vice chair, respectively, of the National Research Council.

www.national-academies.org

SUBCOMMITTEE ON MILITARY WEIGHT MANAGEMENT

RICHARD L. ATKINSON, JR. (*chair*), Obesity Institute, MedStar Research Institute, Washington, D.C.

JOHN E. VANDERVEEN (*vice-chair*), San Antonio, Texas

WILLIAM H. DIETZ, Division of Nutrition and Physical Activity, Centers for Disease Control and Prevention, Atlanta, Georgia

JOHN D. FERNSTROM, UPMC Health System Weight Management Center, University of Pittsburgh School of Medicine, Pittsburgh, Pennsylvania

ARTHUR FRANK, Weight Management Program, The George Washington University, Washington, D.C.

BARBARA C. HANSEN, Obesity and Diabetes Research Center, University of Maryland School of Medicine, Baltimore

STEVEN B. HEYMSFIELD, Human Body Composition Laboratory and Weight Control Unit, St. Luke's-Roosevelt Hospital, New York

ROBIN B. KANAREK, Graduate School of Arts and Sciences, Tufts University, Medford, Massachusetts.

BARBARA J. MOORE, Shape Up America!, Washington, D.C.

Staff

MARY I. POOS, Study Director

LESLIE J. VOGELSANG, Research Assistant (from October 2001)

HARLEEN K. SETHI, Senior Project Assistant (from February 2002)

TAZIMA A. DAVIS, Senior Project Assistant (through November 2001)

COMMITTEE ON MILITARY NUTRITION RESEARCH

JOHN E. VANDERVEEN (*chair*), San Antonio, Texas
BRUCE R. BISTRIAN, Department of Medicine, Harvard Medical School, Boston, Massachusetts
JOHANNA T. DWYER, Frances Stern Nutrition Center, Tufts New England Medical Center, Boston, Massachusetts
HELEN W. LANE, Johnson Space Center, National Aeronautics and Space Administration, Houston, Texas
MELINDA M. MANORE, Department of Nutrition and Food Management, Oregon State University, Corvallis
WILLIAM P. MORGAN, Sport Physiology Laboratory, University of Wisconsin, Madison
PATRICK M. O'NEIL, Weight Management Center, Medical University of South Carolina, Charleston
ESTHER M. STERNBERG, Neuroendocrine Immunology and Behavior Section, National Institute of Mental Health, Bethesda, Maryland
BEVERLY J. TEPPER, Department of Food Science, Rutgers University, New Brunswick, New Jersey

U.S. Army Grant Representative
LTC KARL E. FRIEDL, USA, Military Operational Medicine Research Program, U.S. Army Medical Research and Materiel Command, Fort Detrick, Frederick, Maryland

Staff
MARY I. POOS, Project Director
LESLIE J. VOGELSANG, Research Assistant
HARLEEN K. SETHI, Senior Project Assistant

FOOD AND NUTRITION BOARD

Reviewers

This report has been reviewed in draft form by individuals chosen for their diverse perspectives and technical expertise, in accordance with procedures approved by the NRC's Report Review Committee. The purpose of this independent review is to provide candid and critical comments that will assist the institution in making its published report as sound as possible and to ensure that the report meets institutional standards for objectivity, evidence, and responsiveness to the study charge. The review comments and draft manuscript remain confidential to protect the integrity of the deliberative process. We wish to thank the following individuals for their review of this report:

Catherine M. Angotti, Occupational Health, National Aeronautics and Space Administration; George A. Brooks, Department of Integrative Biology, University of California, Berkley; Anthony G. Comuzzie, Department of Genetics, Southwest Foundation for Biomedical Research; James L. Early, Department of Preventive Medicine, University of Kansas-Wichita; Esther F. Myers, Scientific Affairs and Research, American Dietetic Association; Janet Rankin, Department of Human Nutrition, Foods, and Exercise, Virginia Polytechnic Institute and State University.

Although the reviewers listed above have provided many constructive comments and suggestions, they were not asked to endorse the conclusions or recommendations nor did they see the final draft of the report before its release. The review of this report was overseen by Shiriki Kumanyika, Center for Clinical Epidemiology and Biostatistics, University of Pennsylvania School of Medicine. Appointed by the Institute of Medicine, she was responsible for making certain that an independent examination of this report was carried out in accordance with institutional procedures and that all review comments were carefully considered. Responsibility for the final content of this report rests entirely with the authoring subcommittee and the institution.

Preface

This publication is the latest in a series of reports based on reviews of the scientific literature and workshops sponsored by the Committee on Military Nutrition Research (CMNR) of the Food and Nutrition Board (FNB), Institute of Medicine, the National Academies. A subcommittee of CMNR, the Subcommittee on Military Weight Management, was appointed to organize a workshop and prepare a report based on information presented at a workshop, a review of the scientific literature, and the subcommittee's expertise and deliberations. Other workshops or symposia conducted by CMNR have dealt with topics such as food components to enhance performance; nutritional needs in hot, cold, and high-altitude environments; body composition and physical performance; nutrition and physical performance; cognitive testing methodology; fluid replacement and heat stress; and antioxidants and oxidative stress. These workshops form part of the response that CMNR provides to the Commander of the U.S. Army Medical Research and Materiel Command (USAMRMC) regarding issues brought to the committee through the Military Operational Medicine Research Program at Fort Detrick, Maryland, and the Military Nutrition Division of the U.S. Army Research Institute of Environmental Medicine at Natick, Massachusetts.

HISTORY OF THE COMMITTEE

The CMNR was established in October 1982 following a request by the Assistant Surgeon General of the Army that the Board on Military Supplies of the National Academy of Sciences set up a special committee to advise the U.S. Department of Defense (DOD) on the need for and conduct of nutrition research and related issues. This committee was transferred to the oversight of FNB in 1983. The committee's primary tasks are to identify factors that may critically influence the physical and mental performance of military personnel under all environmental extremes; to identify knowledge gaps and recommend research that would remedy these deficiencies; to recommend approaches for studying the relationship of diet to physical and mental performance; and to review and advise on military feeding standards.

As a standing committee of IOM, the membership of CMNR changes periodically. However, the disciplines represented consistently have included human nutrition, nutritional biochemistry, performance physiology, food science, dietetics, psychology, and clinical medicine. For issues that require broader expertise than exists within the committee, CMNR has convened workshops, utilized consultants, or appointed subcommittees with expertise in the desired area to provide additional state-of-the art scientific knowledge and informed opinion to aid in deliberations.

BACKGROUND

Following the release of the 1995 IOM report, *Recommendations for Research on the Health of Military Women,* CMNR was asked to review existing military policies governing body composition and fitness as part of the Defense Women's Health Research Program. In particular, the committee was asked to determine if existing body composition and appearance standards for women were in conflict with body composition requirements for task performance, and whether those same standards might actually interfere with readiness by encouraging chronic dieting, inadequate nutrient intake, or dangerous eating practices. In March 1998, the CMNR Subcommittee on Body Composition, Nutrition, and Health of Military Women released its report, *Assessing Readiness in Military Women: The Relationship to Body Composition, Nutrition, and Health*. This report made a number of key recommendations:

- Incorporate the use of body mass index and fitness assessment into the current two-tiered body composition assessment procedures.
- Increase emphasis on fitness for readiness in military personnel.
- Develop and validate a single service-wide circumference equation for the assessment of women's body fat.
- Develop task-specific, gender-neutral strength and endurance tests and standards for use in determining placements in military occupational specialties requiring moderate and heavy lifting.
- Encourage military personnel to achieve and maintain healthy weights through a continuous exercise and fitness program.
- Provide nutrition education and ongoing counseling if weight loss is a goal.

Similar recommendations had been made in a 1992 CMNR report, *Body Composition and Physical Performance,* which first suggested that a military body composition standard should be based primarily on the ability to perform required physical tasks and secondarily on long-term health implications, and that all the services should develop job-related physical performance standards for accession into military service.

THE COMMITTEE'S TASK

In July 1999, CMNR was requested to review existing data on (1) optimal components of a weight-management program, (2) the role of age, gender, and ethnicity in weight management, and (3) current DOD activities in weight management; and to provide recommendations for military weight-management programs. This request for a review of effective military and civilian weight-loss and weight-management programs originated from the Director of Military Operational Medicine Research at USAMRMC. Subsequently, a subgroup of CMNR participated in a series of conference calls with USAMRMC and CMNR staff to identify the key areas that should be reviewed and to solicit suggestions for names of scientists who were active in the research fields of interest to serve as workshop speakers or as members of the subcommittee.

The subcommittee was appointed in September 1999, and on October 24–27, 1999, it convened a workshop in response to the request from the Army. The purpose of this workshop was to gather a group of experts to:

- Share knowledge and experience in managing weight control within the services,
- Gain relevant knowledge and experience from industry and academia,
- Develop a consensus toward a more standard DOD-wide approach to weight management that utilizes state-of-the-art knowledge and practices,
- Examine current interventions and those under development, particularly in the pharmaceutical industry, and
- Evaluate their appropriateness for military application or the need for further research.

The subcommittee was charged to identify the most effective interventions for weight loss and maintenance, particularly those most effective for the *nonobese* overweight individuals found in the military setting. Specifically, the subcommittee was asked to address the following questions:

1. What are the essential components of an effective weight/fat loss program, and the most effective strategies to *sustain* weight loss?
2. How do age and gender influence success in weight-management programs? Should age be considered in weight/fat standards, and in weight-management programs and interventions?
3. Which strategies would be most and least effective in a military setting? Should military weight/fat loss programs involve direct participation inter-

ventions, or only monitoring and guidance? Should military programs be more proactive in identifying and discouraging ineffective or dangerous weight-loss practices? Is a warning or cautionary zone prior to enrollment into a weight-control program an effective strategy? When should duty time be authorized for participation in intervention strategies for weight/fat loss?

4. To what extent should weight-control programs/policies be standardized across the services, versus tailored to the individual service, installation or unit? What are the advantages and disadvantages of standardization? Is the provision of state-of-the-art techniques and knowledge a rationale for standardization?

5. How can diet be effectively dealt with as a weight-management component in the military setting? Should pharmacological treatment (anorexiants) be considered for use in the military? In what cases? What factors bear on this decision?

6. How should resistiveness for weight/fat control be dealt with?

7. What are the knowledge gaps in weight-management programs relative to the military? What research is needed?

To accomplish this task, the subcommittee's workshop brought together the personnel responsible for both DOD-wide and service-specific weight-control program policies; a representation of military weight-control program leaders and innovators; and key military, academic, and industry researchers.

The subcommittee reviewed the workshop presentations and the relevant scientific literature and developed a consensus statement on the optimal content for a weight-control program that could be utilized across the services. In the extensive interval since the workshop, the subcommittee has updated their report, incorporating recent references and military data where they were available. In November 2002, DOD released its revised Instruction 1308.3, *DOD Physical Fitness and Body Fat Program Procedures*, and has made some important changes, which the subcommittee applauds. These new guidelines are noted throughout the report as appropriate.

ORGANIZATION OF THE REPORT

Chapter 1 of this report provides background information on the current demographics of the U.S. population. It then describes the military's interest in body-weight and body-fat standards and the implications of these standards for health, performance, fitness, and appearance. Weight standards and weight-management programs currently provided by each of the services and issues of concern related to these programs are described in Chapter 2. Chapter 3 briefly reviews the factors that affect body weight, and Chapter 4 reviews the strategies for weight management. Chapter 5 provides the subcommittee's specific responses to the military's questions; Chapter 6 presents the subcommittee's conclusions and recommendations and identifies research needs. The workshop agenda and speaker abstracts are presented in Appendix A, and the biographical sketches of the speakers and subcommittee members appear in Appendixes B and C, respectively.

ACKNOWLEDGMENTS

It is my pleasure as chairman of the Subcommittee on Military Weight Management to acknowledge the contributions of the FNB staff. Their dedication in the planning and organization of the workshop and the editing of this report made it possible for the subcommittee to respond to the Army's request. In particular, I wish to acknowledge the extensive efforts of Mary I. Poos, the senior staff officer for CMNR. She worked diligently with the subcommittee members in securing the expert panel of speakers and organizing the program for the workshop into coherent sessions, and she contributed substantially to the writing and final updating of the report in response to review. I also wish to acknowledge Ms. Leslie Vogelsang, research assistant to CMNR, for her diligence in checking references and finding missing references; and Ms. Harleen Sethi and Ms. Tazima Davis, senior project assistants to CMNR, and Ms. Gail Spears, staff editor to FNB, for their work in preparing the report drafts and final manuscript.

I wish to commend the workshop speakers for their excellent contributions to the workshop: their abstracts, participation in discussions, and their willingness to take time from very busy schedules to prepare and deliver outstanding presentations made it possible for the subcommittee to conduct a review of the topic area and prepare this report. Their thoughtful responses to questions posed by subcommittee members and workshop participants also contributed immeasurably to the quality of the review. It would be neglectful not to mention the many experts who attended this open meeting at their own initiative and expense. Their questions and comments contributed in no small measure to broadening the exchange of scientific information.

I express my deepest appreciation to the members of the subcommittee who participated extensively during the workshop and in discussions and preparation of the summary and recommendations in this report.

RICHARD L. ATKINSON, *Chair*
Subcommittee on Military Weight Management

Contents

Weight Management

State of the Science and Opportunities for Military Programs

Executive Summary

The primary purpose of fitness and body composition standards in the military has always been to select individuals best suited to the physical demands of military service based on the assumption that proper body weight supports good health, physical readiness, and appropriate military appearance. Prior to the Korean Conflict, these standards were used primarily to exclude underweight candidates. Advances in health care and improved nutrition over the past 75 years have resulted in increases in mean height, weight, and fat-free mass of soldiers, and in the U.S. population as a whole. However, increases in food consumption and decreases in daily activity have raised new concerns about the impact of overnutrition and fatness on overall health, physical fitness, and military performance.

BACKGROUND AND CHARGE TO THE COMMITTEE

Considerable attention has been given to the alarming rise in the incidence of overweight and obesity in the U.S. population. The most recent national data (1999–2000 National Health and Nutrition Examination Survey) show the prevalence of overweight and obesity (defined as a body mass index [BMI] of $\geq$ 25 for overweight and $\geq$ 30 for obesity) in adults 20 years of age and older is 64.5 percent overweight and, of these, 30.5 percent are obese. Furthermore, the prevalence of overweight in adolescents (ages 12–19 years) is 15.5 percent.

The epidemic of overweight and obesity affects the military services of the United States in several ways. For example, it decreases the pool of individuals eligible for recruitment into military services, and it decreases the retention of new recruits. Almost 80 percent of recruits who exceed the military accession weight-for-height standards at entry leave the military before they complete their first term of enlistment. This in turn increases the cost of recruitment and training. These issues threaten the long-term welfare and readiness of U.S. military forces.

To aid in developing strategies for the prevention and remediation of overweight in military personnel, the U.S. Army Medical Research and Materiel Command (USAMRMC), through its director of Military Operational Medicine Research Programs, requested the Committee on Military Nutrition Research (CMNR) to review existing data on: optimal components of a weight-management program; the role of age, gender, and ethnicity in weight management; and current Department of Defense (DOD) activities in weight management in order to provide recommendations for military weight-management programs. In response to this request, the Subcommittee on Military Weight Management was appointed in September 1999.

The subcommittee was charged to identify the most effective interventions for weight loss and weight maintenance, particularly those most pertinent to the nonobese overweight individuals (BMI 25.0–29.9) found in the military setting, to evaluate the interventions' appropriateness for military application or the need for further research, and to develop a consensus toward a more standard DOD-wide approach to weight management that utilizes state-of-the-art knowledge and practices. Specifically, the military requested guidance on the appropriate degree of standardization of programs across the services, whether specific aids for weight loss (e.g., drugs) should be considered, how dietary changes would impact successful weight loss, and whether resistiveness to weight loss and maintenance are genetically controlled to the extent that individuals with genetic predispositions for obesity should be identified and automatically excluded.

METHODS

As part of the response to the military request, the subcommittee convened a workshop to bring together a group of experts to share knowledge and experience in managing weight-control programs within the services, to gain relevant knowledge and experience from industry and academia, to examine current interventions and those under development (particularly in the pharmaceutical industry) for their appropriateness for military application, and to identify needs for further research. In addition, the subcommittee performed an extensive review of the scientific literature for data on optimal components of a weight-management program; the role of age, gender, and ethnicity in weight management; and current DOD activities in this arena. From this review, recommendations were developed on the optimal components of a weight-management program that could be utilized across the services.

CURRENT MILITARY WEIGHT STANDARDS AND WEIGHT-MANAGEMENT PROGRAMS

There are significant demographic differences between the military population and the general U.S. population. The general population is almost evenly split with respect to gender (49.1 percent men and 50.9 percent women), while the military population is approximately 85 percent men and 15 percent women. There are also significant age differences in the two populations. Approximately 31.5 percent of the U.S. population is between the ages of 18 and 40 years, while approximately 80 percent of the military population is in this age range. The military also has a higher percentage of ethnic minorities than the general population, especially among women.

The weight-for-height and body-fat standards of the military services were predicated on the need for the highest level of physical performance in adverse environments, to maintain a high level of readiness at all times, and to present a trim military appearance (e.g., the image that the individual may convey of the military). These standards theoretically take precedence even when individuals demonstrate an ability to perform their assigned tasks in an exceptional manner. Typically, the various branches of the military service have had two sets of weight/fat standards: one set to be met by potential recruits for accession into initial entry training and another equivalent or more stringent set to be retained in the service once admitted. The initial body composition screen consists of a weight-for-height assessment. Historically, maximum allowable weight-for-height tables are used.

When only two anthropometric measurements are used to estimate body composition, height and weight have the highest level of association with the percentage of body fat. Height and weight can also be used to compute BMI, a widely accepted index that correlates with percent body fat. A substantial body of evidence shows that BMI is positively associated with both morbidity and mortality. Each of the services screens active duty personnel at least annually or semiannually for fitness and compliance with weight-for-height standards.

Typically, the maximum allowable weights-for-height varied across services for individuals of the same height, age, and gender, and individual service standards were uniformly more stringent than the DOD recommendations. The disparity in maximum BMI between men and women was marked. For example, prior to 2002, the maximum allowable retention weight-for-height for women in any service corresponded to a BMI of 25.1 (Army), for men it corresponded to a BMI of 28.2 (Air Force).

The military uses circumference measurements to estimate body composition. Until the early 1990s, each service employed its own set of measurement equations for estimating body composition. More recently, a single equation for use across all the services has been mandated by DOD. In November 2002, DOD reissued its reference document on implementation policy and procedures for physical fitness and weight/body-fat standards. This policy mandates that the weight-for-height tables for all the service branches will be based on BMI, and that no service may have a standard more stringent than a BMI of 25 or more liberal than a BMI of 27.5. In addition, all branches of the service must use a single, validated equation based on abdominal and neck circumference and height for men;

and one based on abdominal, neck, and hip circumference and height for women to estimate percent body fat. Body-fat standards for men shall not be more stringent than 18 percent and not more liberal than 26 percent. For women, the fat standards shall not be more stringent than 26 percent and not more liberal than 36 percent. Individuals who exceed these limits must be referred to a weight-management program

A review of the weight-loss programs across the military services highlighted significant deficits that could affect success. All of the programs have a strong motivating component that is highly disciplinary in nature, and the penalties for exceeding the body-fat limits are significant. With exception of those in the Air Force program, the majority of participants receive only minimal counseling by a qualified dietitian. The same appears to be true throughout the services in the area of behavior modification. With the exception of the Air Force and some specific sites in the other services, data collection for program evaluation is lacking.

FACTORS THAT INFLUENCE BODY WEIGHT

Maintaining a healthy body weight is an extremely complex issue. Maintenance of fitness and appropriate body-fat standards by military personnel is affected by each individual's genetics, developmental history, physiology, age, physical activity level, diet, environment, and social background. Some of these factors are biologically programmed (e.g., physiology, genetic makeup, age). Other factors can be manipulated by the individual (e.g., physical activity level, diet), while still other factors may require institutional, systemic, or environmental changes (e.g., worksite and community design, availability of facilities).

Genetics

Individuals appear to show significant heterogeneity in their body weight and body fatness responses to altered energy balance, dietary components, and changing activity levels, although little is yet known about the specific causes of heterogeneity.

There is a group of at least 20 Mendelian syndromes in which obesity is a component; these genetic disorders are rare, however, and family studies do not suggest that the genes responsible for these syndromes are involved in the common forms of human obesity. For more than 99 percent of obese individuals, the genetic basis of their obesity is unknown, and genetics may or may not be a causal factor.

The strongest evidence for genetic weight-regulating mechanisms is the recent elucidation of single gene defects that are associated with excessive weight gain in animals. Of the five gene products identified to date as being associated with weight regulation, leptin is the best characterized. Genetic defects in leptin have been associated with extreme obesity in humans. Although extensive efforts have been made to identify mutations in the genes identified as obesity-associated in rodents and in humans, only a handful of individuals have been identified with mutations in any of the genes that have produced obesity in rodents.

Physiology

A number of phenotypic characteristics have been associated with risk of weight gain, notably alterations in nonvolitional components of energy expenditure. Energy expenditure can be divided into three main components: *resting metabolic rate* (RMR), the energy expended at rest, under thermoneutral conditions, and in a postabsorptive state; *thermic effect of feeding*, the incremental increase in energy expenditure after a meal is consumed, associated with absorption and transport of nutrients and the synthesis, storage, and breakdown of protein, fat, and carbohydrate; and the *energy expended for physical activity,* primarily voluntary movement, but also including the involuntary movements associated with shivering, fidgeting, and postural control. The RMR accounts for 60 to 75 percent of total energy expended in most adults. A number of studies have been performed to evaluate the effect of exercise, particularly resistance training, on RMR. Results have been inconsistent, and thus whether exercise training increases RMR remains controversial.

Age

Many weight-management experts agree that body weight becomes progressively more difficult to maintain with age. Some research has indicated that body weight and associated circumferences increase with advancing age unless food intake is significantly reduced or physical activity is substantially increased. However, health risk associated with BMI remains unchanged in older individuals. Thus, there appears to be little rationale for increasing the upper BMI range consistent with good health as individuals become older.

A large number of cross-sectional studies, however, do demonstrate that body fat increases with age. In contrast to body fat, skeletal muscle mass declines with age beginning around the third decade, and losses of skeletal muscle parallel decreases in bone mass. The mechanisms of body composition changes that accompany aging are multifactorial and include physical inactivity, diet, and hormonal alterations. This loss of lean mass and the gain in fat mass occur even with no apparent change in body weight. Since lean mass contributes the larger share of metabolic activity, total energy expenditure decreases proportionally with loss of lean mass.

Physical Activity

The rapid rise in the prevalence of overweight and obesity in the last 20 years likely reflects major environmental shifts in eating habits and exercise, both of which can be controlled. Some of these shifts include changes in the food supply, food availability, food composition, palatability, and affordability, as well as numerous technological advances that have removed the need for physical labor or physical movement (e.g., elevators, escalators, riding lawn mowers, remote controls for televisions and stereos). Physical activity represents an important component of volitional energy expenditure. Reductions in physical activity over the past several decades have likely contributed to the evolution of positive energy balance and the weight gain characteristic of all industrialized societies.

Exercise, especially in bouts of 30 minutes of activity or more, can promote fat oxidation because the substrate that is preferentially oxidized by muscle tissue switches from carbohydrate to fat. Thus, chronic extended bouts of exercise may, in effect, substitute for expansion of the adipose tissue, allowing the physically active individual to achieve fat balance while maintaining a lower body-fat mass than the sedentary individual.

Food Intake

A high energy intake (i.e., energy intake in excess of energy expenditure) or an energy intake that is not adjusted downward with age and declining physical activity is associated with the development of overweight or obesity in susceptible individuals. In addition to total energy intake, the character of the diet may play a role in the etiology of obesity, with high-fat diets potentially promoting increased body weight.

Social and Environmental Factors

Other factors that contribute to overweight both in the military and in civilian populations include meal patterns and eating habits, familial and ethnic factors, cultural norms, socioeconomic status, smoking, alcohol consumption, use of certain common drugs such as anti-allergens, and the use of antidepressants, hypoglycemic agents, and certain antihypertensive agents. Members of the military population with unusually sedentary job responsibilities and a work environment that promotes a combination of high-pressured, hasty, and thoughtless overeating along with inactivity are likely to be particularly at risk for weight gain. Thus, the social and environmental context of the overweight individual needs to be carefully evaluated.

RECOMMENDATIONS

After careful review of the information presented at the workshop and the scientific literature, the subcommittee makes the following specific recommendations.

Prevention

- Each service should provide training on diet and health, including the fundamentals of energy balance, the caloric content of common foods, portion sizes, and the importance of maintaining high levels of daily activity after intensive training periods (e.g., initial entry training) to prevent weight gain.
- An education program on maintaining healthy weight should also include components directed at military spouses and family.
- Programs to reinforce the concept of exercise and activity as part of the military lifestyle should be developed, along with programs to encourage the reduction of alcohol consumption.
- Particular emphasis should be placed on providing or upgrading physical fitness facilities and equipment that encourage exercise.
- The use of rewards for exercise achievement should be reinforced.
- The services should make the incorporation of "heart-healthy" menus a standard for base dining facilities, with continued emphasis on training all military cooks in low-fat cooking techniques.
- Priority consideration should be given to commercial eating establishments that routinely offer reasonable portion sizes and low-fat dining options when these establishments are competing for base contracts.

Assessment

- Assessments for weight-for-height and percent body fat should be conducted quarterly rather than annually or semi-annually. More frequent assessments should be evaluated to determine if they reduce disordered eating and other risky behaviors.
- Individuals at risk of increased weight or body-fat gain should be identified at the time of accession (e.g., those entering service over the standard, those with a family history of obesity) and their evaluations monitored so that interventions may be instituted as soon as adverse changes are identified.
- The incidence of disordered eating behaviors needs to be documented and addressed across all branches of the military.

Weight-Loss Programs

- A weight-loss diet should be energy deficient by 350 to 1,000 kcal/day; should provide a minimum daily intake of at least 800 kcal/day; should provide a minimum of 60 g of protein/day for women and 75 g of protein/day for men; should provide no more than 30 percent of total energy as calories from fat; and should have a carbohydrate content of no less than 130 g/day (excessively low carbohydrate intake can cause dehydration and impact both physical and cognitive function). The daily use of a multivitamin-mineral supplement may be included.
- A combination of aerobic and strength training exercise, along with increased activities of daily living, is recommended. Energy expended in physical activity should be at a minimum of 2,000 kcal/wk, which amounts to 200 to 300 min/wk of moderate-intensity exercise (3.5–5 hr). In keeping with other recent recommendations, 60 min/day of moderate-intensity activity in addition to activities of daily living is suggested.
- Training and support in behavior modification should include stimulus control, relapse prevention, self-monitoring, cognitive restructuring, and mentoring.
- Follow-up should include regular contact with weight-management counselors; routine self-monitoring of diet, weight, and physical activity; and ongoing psychological support that could be provided via the Internet or by telephone.
- Training programs should be established for all personnel associated with implementing weight-control programs. Training standards for a weight-management military occupational specialty should include training in principles of nutrition, portion control, physical activity/exercise, behavior modification, psychological support, and the use of weight-loss aids. The program should also include mandated continuing education requirements.

Research

- Internet-based programs should be developed using models already in use by the military. Emphasis should be given to the development of a number of options, testing their effectiveness overall, and identifying those with high response rates. Also, the range of individual responses of military personnel should be evaluated since there may be subpopulations that respond well to a given intervention when overall response is not consistent.
- An evaluation of military weight-management programs is essential to determine their effectiveness. This evaluation would require following personnel who have completed the program for 2 to 5 years, and perhaps throughout their military career. Recommendations provided in this report are based almost ex-

clusively on data collected in civilian populations, and effectiveness may be quite different in military populations.

- Many nonprescription preparations are undoubtedly being used in the military for weight loss. Very little is known about their effects on body weight, body composition, overall health, and physical performance. It is particularly important to assess the use of such preparations as well as their effects on military performance.

RESPONSE TO THE MILITARY'S QUESTIONS

What are the essential components of an effective weight/fat loss program, and the most effective strategies for sustaining weight loss?

Years of research have demonstrated that a program for weight/fat loss can only be effective when it is closely integrated with a program for sustaining weight loss.

Essential Components of an Effective Weight/Fat Loss Program

- *Exercise.* For overweight adults who are otherwise healthy, increased physical activity is an essential component of a comprehensive weight-reduction strategy.
- *Behavior modification.* The use of behavior and lifestyle modification in weight management is based on a body of evidence that people become or remain overweight as the result of modifiable habits or behaviors and that by changing these behaviors, weight can be lost and weight loss can be maintained.
- *Net dietary energy deficit.* Energy expended must exceed energy consumed on a consistent basis over an extended period of time, the length of which depends on the degree of overweight.
- *Education.* Information on nutrition principles, food portion control, and the need for energy balance is essential for individuals to develop appropriate eating behaviors.
- *Psychological support and counseling.* Any weight-management program is likely to be more successful if it is accompanied by structured support mechanisms (e.g., from professional counselors, commanders, coworkers, family).
- *Environmental changes.* Restructuring the individual's environment to remove factors that promote overeating and underactivity is also a significant part of weight loss and management. The environment includes the home, the workplace, and the community.
- *Structured monitoring.* The long-term success of weight management appears to depend on a specific and deliberate follow-up program. This struc-

tured follow-up should include monitoring body weight with regular weigh-ins at least weekly during the weight-loss phase and monthly during the maintenance phase.

Sustaining Weight Loss

An integrated program that combines the weight-loss procedures described above with weight-maintenance strategies is essential to achieve the best long-term benefits. The use of maintenance strategies with the strong incentive that is provided by the military regulations on weight control should enhance the chances for successful weight maintenance.

- *Physical activity.* An expenditure of at least 2,000 to 3,000 kcal/wk from exercise is essential.
- *Permanent lifestyle and behavior modifications.* Balancing customary daily energy intake with appropriate habitual levels of physical activity is also necessary. This includes portion control, selecting foods lower in fat and calories, and consistently sustaining higher levels of daily physical activity.
- *Self-monitoring.* Individuals need to record their body weight a minimum of once weekly. They also need to periodically keep a 3-day food diary (about every 3 months) and a physical activity diary or use an activity monitor (e.g., a pedometer) to help maintain weight loss.
- *Continuous structured support.* It is also necessary to have follow-up visits or counseling via phone or the Internet every 2 to 4 weeks for the first 3 months and every 1 to 2 months thereafter, depending on the difficulty in maintaining a stable, healthy weight.

How do age and gender influence success in weight-management programs? Should age be considered in weight/fat standards and in weight-management programs and interventions?

Age

Although weight gain with age is a frequent occurrence, it is not inevitable. Increases in weight with age can be avoided if energy intake is adjusted to compensate for decreases in activity and the loss of lean body mass, or if physical activity is increased (including strength or resistance exercises) to maintain lean body mass. For the benefit of long-term health, there should not be age-related increases in weight-for-height standards.

Research indicates that percent body fat increases with age even if weight does not change. The current upper limits of DOD standards of 26 percent fat in men and 36 percent fat in women, however, is well within the limits of the healthy percent body fat range even for those 60 to 79 years of age. While individual services have upper limits of percent body fat that are uniformly more stringent than the DOD maximum, increases in percent body fat with age are appropriate.

Gender

On average, women have a higher percent body fat than men. Weight gain and lifestyle changes during the childbearing and childrearing years, as well as the hormonal and metabolic changes that accompany pregnancy and menopause, are associated with higher body fat. Thus, the gender-specific fat standards are appropriate.

Which strategies would be most and least effective in a military setting? Should military weight/fat loss programs involve direct participation intervention, or only monitoring and guidance? Should military programs be more proactive in identifying and discouraging ineffective or dangerous weight-loss practices? Is a warning or cautionary zone prior to enrollment in a weight-control program an effective strategy? When should duty time be authorized for participation in intervention strategies for weight/fat loss?

The Most and Least Effective Strategies of a Weight/Fat Loss Program in a Military Setting

The effective strategies for a weight/fat loss program would be the same regardless of whether the setting is military or civilian. However, the implementation of some of these strategies could be facilitated in the military environment, particularly physical fitness, exercise, and behavior modification.

The primary difficulty in the military setting would be in providing structured follow-up due to the mobility of the military population. Other difficulties include remoteness or isolation of some work locations, the paucity of low-fat food selections in vending machines and dining facilities, the availability and affordability of foods with low energy density (e.g., fruits and vegetables, low-fat or nonfat milk), and high-pressure environments with short meal breaks that may promote inappropriate dietary patterns.

Direct Participation Interventions versus Monitoring and Guidance

Direct participation interventions have been demonstrated to improve compliance, increase the success rate of weight/fat loss, and support an improved level of weight maintenance.

Identifying and Discouraging Ineffective or Dangerous Weight-Loss Practices

Military weight programs should collect information on weight-loss practices of overweight individuals as a component of their medical evaluation. Military individuals found to be using ineffective or dangerous weight-loss practices such as extensive fasting, purging, the use of diuretics, and the use of commercially available herbal supplements and diet pills, should be counseled on the risks of these practices and strongly encouraged to adopt standard weight-loss practices. One method to reduce the incidence of dangerous practices is more frequent weigh-ins and emphasis on appropriate diet and physical activity patterns at all times as part of a military lifestyle.

Is a Warning or Cautionary Zone Prior to Enrollment into a Weight-Control Program an Effective Strategy?

The warning zone that is now in effect for the Air Force program (3 months) appears to be an excellent strategy. It gives individuals a chance to manage their overweight/body-fat problem by themselves in a timely manner without assignment to a weight control program, with its accompanying career implications.

Authorizing Duty Time for Participation in Intervention Programs for Weight/Fat Loss

Any medical examination and tests that are appropriate before being assigned to a program for weight/body-fat loss, as well as counseling and monitoring, should be accomplished during duty time. A weight-loss program should be viewed as treatment for a medical condition and be given comparable priority as treatment for other medical conditions.

Since current DOD policy dictates regular exercise as a part of duty time, unit commanders should provide (or require) time for regular exercise to ensure a high level of fitness and readiness.

To what extent should weight-control programs/policies be standardized across the services versus tailored to the individual service, installation or unit? What are the advantages and disadvantages of standardization? Is the provision of state-of-the-art techniques and knowledge a rationale for standardization?

Extent of Standardization Across the Services versus Tailored to an Individual Service

The specifics of implementation of weight-control programs and policies may need to be tailored for each service due to the different environments in which the programs will be carried out (e.g., aboard ships, on CONUS military bases, or on overseas bases). However, they could be standardized across the services to a significant extent as indicated below. A limited number of military health centers should be identified to provide scientifically validated body composition evaluations.

- *Standard methodology*. New technologies for measuring body composition should be adopted service-wide as they become available, once they are validated for accuracy and ease of use.
- *Appearance standard.* A waist circumference standard of no more than 40 inches for men and 35 inches for women should be used as an objective measure for appearance standards as these standards are known to be related to long-term health.
- *Weight-management counselors.* Those responsible for weight-control programs should be certified and their training should be standardized.
- *Internet-based weight-management programs.* A standardized program across all services would be more efficient and could be easily accessed by military personnel regardless of their duty assignment.

The advantages of standardization of weight-control programs and policies are that all military personnel would have access to equivalent weight-management assistance and that the incorporation of new technologies for body composition assessment and the adoption of Internet-based services would be facilitated. In addition, the costs of producing education materials (e.g., portion size models, brochures) would be reduced. The disadvantage of standardization is that it might limit innovation within the branches of the armed forces. There is no scientific disadvantage.

Is the Provision of State-of-the-Art Techniques and Knowledge a Rationale for Standardization?

Standardization of weight-control program components would facilitate the incorporation of new technologies and provide a stronger base for program evaluation, which would in turn protect DOD investments in each individual. To date, none of the existing military weight-control programs have been sufficiently evaluated to justify adoption DOD-wide.

How can diet be effectively dealt with as a weight-management component in the military setting? Should pharmacological treatment (anorexiants) be considered for use in the military? In what cases? What factors bear on this decision?

Diet counseling needs to be administered by individuals who are fully trained in weight-management strategies, and it should be supported by appropriate professional personnel. For those military personnel who are on ships or are dependent on mess halls, more healthy, low-fat food choices and sufficient time for meal consumption are imperative. Providing choices of foods (both snack and full-meal foods) that are less energy-dense; increasing the price of foods high in calories, fat, and refined carbohydrates; and subsidizing the price of fresh fruits and low-calorie snacks in vending machines and exchange service facilities should be considered. In any case, nutrition and lifestyle education is paramount and should be provided early in the initial entry training period and reinforced periodically. The development of distance-based education in nutrition and lifestyle modification may prove useful.

Pharmacological treatments should be considered for those who meet the standard criteria for the use of such compounds (i.e., a BMI of ≥ 30 or ≥ 27 with comorbidities such as hypertension or high cholesterol). These individuals would have to be in military occupational specialties that do not preclude the use of drugs that affect the central nervous system.

How should resistiveness to weight/fat control be dealt with?

Resistiveness, as defined by the military, is a condition that generally refers to a genotype and/or a phenotype that is obesity-prone. These individuals can lose weight, but they usually have to work harder and may need additional assistance in a weight-management program and with structured follow-up.

What are the knowledge gaps in weight-management programs relative to the military? What research is needed?

Knowledge gaps concerning weight-management programs relative to the military are extensive. Most published research has been derived from studies on middle-aged men and women or perimenopausal, Caucasian women in clinical settings. These data have limited relevance to the military population where: (1) only about 25 percent of officers and warrant officers and about 6 percent of enlisted personnel are over the age of 40, (2) only 15 percent are women, and (3) approximately 40 percent are minorities. Considerable research is needed in the primary areas of prevention, treatment, and program evaluation. In addition to the research needs highlighted in the recommendations, research should also be conducted on the following topics.

Prevention

Early Identification of Personnel at Risk

To identify those at risk of overweight or obesity, a set of potential risk factors for weight gain (e.g., overweight at the time of accession, family history of obesity, initial performance on the physical training test, a gain of more than 5 percent over initial entry training weight) should be developed. The effectiveness of educating these individuals during initial entry training or whenever they are identified as being at risk of becoming overweight should be evaluated.

Early Education of Initial Entry Trainees and Families

Initial entry training is a time of learning for individuals new to the military. Just as these individuals learn military tasks (e.g., how to fire a weapon), they could also learn nutritional principles, particularly the importance of energy balance, appropriate portion sizes, and the caloric content of frequently consumed foods. Spouses and other family members could also be included in instruction on nutrition, just as they are in classes on military etiquette. Large-scale, randomized trials with alternate classes of recruits, followed over time, would be useful in determining if such preventive efforts are effective.

Exercise (Structured and Unstructured)

All the services should adopt the strategy of promoting physical fitness as a way of life from the first day of initial entry training. Mandating exercise during the duty day regardless of time pressures is one strategy. Scheduling competitions that require participation by the entire unit and that require unstructured exercise to attain peak performance could be tested as a method to improve overall fitness and activity. The usefulness of resistance or strength training and the optimum mix of aerobic and strength training for the purpose of weight management needs to be evaluated among military personnel.

Reduction of Environmental Factors That Promote Overweight

Research is needed that: evaluates the effectiveness of eliminating high-calorie and high-fat snacks in vending machines, or of offering alternatives such as fruit and low-calorie snacks and meal replacements; evaluates the effects of different time allotments for meal consumption; and evaluates the effectiveness of altering the environment to promote physical activity, such as the creation of walking and bike trails on military bases.

Evaluation of Treatment Methods and Programs

Evaluation of Local Initiatives for Effectiveness

Research is needed to identify and evaluate local weight-loss programs, both military and civilian, for effectiveness. A military-wide competition could be established for the most innovative weight-reduction programs, with recognition and meaningful rewards for the most successful.

Evaluation of Ineffective or Dangerous Weight-Loss Practices

Research from the Navy has demonstrated that unhealthy eating and purging behaviors are more prevalent among military personnel compared with the civilian population. Information is needed on the impact of such dangerous or ineffective weight-loss practices on physical and mental performance among military personnel. The prevalence of bulimia, binge eating disorder, and anorexia nervosa in military personnel and whether the military lifestyle and standards promotes such behavior needs to be determined.

Computerized Follow-Up of Personnel at Risk

An independent, computerized database is needed to identify individuals with risk factors for weight gain or overweight as described above, and to maintain routine contact with these individuals to check on their weight or physical fitness status, to identify problems early, and to intervene as needed. Such computerized information should be centrally maintained and used as a source of data for longitudinal studies on the effectiveness of prevention and treatment innovations. This data should *not* be available to unit commanders to avoid the possibility of discrimination against individuals at risk.

Other Areas for Research

Information is needed on whether there are differences both in gender responses to the various components of weight-management programs (e.g., do men and women respond differently to diet, physical activity, or behavioral change interventions) and in race/ethnicity responses to various weight-management strategies.

1

Background and Context of the Overweight Problem

Considerable attention has been given to the alarming rise in the incidence of overweight and obesity in the U.S. population, both in the scientific literature and in the popular press. The prevalence of overweight and obesity, defined as a body mass index (BMI = weight [kg] divided by height $[m]^2$) from 25 to 29.9 and 30 or higher, respectively, was relatively stable from 1960 to 1980. However, data from the Third National Health and Nutrition Examination Survey (NHANES III) from 1988–1994 showed an increase in the prevalence of overweight and obesity from 47 percent to 56 percent and a rise in the prevalence of obesity from approximately 15 percent to 23 percent (Flegal et al., 1998; Kuczmarski et al., 1994). More recent data indicate that these trends have continued.

THE CURRENT NATIONAL SITUATION

The latest NHANES data from 1999–2000 (Flegal et al., 2002) show that 64.5 percent of the U.S. population 20 years of age and older is now classified as overweight or obese. The prevalence of obesity (BMI $\geq$ 30) has risen from 23 percent to 30.5 percent. These trends are seen across both sexes and all ethnic groups, with the greatest increases occurring in non-Hispanic Black females. Furthermore, since 1980, the percentage of adolescents (ages 12–19 years) who are overweight has tripled from 5 percent to 15.5 percent (Ogden et al., 2002). There are some disparities however; overweight and obesity are particularly common among minority groups and those with lower family income and less education (HHS, 2001).

The epidemic of overweight and obesity in the civilian population, which many experts attribute to the ready availability of a vast array of foods combined with an increasingly sedentary lifestyle, affects the military services of the United States in two significant ways. First, it decreases the pool of individuals eligible for recruitment into the military services, and second, it decreases retention—almost 80 percent of recruits who exceed the accession weight-for-height standards at service entry leave the military early (i.e., by year 2 of a 3–4 year term of enlistment).

Another important consideration of the impact of overweight and obesity is their effect on chronic disease. Studies of the relationship between health and disease have used the premise that a BMI of less than 18.5 constitutes underweight, and a BMI of 18.5 to 24.9 constitutes healthy weight.

NOTE: A BMI consistent with overweight (25.0–29.9) does not by itself indicate that an individual is over-fat, nor does a BMI consistent with underweight indicate that an individual is *not* over-fat. There are some instances where an individual could be misclassified as overweight due to body composition (e.g., individuals with a large amount of lean muscle tissue, as might be found in the military). Additional testing must be done to determine whether the excess weight in such individuals consists of fat.

Overweight and Health

The effects of excess body weight are widespread and raise a variety of concerns relevant to the health and performance of members of the military. The major comorbidities associated with obesity and the implications of these comorbidities for the military services are briefly reviewed below. (For an extensive review of the major health effects of overweight, see Bray, 1996 and Must et al., 1999).

Overweight and obesity have also been associated with a variety of adverse social and economic consequences. These appear to be more significant among women than among men. For example, one study showed that obese women completed fewer years of school, married less frequently, and had lower earnings than women who were not obese (Gortmaker et al., 1993). Although these data were obtained before obesity achieved its current prevalence, they suggest a variety of long-term effects on material and psychological well-being.

Obesity also has a variety of adverse physiological effects. The major comorbidities associated with obesity are shown in Box 1-1. It has been observed that the prevalence of type 2 diabetes mellitus, hyperlipidemia, hypertension, and heart disease increased with the severity of obesity, and that prevalence ratios were generally greater in younger than in older adults (Must et al., 1999). Approximately 70 percent of overweight individuals have at least one of these complications, and over 30 percent have two or more (Must et al., 1999).

Obesity is also associated with increased mortality rates. In one study by Allison and colleagues (1999), obesity-related mortality was estimated from data collected in five prospective cohort studies. The estimated number of annual deaths in the United States attributable to obesity ranged from 280,000 to

BOX 1-1 Consequences of Adult Obesity

Psychosocial consequences
- Low self-esteem
- Disordered eating behavior
- Discrimination

Medical consequences
- Cancer
- Diabetes mellitus
- Gall bladder disease
- Gastro-esophogeal reflux disease
- Heart disease
- Hyperlipidemia
- Hypertension
- Osteoarthritis
- Polycystic ovary disease
- Pseudotumor cerebri
- Sleep apnea
- Urinary incontinence
- Increased maternal and fetal complications during pregnancy and postpartum
- Early mortality

325,000, depending on whether the analysis controlled for smoking rates. Approximately 80 percent of the deaths attributable to overweight occurred in persons with a BMI $\geq$ 30, which is the lower limit for obesity. The estimates of the effects of obesity on mortality rates are quite consistent with earlier published estimates by McGinnis and Foege (1993), who suggested that approximately 300,000 deaths per year could be attributed to poor diet and inactivity patterns, which are the major contributors to obesity.

The comorbidities associated with obesity substantially increase health care costs. For example, total costs associated with obesity-related type 2 diabetes mellitus; coronary heart disease; hypertension; gall bladder diseases; breast, endometrial, and colon cancer; and osteoarthritis in 2000 were estimated at almost $117 billion per year (HHS, 2001). Approximately half of these costs were medical costs directly associated with the treatment of obesity and its comorbidities; the other half were indirect costs associated with increased absenteeism and decreased economic productivity. In one managed care organization, obesity was clearly associated with increased outpatient visits, inpatient days, and use of pharmacy and radiology services (Quesenberry et al., 1998).

Upper Body Adiposity

BMI does not account for all of the increased morbidity associated with obesity; the distribution of adipose tissue also influences the risk of excess weight. Upper body, or more specifically, visceral adipose tissue, carries a higher morbidity risk than adipose tissue deposited in the subcutaneous compartments of the buttocks, thighs, and lower extremities (NHLBI, 1998).

Individuals with upper body adiposity may be predisposed to other obesity-related conditions such as insulin resistance, glucose intolerance, dyslipidemias, and high blood pressure, often referred to collectively as "Syndrome X" or the "metabolic syndrome" (Bjorntorp, 1992a, 1992b; Hjermann, 1992). Factors that increase the deposition of visceral adipose tissue include male gender, lack of physical activity, alcohol use, and smoking (Emery et al., 1993; Han et al., 1998). The distribution of upper body adipose tissue may also impact appearance, which is relevant to military standards.

In order to clinically evaluate adipose tissue distribution, an individual's waist circumference (W) is evaluated as a measure of visceral obesity, with $W > 102$ cm (40 in) in men and $W > 88$ cm (35 in) in women considered high risk for heart disease (NHLBI, 1998). Waist circumference measurements are supplementary to BMI when diagnosing overweight and obesity; waist measurements lose their predictive value for increased risk of heart disease with a BMI ≥ 35.

UNIQUENESS OF THE MILITARY ENVIRONMENT

Among active duty military personnel, diabetes, hypertension, and ischemic heart disease accounted for less than 1 percent of visits made to ambulatory care clinics in 1998. These findings should not be surprising given that active duty personnel are younger, are less likely to be obese, and are more physically fit than the average civilian adult. However, overweight and obesity do exist in the military, and chronic health risk is a concern, especially among older, more senior personnel. For example, Robbins and coworkers (2002), in a retrospective cohort study design of active duty Air Force personnel, found that approximately 20 percent of these men and women exceeded their official maximum allowable weight-for-height. Based on a review of health records, they estimated excess weight-attributable medical costs were $19.26 million, with an additional $3.5 million attributable to lost productivity and 28,351 lost workdays. Although the primary concern of the Department of Defense (DOD) has been the effects of weight and body composition on the fitness and performance of military personnel, recent changes in the laws regarding health care for veterans have added the costs of obesity-related comorbidity coverage as another area of concern.

Also of special relevance to the military are the effects of fatness and of the lack of fitness on injury rates during initial entry training. In several small studies, an increased BMI was associated with an increased injury rate during initial entry training and with performance in the 1- and 2-mile runs, sit-ups, and push-ups by men (Jones et al., 1992).

Demographics

There are a number of important demographic differences between the military and the general population. While the general population is fairly evenly split between genders (49.1 percent men versus 50.9 percent women) (U.S. Census Bureau, 2003), the military is largely comprised of men (85 percent versus 15 percent women) (Personal communication, B. Maxfield, Office of the Deputy Chief of Staff for Personnel, March 7, 2003), although this varies somewhat with the individual services. For example, the Air Force is comprised of 80.6 percent men and 19.4 percent women, while the Marine Corps is comprised of 94 percent men and only 6 percent women (Personal communication, B. Maxfield, Office of the Deputy Chief of Staff for Personnel, March 7, 2003).

Ethnic demographics also differ somewhat between the general U.S. population and the active-duty military population. Although the proportion of Whites, American Indian/Alaska Natives, and Asian American/Pacific Islanders in the military tend to reflect the general U.S. population, the percentage of Black men is higher in the military than in the general population (17.7 percent vs. 12.3 percent), while the percentage of Hispanic men is lower (9 percent vs. 13.4 percent) (Tables 1-1 and 1-2). There is also a notable difference in the distribution of ethnicity by gender in the military compared with the general population. A greater proportion of women in the military are ethnic minorities. For example, 41.7 percent of Army women are Black and 9.7 percent are Hispanic, while 21 percent of Marine Corps women are Black and 16.6 percent are Hispanic (Table 1-2).

Another significant demographic that differs between the general U.S. population and the active-duty military population is that of age. While only 31.5 percent of the U.S. population is between the ages of 18 and 40 years (U.S. Census Bureau, 2003), this age range encompasses nearly 80 percent of the active-duty military population.

Health and Fitness

Table 1-3 presents a comparison of the percentage of the general population (Flegal et al., 2002; Freedman et al., 2002) versus the military service population in four BMI categories. While the percentage of military men and women in the BMI category of 25 to 29.9 is higher than the general population, the percentage in the BMI category of ≥ 30 is much lower. Also, the percentage of women with a BMI of less than 25 is higher for military women than for civilian women. The

TABLE 1-1 Percent Gender and Race/Ethnicity of the U.S. Population Compared with the Department of Defense (DOD) Population

Gender/Race/Ethnicity[a]	U.S. Population (%)	DOD Population (%)
Men (% of total population)	49.1	85
Race/Ethnicity		
White	68.7	66.4
Black	12.3	17.7
Hispanic	13.4	9.0
AA/PI	4.0	4.0
AI/AN	0.9	1.0
Women (% of total population)	50.9	15
Race/Ethnicity		
White	69.1	51.6
Black	13.1	31.4
Hispanic	12.2	9.2
AA/PI	3.8	4.0
AI/AN	1.2	1.1

[a] AA = Asian American, PI = Pacific Islander, AI = American Indian, AN = Alaska Native.

SOURCE: U.S. data: 2001 U.S. population estimates, U.S. Census Bureau (2003); DOD data: 2002 Distribution of Active Duty Forces, Personal communication, B. Maxfield, Office of the Deputy Chief of Staff for Personnel, March 7, 2003.

high prevalence of military personnel in the 25 to 29.9 BMI category reflects the fact that until late 2002, the military maximum weight-for-height standards were not based on the standard BMI categories (NHLBI, 1998).

The military environment has both positive and negative aspects associated with it in terms of maintaining physical fitness and healthy weight. On the positive side, military personnel have ready access to health care providers. In addition, DOD has the potential for centralized, longitudinal record-keeping on all active duty personnel, the unusual ability to provide incentives and consequences for weight change, and the potential ability to modify environmental factors that are important for weight control. Possible negative aspects of the military environment include a very mobile population and the potential for inappropriate weight-loss activities fostered by the need to meet weight, fitness, and fatness standards.

Weight and Body Composition

At present, all active-duty personnel must be weighed and assessed for physical fitness annually or semiannually. If an individual's weight exceeds the maximum for his or her height according to the screening tables for his or her

TABLE 1-2 Percent Gender and Race/Ethnicity of the Military Branches

Military Branch	White	Black	Hispanic	AA/PI[a]	AI/AN[b]	Total
Men						
Army	61.9	22.1	9.5	3.2	0.8	84.6
Navy	63.3	17.4	9.8	6.5	1.9	85.6
Marine Corps	68.2	13.9	13.1	2.6	0.9	94.0
Air Force	75.4	13.8	5.2	2.9	0.5	80.6
Women						
Army	41.2	41.7	9.7	3.8	1.2	15.4
Navy	51.6	28.1	11.1	5.2	2.8	14.4
Marine Corps	55.6	21.0	16.6	3.2	1.7	6.0
Air Force	61.8	24.7	6.0	3.8	0.7	19.4

[a] AA = Asian American, PI = Pacific Islander.

[b] AI = American Indian, AN = Alaska Native.

SOURCE: 2002 Distribution of Active Duty Forces, Personal communication, B. Maxfield, Office of the Deputy Chief of Staff for Personnel, March 7, 2003.

service, the individual is referred for a second-tier assessment (a determination of percent body fat), to ascertain whether the increased weight is due to fat or to lean tissue. In addition, a commander may order an individual in his or her command to be weighed at any time if the commander believes that the individual presents an overweight appearance in uniform. Personnel whose percent body fat exceeds the limit for their service and who do not qualify for a medical waiver are referred to a weight-management program (at the discretion of the commander), which carries professional consequences.

Administration of military weight-management programs is left to each service individually. These programs, which are described in greater detail in Chapter 2, generally require a single visit to a health professional followed by regular weigh-ins until weight and/or body fat goals are reached. Individuals are required to demonstrate continuing progress toward these goals by losing a prescribed number of pounds per month. Failure to show continued progress in weight loss or continued failure to comply with body-fat standards without a medical waiver can result in separation from the service. Similar attention is not devoted to personnel who are underweight.

Appearance

The DOD appearance standard is articulated by DOD (1995) Directive 1308.1, *DOD Physical Fitness and Body Fat Programs*. This policy is shared, but described slightly differently, by each of the service branches. According to the Directive, "maintaining desirable body composition is an integral part of

TABLE 1-3 Percent Body Mass Index (BMI) of Military Branches[a] by Gender Compared with the General U.S. Population

	Army		Navy	
BMI	Men	Women	Men	Women
< 18.5	0.3	0.6	0.5	1.8
18.5–24.9	39.6	58.8	30.4	52.2
25.0–29.9	46.0	34.4	52.9	38.6
30.0–34.9	13.2	5.6	14.3	6.5
35.0–39.9	0.9	0.5	1.7	0.8
≥ 40	< 0.1	< 0.1	0.2	0.1

[a] No data available for U.S. Marine Corps.

[b] Adapted from Flegal et al. (2002); Freedman et al. (2002). BMI categories for U.S. population data are < 25, 25.0–29.9, 30.0–39.9, ≥ 40.

SOURCE: Army data: Personal communication, G. Bathalon, U.S. Army Medical

physical fitness, general health, and military appearance" (p. 2), and the first line of body composition evaluation is by weight-for-height and appearance. For example, according to Army Regulation 600-9 (U.S. Army, 1987), one of the two goals of military weight standards is for soldiers to present a physical appearance in uniform "which is neat and trim." The regulation goes on to describe the standard further by emphasizing that "excessive body fat connotes a lack of personal discipline, detracts from military appearance, and may indicate a poor state of health, physical fitness, or stamina." No objective criteria (rating scales) have been associated with the appearance standard as it is enforced, although development of objective criteria has been recommended previously (IOM, 1992a, 1998).

Although appearance is associated slightly with percent body fat, it is associated more significantly with abdominal circumference (Hodgdon et al., 1990; U.S. Army, 1987; Vogel and Friedl, 1992). Army and Marine Corps personnel must supply recent photos of themselves to their promotion boards (this practice has been eliminated by the Air Force and Navy), but appearance judgments can be rendered by commanding officers at any time. When these judgments involve a suspicion of overweight (as opposed to an untidy uniform or other details of appearance), the individual must be weighed and may be required to have a body-fat determination and enter a weight-management program if standards are exceeded. In essence, the Directive considers appearance as important as weight-for-height standards, but it does not provide any objective criteria for assessing appearance. Instead, the Directive defers implementation of the policy to the individual services, which in turn defer to the individual units to establish criteria and implement the policy. This results in uneven application of the policy among units and across the services.

Air Force		U.S. Population[b]	
Men	Women	Men	Women
0.9	3.0	—	—
6.7	62.2	32.8	38.1
52.7	31.4	39.8	28.5
10.5	2.8	26.0	30.6
0.7	0.4	—	—
< 0.1	< 0.1	1.5	2.8

Research and Materiel Command, 2003; Navy data: Personal communication, T. Cepak, Navy Physical Readiness Program, April 25, 2003; Air Force data: Personal communication, J. Spahn, Population Health Support Branch, May 15, 2003.

The relative role that appearance should play in relation to weight and body-fat programs in the military is a multifaceted issue. The military embraces a policy on appearance for several psychosocial reasons:

- It is perceived to be an indication of fitness.
- It may affect how the general public views the military.
- The appearance of military personnel is believed by some to be a factor in esprit de corps (Bauer et al., 1976; USMC, 1995).
- It may have some impact on how a country's military is perceived internationally.

The issue of appearance also influences the individual's self-esteem and acceptance by peers.

PREVIOUS RECOMMENDATIONS ON BODY FAT AND FITNESS

In 1992, the Committee on Military Nutrition Research (CMNR) was asked to evaluate whether the body composition, fitness, and appearance standards of the military were consistent with optimum job performance. Their report, *Body Composition and Physical Performance: Applications for the Military Services* (IOM, 1992a), provided five major recommendations:

1. All the services should develop job-related physical performance tests.
2. The differences between accession and retention standards need reevaluation for all services.
3. The inequities in the body composition standards for men and women need to be addressed.

4. Body composition standards need to be validated relative to the ethnic diversity of the military population.

5. If the military deems appearance standards necessary (although no relationship between military appearance and military performance could be identified), these standards should be objective.

Following the lifting of the combat exclusion rule in 1993 (which opened to women a large number of occupational specialties that were previously closed to them) and the increased frequency of deployments, the percentage of female active-duty personnel has steadily increased. Concerned that the body composition, appearance, and fitness policies might be negatively impacting the health of female service personnel, the U.S. Army Medical Research and Materiel Command (USAMRMC) requested that CMNR revisit these issues specifically as they pertained to military women. In response to this request, the CMNR Subcommittee on Body Composition, Nutrition, and Health of Military Women published a report (IOM, 1998). This report examined the body composition and fitness standards of the four service branches in light of recent research that explored the relationships among body composition, fitness, performance, nutrition status, and health. To assess the implications of meeting the body composition and appearance standards for women, military weight-management programs and dieting practices were examined and compared with those in the civilian sector. The report also explored the potential health risks of chronic dieting in light of the high performance level expected of military personnel since underweight may be as much of a medical concern as overweight. This review (IOM, 1998) provided several key recommendations for military women:

- BMI and fitness assessment should be incorporated into the current two-tiered system of body composition assessment procedures.
- The maximum allowable BMI should be set at 25, based on considerations of health and chronic disease risk, with a maximum body fat of 36 percent for women if the fitness test is passed.
- A single, service-wide circumference equation should be developed and validated for the assessment of women's body fat.
- Military women should be strongly encouraged to achieve and maintain healthy weights through a continuous exercise and fitness program and should be provided nutrition education and ongoing counseling if weight loss is a goal.

THE CURRENT TASK

In July 1999, CMNR was requested to (1) review the data on optimal components of a weight-management program, (2) review the data on the role of age, gender, and ethnicity in weight management, (3) review current DOD activities in weight management, and (4) provide recommendations for military weight-management programs. This request originated from the Director of Military Operational Medicine Research at USAMRMC. The Subcommittee on Military Weight Management was appointed in September 1999; on October 24–27, 1999, the committee convened a workshop in response to a request from Army representatives. The workshop brought together the personnel responsible for both DOD-wide and service-specific weight-control program policies; a representation of military weight-control program leaders and innovators; and key military, academic, and industry researchers to:

- Share knowledge and experience in managing weight-control programs within the services.
- Gain relevant knowledge and experience from industry and academia.
- Examine current interventions and those under development for weight loss, particularly in the pharmaceutical industry.
- Evaluate the appropriateness of weight-loss interventions for military application or the need for further research.
- Develop a consensus toward a more standard DOD-wide approach to weight management that utilizes state-of-the-art knowledge and practices.

The subcommittee was charged to identify the most effective interventions for weight loss and maintenance, particularly those most effective for the non-obese overweight individuals found in the military setting. Specifically, this subcommittee was asked to addresses the following questions:

1. What are the essential components of an effective weight/fat-loss program, and the most effective strategies for sustaining weight loss?
2. How do age and gender influence success in weight-management programs? Should age be considered in weight/fat standards and in weight-management programs and interventions?
3. Which strategies would be the most and least effective in a military setting? Should military weight/fat loss programs involve direct participation interventions or only monitoring and guidance? Should military programs be more proactive in identifying and discouraging ineffective or dangerous weight-loss practices? Is a warning or cautionary zone prior to enrollment into a weight-control program an effective strategy? When should duty time be authorized for participation in intervention strategies for weight/fat loss?
4. To what extent should weight-control programs/policies be standardized across the services versus tailored to the individual service, installation, or unit? What are the advantages and disadvantages of standardization? Is the provision of state-of-the-art techniques and knowledge a rationale for standardization?
5. How can diet be effectively dealt with as a weight-management component in the military setting? Should pharmacological treatment (anorexiants)

be considered for use in the military? In what cases? What factors bear on this decision?

6. How should resistiveness to weight/fat control be dealt with?
7. What are the knowledge gaps in weight-management programs relative to the military? What research is needed?

SUMMARY

The rise in prevalence of overweight and obesity in the general population as defined by specific BMI cut-off of ≥ 25 for overweight and ≥ 30 for obesity has been associated with a significant increase in chronic diseases and mortality. However, among active-duty military personnel, 80 percent of whom are between 18 and 40 years of age, chronic obesity-related diseases are less of an issue than the impact of overweight on physical fitness, performance of jobs that require physical exertion, injury rates, and appearance.

2

Military Standards for Fitness, Weight, and Body Composition

"The physical characteristics of the U.S. fighting soldier have long proved to be a significant factor in the maintenance of a strong military force. Throughout history it has been demonstrated that the stronger, more fit, mentally sound soldier is better able to perform his or her assigned duties at optimal levels of proficiency. This proficiency has been measured in various ways, by quality of work, productivity, promotion success, and test scores. It may also have been measured, at times simply by survival (Wheeler, 1965). Measurable attributes affecting performance include physical characteristics, medical and mental illness, behaviors of risk, intelligence level (Altus, 1949), athletic ability, and endurance (Gould, 1979)" (Johnson, 1997).

This chapter provides a brief background on the relationship of body fat and fitness and the current policies of each branch of the military with respect to weight and body composition standards and weight-management programs.

INTRODUCTION

The primary purpose of fitness and body composition standards in the military has always been to select soldiers best suited to the physical demands of military service, based on the assumption that proper body weight supports good health, physical readiness, and appropriate military appearance. The idea of a strong, trim military soldier is certainly not a new concept. Weight-for-height has been used as a key measure of a potential recruit's fitness for military service for almost 150 years. The first height and weight tables for the U.S. military were created during the Civil War. Anthropometric measurements of Civil War draft recruits were collected at the end of the war by Colonel Jedediah H. Baxter, chief medical officer in the Office of the Provost Marshall General (Johnson, 1997). These data were later published in *Statistics, Medical and Anthropological* (1875, as reported by Love et al., 1958). Prior to the Korean Conflict, these standards were used primarily to exclude underweight candidates. Advances in health care and improved nutrition over the past 75 years have resulted in increases in mean height, weight, and fat-free mass of soldiers. However, the likelihood of overnutrition leading to overweight and obesity and increases in inactivity have raised new concerns about the impact of fatness on health and military performance.

FITNESS VERSUS FATNESS

Assessing Fitness versus Fatness

One of the considerations most relevant to the issue of fitness in the military is how fitness should be assessed. As described in the recently revised Department of Defense (DOD) *Physical Fitness and Body Fat Program Procedures* (DOD, 2002), the four components of fitness assessment are: (1) aerobic capacity, (2) muscular strength, (3) muscle endurance, and (4) body composition, which is influenced by other measures of fitness. Fatness, as defined by DOD, means a body-fat content in excess of 26 percent of total weight for men and 36 percent of total weight for women.

Fitness and fatness are frequently confused due to the methods used to express data related to fitness. For example, the definitive measure of cardiorespiratory (i.e., aerobic) fitness is the determination of maximal oxygen consumption (VO_{2max}). VO_{2max} is usually measured while the subject is exercising on a treadmill, according to a defined protocol that gradually increases speed and incline, until voluntary exhaustion and maximal heart rate are achieved. Maximal heart rate is usually estimated as a heart rate of 220 minus the subject's age. The most appropriate expression of VO_{2max} is as ml O_2/min, or as ml O_2/kg fat-free mass/min. The effects of training on cardiovascular endurance may increase VO_{2max} by approximately 20 percent. Unfortunately, however, in many studies VO_{2max} is expressed as ml O_2/kg body weight. Because this expression includes fat, which does not increase oxygen consumption in response to exercise, VO_{2max} expressed as ml O_2/kg body weight may reflect differences in performance, but does not allow comparisons of cardiovascular fitness.

Fitness, Fatness, and Injury

Jones and colleagues (1992) studied the relationship of fitness and fatness (percent body fat) on injury rates of recruits during entry training at Fort Jackson, South Carolina, in 1984 and 1988. Fitness was defined on the basis of 1- or 2-mile run times and the number of sit-ups and push-ups completed during a 2-minute interval. All three fitness measures were highly correlated to fatness in both men and women. In men, percent body fat, determined from four skin-fold measures, was significantly and positively correlated with 1- and 2-mile run times and inversely correlated with the number of sit-ups and push-ups. Fitness was positively correlated with body mass index (BMI) as well, except no significant relationship was found for number of push-ups. Among women, the results of the three fitness tests were also positively correlated with percent body fat, although the strength of the relationships was weaker. BMI was positively, but weakly, correlated with 1-mile run and weakly, but inversely, correlated with push-ups. However, in a subsequent study of female Army initial entry trainees, Sharp and colleagues (1994) found that women who failed the percent body fat standard performed significantly better on physical performance measures of strength. For men, injury rates were directly correlated with percent body fat; for women, the highest rates of injury occurred in the leaner groups. Among both men and women, faster run times were associated with increased injury rates. In a multivariate analysis, the odds ratio for injuries to women was 2.5 times those for men. In analyses stratified by gender, both fatness and fitness independently accounted for significant proportions of the variance in injury rates.

Fitness, Fatness, and Mortality

Fitness may be an independent predictor of mortality. In a series of studies, Blair and coworkers (1989) have shown that fitness, defined as maximal treadmill time, was inversely associated with mortality, even after control for a variety of other variables linked to early mortality, such as serum cholesterol, blood pressure, and blood glucose. However, the highest mortality rates occurred in the least fit individuals with the lowest BMIs. In subsequent studies, Caucasian men who maintained or improved adequate levels of fitness had lower mortality rates than men who were persistently unfit (Blair et al., 1995). In more detailed studies of the relationship of obesity and fitness, low fitness appeared to increase mortality rates among men in all weight categories and carried a risk comparable to other cardiovascular risk factors (Wei et al., 1999). In another study (Lee et al., 1999), men who were lean and unfit had a higher mortality rate than men who were obese and fit. These results suggest that fatness and fitness may have independent effects on mortality.

Caution is needed, however, in applying the data related to fitness and fatness reviewed above. First, the most comprehensive studies derive from a single patient population (Caucasian men). Therefore, the generalizability of these observations to other populations may be limited. Second, in many of the earliest papers, VO_{2max} was measured during submaximal exercise, but it was expressed as ml O_2/kg body weight. Because obesity was defined on the basis of BMI, individuals with increased BMIs may have been spuriously classified as obese. This difficulty was only partially addressed by the analyses of the effect of fitness within BMI categories. A more recent study examined the relationship of BMI, cardiorespiratory fitness, and all-cause mortality in women (Farrell et al., 2002). After adjusting for age, smoking, and baseline health status, the authors found that compared with normal-weight women, overweight and obesity did not significantly increase all-cause mortality. However, women with moderate and high cardiorespiratory fitness had significantly lower mortality risk compared with those with low cardiorespiratory fitness. These highly promising

TABLE 2-1 U.S. Army Maximum Weight (lb)-for-Height Accession Standards by Age

Height	Men (y)				Women (y)			
(in)	17–20	21–27	28–39	40+	17–20	21–27	28–39	40+
58					112	115	119	122
59					116	119	123	126
60	139	141	143	146	120	123	127	130
61	144	146	148	151	124	127	131	135
61	148	150	153	156	129	132	137	139
63	153	155	158	161	133	137	141	144
64	158	160	163	166	137	141	145	148
65	163	165	168	171	141	145	149	153
66	168	170	173	177	146	150	154	158
67	174	176	179	182	149	154	159	162
68	179	181	184	187	154	159	164	167
69	184	186	189	193	158	163	168	172
70	189	192	195	199	163	168	173	177
71	194	197	201	204	167	172	177	182
72	200	203	206	210	172	177	183	188
73	205	208	212	216	177	182	188	193
74	211	214	218	222	183	189	194	198
75	217	220	224	228	188	194	200	204
76	223	226	230	234	194	200	206	209
77	229	232	236	240	199	205	211	215
78	235	238	242	247	204	210	216	220
79	241	244	248	253	209	215	222	226
80	247	250	255	259	214	220	227	232

SOURCE: U.S. Army (1998).

results suggest that the military focus on the physical fitness of personnel is appropriate not only for performance, but also for overall health.

WEIGHT STANDARDS FOR ACCESSION AND RETENTION

Typically, the various branches of the military have had two sets of weight standards: one set of standards to be met by potential recruits for accession into initial entry training, and another equivalent or more stringent set of standards in order to be retained in the service.

TABLE 2-2 Maximum Body Mass Index (BMI) (kg/m^2) for Height for Accession

	Men				Women			
Height (in)	Army	Navy	Marine Corps	Air Force	Army	Navy	Marine Corps	Air Force
64	28.0	27.5	27.5	28.2	24.9	26.8	25.1	25.1
65	28.0	27.5	27.5	28.0	24.8	26.7	25.0	25.0
66	27.9	27.5	27.5	28.1	24.9	26.4	25.1	25.1
67	28.0	27.6	27.5	28.1	24.9	26.2	25.1	25.0
68	28.0	27.6	27.6	28.0	24.9	25.9	25.0	25.0
69	27.9	27.5	27.5	28.0	24.8	25.7	25.0	24.9
70	28.0	27.6	27.6	27.9	24.8	25.4	25.0	24.9
71	28.0	27.5	27.5	27.8	24.7	25.3	25.0	24.7
72	27.9	27.6	27.6	27.9	24.8	25.1	25.0	24.7
73	28.0	27.5	27.6	27.9	24.8	25.0	25.0	24.9
74	28.0	27.5	27.5	28.0	24.9	25.0	25.1	25.0
75	28.0	27.6	27.4	28.1	25.0	25.0	25.0	24.9
76	28.0	27.6	27.4	28.1	25.1	25.0	25.0	25.0
77	28.0	27.6	27.3	28.0	25.0	25.1	25.1	25.0
78	28.0	27.6	27.2	28.0	25.0	25.0	25.0	24.9
79	27.9	27.5	27.2	28.0	25.0	25.1	25.1	24.9
80	28.0	27.5	27.2	28.0	24.9	25.0	25.1	24.9

NOTE: Navy, Marine Corps, and Air Force accession standards are the same as their retention standards. Army BMI was calculated from age group 28–39 y weight-for-height accession standards. The new Department of Defense Instruction 1308.3 (DOD, 2002) sets BMI standards between a lower limit of 25 and an upper limit of 27.5.
SOURCE: USAF (2002); U.S. Army (1998); USMC (2002); U.S. Navy (2002).

Accession Standards

Each of the services maintains gender-specific, weight-for-height and body-fat standards for accession (entry) into active military service in order to prevent the entry of overfat individuals. In the Army and Navy, accession standards are more liberal than retention standards, and the Army accession weight-for-height standards change with increasing age (see Table 2-1). Accession standards for all the services, based on BMI, are presented in Table 2-2. Body-fat standards for accession and retention are presented in Table 2-3. Currently, the Navy's body-fat accession standard is 1 percent higher than its retention standard. The Army accession standard is more liberal relative to the retention standard for men than it is for women. This is based on evidence that male recruits lose weight during initial entry training and early in their enlistment and maintain the weight loss, while women may lose weight during initial entry training, but tend

TABLE 2-3 Maximum Body Fat (%) for Accession and Retention

Service	Gender	Age (y) 17–20	21–27	28–39	40+
Army	Male	20	22	24	26
	Female	28	30	32	34
Navy[a]	Male	22	22	22	23
	Female	33	33	33	34
Marine Corps	Male	18	18	18	18
	Female	26	26	26	26
Air Force	Male	20 (17–29 y)		24 (30+ y)	
	Female	28 (17–29 y)		32 (30+ y)	

NOTE: The body fat % is dependent upon age group, except for the Marine Corps, which does not distinguish between age groups.

[a] The Navy accession standard for body fat is 1% higher than retention standards. Specifically, the Navy accession standard for women is 34 percent body fat with a retention standard of 33 percent, for men the accession standard is 23 percent body fat and the retention standard is 22 percent.

SOURCE: GAO (1998); Singer et al. (2002).

to regain some of it (Friedl et al., 1989). Accession standards for the Air Force and Marine Corps are the same as their retention standards.

Because an accurate measurement of height and weight is considerably easier than an accurate measurement of percent body fat, the initial body composition screen for accession consists of a weight-for-height assessment using service-specific maximum allowable weight-for-height tables. Height and weight can be used to compute BMI, a widely accepted surrogate index of percent body fat (Gurrici et al., 1998; IOM, 1992a; NHLBI, 1998; Strain and Zumoff, 1992; Wang et al., 1996). It should be noted, however, that the military standards for maximum weight-for-height were established long before the science supporting the use of BMI was developed.

When only two measurements are used, height and weight have the highest level of association with the percentage of body fat. However, each service has conducted extensive anthropometric measurements of service personnel and used these data, together with data on body composition, to assess the best single additional measurement for estimating body fat (Friedl, 1992; Hodgdon, 1992). Until quite recently (DOD, 2002), none of the services had adopted the BMI per se as an alternative to maximum weight-for-height standards. However, the Air Force has considered BMI as part of the evaluation process before assigning an overweight individual to a weight-control program.

The maximum allowable weights-for-height have varied across services for individuals of the same height, age, and gender. The individual service standards were uniformly more stringent than the DOD recommendations. For example, as reviewed by the General Accounting Office (GAO, 1998), in 1998 the maximum allowable weight-for-height corresponded to a BMI of 25.1 for women in the Army, whereas for women in the Marine Corps, it corresponded to a BMI of 23.8. The disparity in maximum BMI between men and women was marked: while the maximum allowable weight-for-height for women in any service corresponded to a BMI of 25.1 (Army), for men it corresponded to a BMI of 28.2 (Air Force) (GAO, 1998).

However, in the recent revision of DOD Instruction 1308.3 (DOD, 2002), the weight-for-height tables have been revised to correspond to an upper-limit BMI of 27.5 and a lower limit BMI of 25, and it specifies that no service shall set more stringent screening weights than those corresponding to a BMI of 25. Thus, the Marine Corps had to raise its previous standard of 23.7 for women, while the Air Force had to decrease its previous standard of 28.2 for men.

Prospective recruits who exceed the accession weight limit for their height must undergo a body-fat assessment. The maximum allowable percentage of body fat for women on entry into the service ranges from 26 percent to 34 percent, depending on the service and for the Army, age. The maximum allowable percentage of body fat for men on entry into the service ranges from 18 percent to 26 percent depending on service and age (USAF, 2002; U.S. Army, 1987; U.S. Navy, 2002; USMC, 2002) (see Table 2-3). Each service uses circumference measurements to estimate body composition and, until recently, each employed its own set of measurement equations. However, as of November 2002, DOD has mandated a single circumference equation to be used across all the services for assessing percent body fat in men, and a different equation to be used in women.

In 1998, the Navy adopted a maximum standard of 23 percent body fat for men and 34 percent for women (Hodgdon, 1999). In setting these standards, the Navy consensus panel recognized that measures of height and weight "only approximate the precise magnitude of fatness," and that lack of a strong relationship may lead to inaccurate classifications. However, height and weight were the only measurements for which a great deal of epidemiological data were available (Hodgdon, 1999). Ideally, more sophisticated body-fat measurements should augment the weight-for-height indices.

Setting accession standards has implications for recruiting. When the services set restrictions on recruitment eligibility based on weight-for-height and estimated percent body fat, they eliminate a portion of individuals who might otherwise qualify for service. In the Third National Health and Nutrition Examination Survey (NHANES III), 59 percent of the men and 51 percent of the women in the survey over age 20 years exceeded recent guidelines (NHLBI, 1998) that suggest that men and women are overweight when they exceed a BMI of 25 (Flegal et al., 1998; Kuczmarski et al., 1997).

Nolte and coworkers (2002) recently examined NHANES III data to determine the percentage of the U.S. population between the ages of 17 and 20 years that would meet the military weight-for-height standards that were in effect at

TABLE 2-4 Maximum Permissible Body Mass Index (BMI) (kg/m^2) for Given Height for Retention

	Men				
Height (in)	DOD	Army	Navy	Marine Corps	Air Force
64	27.5	26.5	27.5	27.5	28.2
65	27.5	26.5	27.5	27.5	28.2
66	27.5	26.4	27.5	27.5	28.1
67	27.5	26.5	27.5	27.6	28.1
68	27.5	26.5	27.6	27.6	28.0
69	27.5	26.5	27.5	27.5	28.0
70	27.5	26.6	27.5	27.6	27.9
71	27.5	26.4	27.4	27.5	27.8
72	27.5	26.5	27.3	27.6	27.9
73	27.5	26.4	27.2	27.5	27.9
74	27.5	26.5	27.1	27.5	28.0
75	27.5	26.6	27.0	27.5	28.1
76	27.5	26.5	27.0	27.6	28.1
77	27.5	26.5	26.9	27.6	28.0
78	27.5	26.5	26.8	27.6	28.0
79	27.5	26.5	26.6	27.5	28.0
80	27.5	26.4	26.5	27.5	28.0

NOTE: Navy, Marine Corps, Air Force, and Department of Defense (DOD) standards are the same as their accession standards. Army BMI was calculated from age group 28–39 y weight-for-height retention standards.

the time the study was conducted. Their analysis indicated that 13 to 18 percent of men and 17 to 43 percent of women in this age range exceeded the military standards. The authors concluded that these data indicated a need for the military to reassess their standards. Perhaps a more appropriate conclusion (particularly for long-term health) would be to highlight the need for weight-gain prevention strategies targeted towards adolescents, particularly minority women. Data from the 1999–2000 NHANES indicate that BMI continues to increase, with the most recent data indicating that the prevalence of overweight and obesity in all men over the age of 20 years has now increased to 67.2 percent, while prevalence in women over the age of 20 years has risen to 61.9 percent (Flegal et al., 2002).

Women				
DOD	Army	Navy	Marine Corps	Air Force
27.5	23.6	26.8	25.1	25.1
27.5	23.5	26.7	25.0	25.0
27.5	23.6	26.4	25.1	25.1
27.5	23.4	26.2	25.1	25.0
27.5	23.5	25.9	25.0	25.0
27.5	23.4	25.7	25.0	24.9
27.5	23.4	25.4	25.0	24.9
27.5	23.3	25.3	25.0	24.7
27.5	23.4	25.1	25.0	24.7
27.5	23.4	25.0	25.0	24.9
27.5	23.5	25.0	25.1	25.0
27.5	23.5	25.0	25.1	24.9
27.5	23.7	25.0	25.0	25.0
27.5	23.6	25.1	25.1	25.0
27.5	23.6	25.0	25.0	24.9
27.5	23.6	25.1	25.1	24.9
27.5	23.6	25.0	25.1	24.9

SOURCE: DOD (2002); USAF (2002); U.S. Army (1987); USMC (2002); U.S. Navy (2002).

Retention Standards

The retention standards are the maximum weights-for-height and percent body fat that military personnel are allowed to avoid referral to a weight-management program (DOD, 1995). The current BMI retention standards for men and women for each military service are presented in Table 2-4. The maximum allowable percentage of body fat for men ranges from 18 to 26 percent depending on service and age, while for women it ranges from 26 to 34 percent (See Table 2-3).

Each of the services screens active duty personnel either annually or semi-annually for fitness and compliance with weight-for-height standards. Personnel may be screened several times a year in the course of medical examinations, physical fitness tests, or training school examinations. Thus, personnel receive regular feedback on how well they meet the standards of weight-for-height. The consequences of these practices are clear. In the NHANES III study, 34 percent of civilian men and 36 percent of civilian women over age 20 years exceeded a

BMI of 27 (NCHS, 1998). In contrast, in a 1998 worldwide survey of active duty military personnel from all four services (n = 17,264), only 21 percent of active duty men and 9 percent of active duty women exceeded a BMI of 27. Additionally, 57 percent of active duty men and 25 percent of active duty women exceeded the newer overweight standard of 25, compared with 59 percent and 51 percent of civilian men and women, respectively (Bray et al., 1999; Flegal et al., 1998).

Because the data from Bray and coworkers (1999) are self-reported rather than actual measurements, some bias may exist. However, investigators who collected both self-reported data and actual measurements concluded that such biases were small. They found that correlation between self-reported data and actual measurements was high ($R \geq 0.82$), and that self-reported data enabled investigators to classify weight category correctly 94 percent of the time (Jeffery, 1996; Strauss, 1999). Moreover, the data of Bray and coworkers (1999) were taken from surveys completed anonymously and collected by personnel who were outside the military chain of command of the respondents. Thus, these data most likely accurately portray the scope of the problem of overweight in the military services.

THE IMPACT OF WEIGHT AND BODY-FAT STANDARDS

One way to assess the impact of body-fat standards on the military is to look at the cost in terms of personnel management, namely the proportion of personnel enrolled in weight-management programs at any given time. Assignment to these programs requires paperwork and other administrative costs and may involve lost duty time. As of December 1999, 0.5 percent of male officers, 1.3 percent of female officers, 1.6 percent of male enlisted personnel, and 3.0 percent of female enlisted personnel were enrolled in the Air Force Weight Management Program. Data on weight-management programs recidivism or long-term success are not systematically compiled by any of the services, a situation that is, at least in part, intentional. The services attempt to minimize the stigma associated with participation in these programs by purging records.

The Impact on the Health Care System

Another way to assess the impact of body-fat standards on the military is to estimate their cost to the health care system. In 1998, according to the Defense Medical Epidemiology Database (DMED)[1], active duty personnel made 9.1 million visits[2] to ambulatory care clinics. Just over 40,000 of those visits were for a

---

[1] http://www.amsa.army.mil. The Army maintains the database, but it contains data from all four services.

[2] International Classification of Disease, 9th revision (ICD9) codes 001 through V99.

primary diagnosis of "obesity" or "localized adiposity."[3] An additional 2,700 visits were for a primary diagnosis of "anorexia," "bulimia," or other "eating disorder."[4] That is, less than one-half of 1 percent of all ambulatory visits made by active duty personnel were recorded as being primarily for concerns about body weight, body composition, or dysfunctional weight-loss practices. A different approach was reported by Robbins and colleagues (2002), who examined anthropometrics, demographics, and health behaviors of 4,974 active duty Air Force men and women. This analysis found that more than 20 percent exceeded their maximum allowable weights and that this was associated with an increased cost of $22.8 million per year for medical care and lost workdays (especially among men). Unfortunately, the statistics on visits to military clinics for weight-related matters do not provide a complete picture. Military personnel are likely to enroll in commercial weight-reduction programs or to self-treat with supplements or over-the-counter medications rather than call attention to their weight, which invites possible disciplinary action or separation from the service with loss of benefits.

Diabetes, hypertension, and ischemic heart disease accounted for less than 1 percent of the visits made to ambulatory care clinics by active duty personnel in 1998. Taken together, all visits for "endocrine, nutritional, and metabolic diseases and immune disorders" and "diseases of the circulatory system" accounted for 4.5 percent of the total visits (in contrast, musculoskeletal disease and injuries/poisonings accounted for 26 percent and 16 percent of all visits, respectively). Thus, since the military is made up predominately of young, healthy individuals who exercise with some regularity, it appears that they are far more likely to suffer musculoskeletal injuries than they are to present health problems associated with obesity.

The Impact on Weight-Loss Behavior and Disordered Eating

Eating disorders have been widely studied among civilian women and among select groups of men (e.g., athletes, wrestlers). Gross disturbances in eating behavior characterize the conditions of anorexia nervosa currently seen in 1 to 2 percent of females in the general population, and bulimia nervosa, which has a prevalence of 1 to 3 percent in this population. Both disorders have a female-to-male ratio of occurrence of 10:1. Another category of eating disorders, known as not otherwise specified (NOS), has been reported in the literature to occur in 3 to 35 percent of the population.

The need to maintain weight-for-height and body composition standards does place pressure on military personnel, particularly those who may find themselves in more sedentary occupations after completing initial entry and advanced individual training. The military policy of testing personnel annually or

[3] ICD9 codes 278-0 and 278-1, respectively.
[4] ICD9 codes 307-1, 307-51, and 307-51, respectively.

semi-annually can lead to undesirable and potentially unhealthy practices. For example, Peterson and coworkers (1995) examined the incidence of bulimic weight-loss behaviors in individuals in a military weight-management program, a civilian weight-loss program, and military personnel not in a weight-loss program. Military personnel in a weight-management program engaged in significantly more bulimic behaviors than either of the other two groups. Behaviors such as vomiting, strenuous exercise, and use of saunas or steam rooms was four times more common in those assigned to the military weight-management program. These results are more notable in that this group of individuals was predominantly male (65 percent).

In a series of studies of Navy personnel and of military women in all services, McNulty used the Stanford Eating Disorders Questionnaire with 706 active-duty Navy nurses (McNulty, 1997a), 1,425 active-duty Navy men (23.7 percent officers and 76.3 percent enlisted men, McNulty, 1997b), and 1,278 active-duty women in the Army, Navy, Marine Corps, and Air Force (McNulty, 2001).

The existence of eating disorders was found to be wide-spread in the Navy nurses, even among normal-weight women within the standard of 30 percent body fat. The prevalence of bulimia nervosa was 12.5 percent in this population, more than six times the prevalence reported in the civilian literature (McNulty, 1997a). Among the top five reasons given by these women for engaging in these practices were: being overweight, command morale, and maintaining the Navy fitness standards.

Among Navy men, 50.1 percent of the men across all ranks were classified as having an eating disorder (6.8 percent bulimic, 2.5 percent anorexic, and 40.8 percent NOS). While the use of diuretics, vomiting, diet pills, laxatives, and fasting all had a 2 to 4 percent prevalence under normal conditions (binge eating at 14 percent), these behaviors increased to a prevalence of 14 to 15 percent at the time of weigh-ins and fitness testing (binge eating at 26 percent). The top four reasons for engaging in these behaviors were: feeling overweight, rotating shifts, shipboard assignments, and no time allowed for physical fitness except during off-duty hours (McNulty, 1997b).

In another study focused on women in all branches of the service (McNulty, 2001), data were gathered from 235 Army women, 443 Navy women, 355 Air Force women, and 245 Marine Corps women. For the combined sample of 1,278 service women, the prevalence of eating disorders was 1.1 percent for anorexia nervosa, 8.1 percent for bulimia nervosa, and 62.8 percent NOS; 28 percent reporting normal eating. Marine Corps women scored significantly higher for all disorders than women in other service branches, although they had the lowest reported percent body fat (91.3 percent of Marine Corps women had body fat less than 26 percent, compared with 60 percent of Army women, 69 percent of Navy women, and 67 percent of Air Force women). Of the Marine Corps women surveyed, 22.3 percent reported being amenorrheic, compared with 10.2 percent of Army women, 9.9 percent of Navy women, and 7.4 percent of Air

TABLE 2-5 Percent of Military Women Using Purging Behaviors to Meet Weight/Height Standards

Behavior	Army	Navy	Marine Corps	Air Force
Diuretics	1.3	4.4	6.3	2.9
Vomiting	2.6	2.3	3.3	3.2
Fasting	18.8	18.3	38.0	20.2
Diet pills	8.6	11.2	28.6	13.4
Laxatives	2.2	2.3	12.4	3.4
Exercise (> 2×/d)	3.4	3.9	13.1	2.3

SOURCE: McNulty (2001).

Force women. The prevalence of use of various purging behaviors across the services are shown in Table 2-5. The top five reasons given for engaging in these types of behaviors were: competitiveness for advancement, concern for weight, being forced into a weight-control program, being harassed by supervisors for weight, and for Marine Corps women—lack of availability of low-fat meals. Clearly, these types of behaviors, coupled with the high prevalence of amenorrhea, could have significant long-term health implications for military women.

The Impact on the Loss of Personnel

The impact of body-fat standards on the military also can be assessed in terms of the separation of personnel. In 2002, almost 1.4 million men and women served on active duty in the four military services. The data of Lindquist and Bray (2001) suggest that 54 percent of active duty personnel are in danger of being assigned to a weight-control program, and some of these may be at risk of separation from the service due to overweight (based on self-reported BMIs). As shown in Table 2-6, over 4,600 individuals were discharged from the military for being overweight in 1999, but the numbers show a steady decline. (A large part of the decline is due to the Navy's decision to halt discharges for overweight. Navy personnel who fail to meet the standards are now allowed to serve out their current term of enlistment, but they are not permitted to re-enlist.) In 2002, total early separations for persistent failure to meet weight and body composition standards totaled just over 1,400 individuals. This is approximately 0.1 percent of the active duty force of 1.4 million personnel and represents a lost investment of approximately $57 million (in 1995 dollars), based on an estimated cost of recruitment and training of $40,283 per person (DOD PEC, 1997).

MEETING THE WEIGHT AND BODY-FAT STANDARDS

The past decade has brought considerable progress in developing new technologies (efforts that were funded substantially by DOD) and scientifically sound

TABLE 2-6 Number of Military Personnel Separated for Failure to Meet Weight and Body Composition Standards

	Year			
Service	1999	2000	2001	2002
Army (total)	1,703	1,202	1,013	953
Men	1,448	1,004	847	776
Women	255	198	166	177
Navy[a] (total)	2,190			
Men	1,768	Not	Not	Not
Women	422	applicable	applicable	applicable
Marine Corps (total)	156[b]	107	94	74
Men		94	88	67
Women		13	6	7
Air Force (total)	600	537	486	392
Men	389	364	333	237
Women	211	173	153	155
Total	4,649	1,846	1,593	1,419[c]

NOTE: In 1999, there were a total of 1,370,963 (DOD, 1999) enlisted personnel and officers in the services. In 2002, there were total of 1,402,120 active duty personnel.

[a] Navy data is from 1997. In 1998, the Navy placed a moratorium on administrative discharges for overweight.

[b] Marine Corps data is from 1998.

[c] Represents 0.1 percent of active duty forces.

SOURCE: Army data: personal communication, J. Sloan, Office of the Deputy Chief of Staff, May 19, 2003; Navy data: personal communication, T. Cepak, Navy Physical Readiness Program, 1999; Marine Corps data: personal communication, B. McGuire, Training Command, April 30, 2003; Air Force data: personal communication, J. Spahn, Population Health Support Branch, May 15, 2003.

methods of assessing body fat and setting appropriate weight and body-fat standards in support of the military's body composition, fitness, and readiness goals. DOD-wide uniformity in the use of these methodologies and standards is being sought to promote maximum objectivity and fairness to service members across the four services. As discussed earlier, a revised DOD Instruction has been issued that presents new DOD standards for maximum weight-for-heights corresponding to a minimum BMI of 25 and a maximum BMI of 27.5 (DOD, 2002). In addition, this policy also mandates the implementation of a single circumferential equation to estimate percent body fat for men and one for women to be used by all the services.

The weight and body-fat standards of the military services were predicated on the need for the highest level of physical performance in adverse environments, and to a lesser degree on the image that the individual may convey of the military. These standards theoretically take precedent even when individuals demonstrate an ability to perform their assigned tasks in an exceptional manner.

There are a number of problems created by these standards. First, many occupational specialties of today's military services do not require demanding physical performance and, in fact, may foster adverse changes in body composition due to their sedentary nature. Second, there is a high cost for recruiting, training, and assimilating individuals with needed skills into some highly technical positions. Third, the pool of potential applicants is small during good economic times. Finally, once trained by the military, many of these individuals in critical career fields can find higher-paying jobs in the civilian community where their body composition presents no problem.

Alternatively, the case can be made that all military personnel are potentially needed for duty in situations of armed conflict and thus even individuals that have occupational specialties that foster sedentary activity may be required to perform other tasks that demand physical strength and endurance. There is also the perception that individuals who have a low body-fat mass are likely to have less illness, which is important in hostile environments. Unfortunately, there are few data available on the relationship of body composition and performance of occupational specialties that do not require significant physical activity. There is an abundance of data on the relationship of body composition and long-term health, but less is known about this relationship in young individuals in the short term. Compliance with the military weight and body-fat standards may provide significant benefits to individuals after they retire from active duty, but it may not provide significant benefit to the services in terms of increased reliability of performance in many occupational specialties.

WEIGHT-MANAGEMENT PROGRAMS

The emphasis on methods and standards stands in sharp contrast to the lack of effort being devoted to improving policies and programs to assist service members who do not meet these standards, that is, programs for weight and fat loss and sustainment of these losses. While DOD and each of the services provide general guidance on body-weight management, the specifics of most weight/fat loss programs are unique to particular installations or units. The services have done relatively little medical and physiological research in this area, a deficiency that is particularly evident considering private industry's current effort to develop pharmacological and other novel weight-loss and maintenance interventions. In an era of recruitment and retention difficulties, the military could decrease the loss of trained personnel by capitalizing on these developments, improving existing programs, and attempting to provide more uniformity to weight-management programs across the services. More importantly, DOD needs to develop a strong focus on prevention programs, as well as on remedial programs.

Several factors have encouraged the military services to expand and refine their weight-control programs:

- The elimination of the draft and the conversion to an all-volunteer military has reduced the number of new recruits.
- The impact of obesity on long-term health has been more fully defined by epidemiological studies.
- Increases in manpower costs due to duty restriction or separations have been found to be significant.

Where the services diverge most is in their approach to weight management (see Table 2-7). The programs differ in a variety of ways, including:

- the amount of central control,
- the extent of medical evaluation given each individual,
- the existence of cautionary zones,
- the amount of counseling provided,
- the scope of the program (e.g., diet, exercise, behavioral modification),
- the qualifications of the staff administering the program,
- the procedures for data collection and evaluation of effectiveness, and
- the organizational setting of the program.

The Air Force has the most extensive weight-management program and maintains the most central control. A uniform set of procedures is prescribed by regulations that apply to all major Air Force installations. Air Force personnel assigned to remote locations are sent to the nearest clinic for evaluation and counseling or, in some instances, the program staff travels to the remote site. Programs in the other services are less standardized and employ more local innovation. Although the Army, Navy, and Marine Corps have centrally mandated programs, the details of the programs' content vary from one site to another. This is particularly true of the Army program, in which various sites have incorporated very different levels of counseling and the use of therapy. Some Army and Air Force sites have instituted innovative communication techniques, such as the use of Internet web sites. The Air Force is the only service that has adopted what might be considered a cautionary zone in which overweight individuals are given a 3-month opportunity to achieve weight compliance without administrative action.

No service has engaged in a preventive program applicable to all personnel, although the requirement to maintain body weight below upper limits is part of general indoctrination. The Air Force has reported on studies that have evaluated the effects of diet counseling using the Dietary Guidelines and the Food Guide Pyramid to improve responses in a 90-day fitness program (Gambera et al., 1995) and on a pilot study that evaluated the effects on new recruits of providing

TABLE 2-7 Current Military Weight-Management Policies and Procedures

	Army[a]	Navy[b]	Marine Corps[c]
How often/when weighed	Semiannual and at specific times	Semiannual PFA, risk factor screening Height/weight measurement includes body-fat assessment (only for members over maximum weight) PRT: Each PFA is conducted no later than 8 mo apart but no sooner than 4 mo apart	Semiannual
Body-fat measure reason	Overweight (per screening table), appears overweight	Exceeds maximum weight-for-height measurement	Exceeds height/weight standards

TABLE 2-7 Continued

	Army[a]	Navy[b]	Marine Co
Sites measured	Females: neck, hip, forearm, wrist Males: neck, abdomen	Females: neck, hips, waist Males: neck, abdomen	Females: n (greates ance of abdome waist) Males: nec (at nave
Personnel responsible for body-fat assessment	Company (or similar level) commander or designee	CFL, graduated from a 1-wk Physical Fitness Specialist course provided by the Cooper Institute	Command tative
Weight-management program execution	Weight-reduction counseling by health care personnel prior to or shortly after soldier is entered in the Weight Control Program Soldier is flagged under provisions of AR 600-31	If a service member fails a PFA, then it is mandatory for the CFL to personalize their fitness regimen and track their progress until they pass two consecutive PFAs Each member must receive nutrition counseling by a registered die-	MO evalua If no under cal cond signed t trition e program

		titian and receive a Navy Nutrition and Weight Control Self-Study Guide Each member can participate in SS	
Fails fitness test	Remedial PT	Failure to pass the body composition and/or the PRT constitutes a PFA cycle failure Mandatory FEP at unit level until sailor passes two consecutive PFAs Fails three PFAs in a 4-y period then denied reenlistment and mandatory punitive comments on fitness report	Assigned to RPCP

TABLE 2-7 Continued

	Army[a]	Navy[b]	Marine Co
Medical evaluation	Health care personnel when requested by the unit commander or prior to separation due to failure to make satisfactory progress	Must receive clearance from appropriate medical authority to participate in FEP (MD, PA, NP, IDC)	MO
Exemptions/deferrals (profile)	Pregnancy, postpartum recovery Documented medical condition	Pregnancy, waived from PRT/BCT until 6-mo postpartum Well-documented medical condition may be given a medical waiver from participation in body composition assessment, PRT, or physical conditioning	Pregnancy
Required weight loss ("progress")	3–8 lb/mo	No minimum exists CFL monitors progress of individual on FEP Stays on mandatory FEP until two consecutive PFAs have been passed	Normally: goal)/(6 n Case-by-ca mined by

		Bimonthly mock PRT and body-fat assessments are conducted to ensure progress	
Program structure	Soldier is entered into program Weight-reduction counseling (follow-up is established at the discretion of the health care personnel) Monthly weigh-ins (unit level) to assess progress (body-fat measurements may be made at this time) Removal from program when body-fat standard is achieved	Mandatory participation in FEP tailored to individuals needs CFL utilizes MWR fitness instructors to assist with exercise program CFL supplies Navy Nutrition and Weight Control Manual, self paced Nutrition counseling given by RD, possible participation in local weight-management program	6-mo initial assignment/6-mo extensio permissible if progr is being made Second assignment 6 mo, no extension available

TABLE 2-7 Continued

	Army[a]	Navy[b]	Marine Co
Program structure (continued)		Referral to SS, 10-wk weight-management program officially sanctioned program by BuMed SS is only offered by MTFs that choose to participate; not mandatory	
Completion of program	When body-fat standard is achieved	Remains in FEP until two consecutive PFAs are passed If a member graduates from SS, there is no requirement to be back within standards Three-failure rule in a 4-y period is still in effect	Self-mainte standards,

Administrative actions (grounds for separation)	36-mo probation 6 mo without meeting body-fat standards Exceeding body-fat standard within 12 mo of program completion	Members no longer separated for PRT/body composition failures No punitive administrative marks until third failure in a 4-y period Enlisted: May not reenlist, advance or redesignate until three consecutive PFAs are passed and within standards on day of action Officers: May not promote or redesignate until three consecutive PFAs are passed and within standards on day of action	No progress during initial assignment (to lack of effort) or meeting weight sta dard or body-fat go during 2-d assignm

TABLE 2-7 Continued

	Army[a]	Navy[b]	Marine Corp
Remedial action in basic combat training		Measuring outside of body composition standards constitutes a PFA cycle failure and all above actions apply	See administ tions

[a] AR = army regulation , PT = physical training.
[b] PFA = physical fitness assessment, PRT = physical readiness test, CFL = command fitness leader, ment program, MD = medical doctor, PA = physicians assistant, NP = nurse practitioner, IDC = inde combat training, MWR = morale, welfare, and recreation, RD = registered dietitian, BUMED = Bur medical treatment facilities.
[c] PT = physical training, MO = medical officer, RPCP = remedial physical conditioning program.
[d] PCS = permanent change of station, TDY = temporary duty away, BOTS = basic officer training sc cation, MAW = maximum allowable weight, HAWC = health and wellness center, HPM = health pr command, MD = medical doctor, UC = unit commander, TMD = temporary medical deferral, IC = i weight body fat management program, EDP = exercise and dietary period.
SOURCE: USAF (2002); U.S. Army (1987); USMC (2002); U.S. Navy (2002).

"heart-healthy" dining hall menus (Fiedler et al., 1999). A recent Army study (Arsenault and Cline, 2000) reported the positive effects of the regular consumption of reduced-fat food items on total nutrient consumption and BMI in 50 women in a U.S. Army Medical Department Officer Basic Course.

Each of the services performs medical evaluations to rule out possible medical causes of overweight before referring an individual to a weight-management program. A medical officer evaluates the individual's records and physical health to ensure that participation in a weight-management program will be safe. However, the extent of this medical evaluation is not well defined, except by the Air Force. In some programs, specific tests are conducted for underlying disease; the Air Force also assesses psychosocial factors such as readiness and stress levels.

Army

The Army program, "Weigh to Stay," is managed by physical fitness trainers who must complete a course on weight loss and weight-control counseling. The Army also runs a number of hospital weight-loss and weight-management programs that are overseen by physicians as part of preventive medicine research efforts. The Hawaii-based program is highly innovative in its reliance on behavior modification and use of the Internet to maintain support of individuals at remote locations (James LC et al., 1997; James et al., 1999b). Monthly weigh-ins are required, and those who fail to make satisfactory progress (loss of 3 to 8 lb/mo) for 2 consecutive months can face separation. Exemptions from the program are granted for prolonged illness, pregnancy (up to 180 d postpartum), hospitalization, or a medical profile waiver (U.S. Army, 1987).

Navy

According to the *Physical Readiness Program* (U.S. Navy, 2002) the Navy's Command-Directed Physical Conditioning Program (CDPCP) is required for all individuals who fail the physical fitness test or who do not meet body fat standards. It is a 6-month program managed by a command-trained, physical-fitness coordinator (an enlisted person who has undergone 2.5 days of training). The program includes mandatory supervised exercise three times per week. Each individual who exceeds body-fat standards is issued a self-study nutrition and weight-control guide. A more rigorous, second phase program is the Bureau of Medicine-Approved Weight Management Program, an intensive 2-week outpatient program that requires the commanding officer's endorsement and 6-months prior participation in the CDPCP. Individuals with three fitness or body fat failures are not eligible (three failures in 4 years results in administrative action and although individuals are no longer separated from the service, they are not permitted to reenlist and are not eligible for promotion for the duration of their enlistment term). Successful completion of the Bureau of Medicine program and 1 year of follow-up in which progress continues toward meeting body fat standards result in a clear record. The Navy also conducts a 2-day course on recipe modification for mess specialists. The Navy has some innovative, small-scale weight-control programs to which selected individuals can be assigned. These include a 10-week program on nutrition, behavior modification, and exercise, with monthly support-group follow-up at the Norfolk Navy Environmental Health Center; a shipboard weight-control program (Dennis et al., 1999); and a program at San Diego Naval Medical Center that is regarded as a model for programs used at other locations (Carlson and Burman, 1984; Trent and Stevens, 1993, 1995). The challenge for the Navy has been to devise a single program that would address the needs of personnel at diverse duty stations and that could be taught by minimally trained personnel (Hoiberg and McNally, 1991).

Marine Corps

The Marine Corps' physical fitness/weight-control program, "Semper Fit," similar to that of the Army, is managed by physical fitness trainers. Diet counseling is administered by self-study or by a dietitian if the individuals are close to an installation with an available dietetic service. Individuals who fail to meet the body fat standards and who do not receive a medical waiver are enrolled for an initial period of 6 months. If the individual is progressing but has not yet reached the target weight or percent body fat at the 6-month point, he or she may be allowed to continue for another 6 months. If after reaching the goal, the individual fails again during the rest of his or her career, he or she is allowed another 6 months to achieve compliance or face separation (USMC, 2002).

Air Force

The Air Force Weight and Body Fat Management Program (WBFMP) operates from a health and wellness center (HAWC) located on each base, which is responsible for assessment of weight, body fat, fitness, and data recording. Personnel who exceed the body-fat standards undergo clinical, laboratory, and psychological assessment to determine their qualification for the WBFMP. Those deemed unqualified are sent to an appropriate practitioner for care. The program consists of three phases. Medically cleared personnel are admitted to a 3-month initial program that provides counseling on diet and behavior modification by an Air Force dietitian or other authorized medical personnel, as well as exercise instruction provided by the HAWC staff. All individuals assigned to the program must attend a series of four classes concerning diet, behavior modification, and exercise. Personnel enrolled in the initial program are not penalized by administrative actions during the 3-month enrollment, although they are restricted from some professional activities. Personnel who meet their weight/body fat standard after completion of the 3-month program proceed to Phase II, a 6-month maintenance/monitoring program. Following successful completion of

Phase II, the individual's WBFMP records are expunged. Personnel who fail to meet their goal within the first 3 months of the initial program are enrolled in Phase I, a more intense weight-management program in which monitoring is conducted monthly and the individual is subject to significant administrative restrictions relating to assignments, training, and promotions. Each Air Force installation has the authority to select programs approved by the Major Command dietitian for use in counseling on diet and exercise (USAF, 2002), for example, "The Sensible Weigh" or "Shape Your Future Your Weigh."

SUMMARY

Accession and retention weight-for-height and percent body fat standards vary across the four services, as does the comprehensiveness of weight-loss programs. A review of the weight-loss programs across the military services highlights some significant deficits that could affect success. All of the programs have a strong motivating component that is highly disciplinary in nature—the penalties for exceeding the body fat limits are significant. The majority of participants receive only minimal counseling by a qualified dietitian (with the exception of those in the Air Force program). The same appears to be true throughout the services for the area of behavior modification. With the exception of the Air Force (Spahn, 1999) and some specific sites in the other services, data collection for program evaluation is lacking.

3

Factors That Influence Body Weight

There are numerous factors that can influence body weight. The individual has no control over some of these factors, including developmental determinants, genetic makeup, gender, and age. Other factors that influence body weight over which the individual has potential control include level of physical activity, diet, and some environmental and social factors. This chapter explores the relationship between each of these factors and body weight.

DEVELOPMENTAL DETERMINANTS

It has been postulated that there are times during people's lives when exposure to certain factors may increase their risk for the onset of obesity. These times have been termed "critical periods." If these critical periods, along with the influential factors, can be clearly defined, it may be possible to identify individuals at increased risk for the development and persistence of overweight and obesity in adulthood. The prenatal period, the period of adiposity rebound, and adolescence have been proposed as critical periods in childhood (Dietz, 1994); pregnancy and the immediate postpartum period have been proposed as critical periods for women in adulthood.

Prenatal Factors

Although the data are subject to a variety of interpretations, it has been documented in both animals and humans that females who are severely food restricted during the first one to two trimesters of pregnancy have progeny who have a higher prevalence of obesity, diabetes, insulin resistance, and hypertension later in life. Progeny of survivors of the Dutch famine in World War II demonstrated a higher prevalence of obesity and diabetes (Ravelli et al., 1976), although this conclusion was questioned by later studies (Jackson et al., 1996; Susser and Stein, 1994). Malnutrition in utero also has been reported to result in increased obesity and its complications later in life (Stanner et al., 1997). Lower birth weights also seem to be associated with increased upper body visceral adiposity in later life with its attendant increased risk of cardiovascular disease (Oken and Gillman, 2003; Rogers, 2003). Since individuals from a lower socio-economic background are more likely to be exposed to malnutrition during gestation or early childhood, the prevalence of obesity in such subgroups might be expected to be higher.

Adiposity Rebound

Adiposity increases from birth until approximately 1 year of age, then declines to a minimum at approximately 6 years of age. The term "adiposity rebound" refers to the increase in body mass index (BMI) and body fat that occurs after this nadir in children between the ages of 5 and 7 years. Children experiencing adiposity rebound at an earlier age appear to have a three- to sixfold greater risk of increased adult BMI than do other children (Whitaker et al., 1998). He and Karlberg (2002) demonstrated, through the development of probability charts based on 3,650 children followed from birth to 18 years of age, that children who experienced this rebound before 8 years of age have a higher risk of adulthood obesity. However, Guo and coworkers (2000), using serial BMI data from the Fels Longitudinal study demonstrated that while there was no association between early age at adiposity rebound and adult BMI status in men, after controlling for effects of birth weight, adult physical activity, alcohol and cigarette use, there was approximately twice the risk for overweight with early rebound in women.

Causes of early adiposity rebound have been variously attributed to advanced skeletal maturity (Roland-Cachera et al., 1984; Williams and Dickson, 2002), high protein intake (Roland-Cachera et al., 1995), and parental BMI (Dorosty et al., 2000). Cameron and Demerath (2002) concluded after extensive review of the available scientific literature that the evidence is still not clear about whether age at adiposity rebound is a critical period for the development of obesity, but that early adiposity rebound might well be a statistical predictor of later obesity because of its strong relationship with early adiposity and accelerated maturation, both of which are established markers of later risk of obesity.

Adolescence

Although only 30 percent of adult obesity begins during childhood, 70 percent of the adult obesity that begins in childhood may start during adolescence (Dietz, 1994). Adolescent obesity is associated with a variety of adverse health effects in adulthood, including early mortality in men and increased risks of coronary heart disease, diabetes, and colorectal cancer (Miller, 1988; Must et al., 1992; Wylie-Rosett, 1988). Most of these risks were only slightly attenuated by adjustment for adult obesity, which suggests that obesity during adolescence may determine the risk of these later complications regardless of whether or not the individuals are obese adults.

While total fatness is an important consideration when evaluating developmental aspects of obesity, an additional consideration is adipose tissue distribution. Visceral adipose tissue has an independent effect on obesity-associated comorbidities (Emery et al., 1993) that is separate from that of total body fat, although the developmental aspects of visceral adipose tissue deposition have not been well studied. Among children, visceral adiposity appears to be associated with an increased risk of cardiovascular risk factors such as elevated triglycerides and reduced high-density lipoproteins that are independent of total body fat (Caprio et al., 1996; Gutin et al., 1994). However, the ages at which these relationships appear remain unclear. Cross-sectional studies suggest that visceral adipose tissue deposition is not marked before adolescence, but increases rapidly at that time.

Adulthood

The period after adolescence has not been intensively studied, although approximately two-thirds of adult obesity begins after adolescence. Whether additional critical periods exist in adulthood is less certain, but pregnancy and postpartum may constitute one such period for a subset of women (Williamson et al., 1994). Postpartum weight retention appears to range from 0.5 to 4.8 kg for most women (Johnston, 1991), but African-American mothers may be twice as likely to retain 9.1 kg (20 lb) or more postpartum than Caucasian mothers (Parker and Abrams, 1993). Boardley and colleagues (1995) found that African-American women ate more and were less physically active postpartum than were the Caucasian women in their sample. When the possible confounding factors of prepregnancy weight, gestational weight gain, prenatal physical activity, parity, and socioeconomic status were controlled, African-American women still retained more weight in the postpartum period than did Caucasian women. Results of several recent studies suggest that possible genetic factors may be involved in the tendency to retain weight postpartum. One study found that in women with normal prepregnancy BMIs, high first-trimester serum leptin concentrations (a protein hormone encoded by the *obese* gene) correlated with increased gestational weight gain and postpartum weight retention (Stein et al., 1998). In another study, women within 12 months of the birth of their first child who were homozygous for the 825T allele of the G-protein ß3, considered a "thrifty" genotype, had significantly higher BMIs and postpartum weight retention than women who did not carry the genotype (Gütersohn et al., 2000). No effect of the genotype was observed among women who had never given birth, suggesting a pregnancy-specific phenomenon. In addition, this relationship was only observed among women who engaged in low levels of physical activity, supporting the idea that physical activity may mitigate effects of genetic endowment on the potential for postpartum weight retention. Whether this particular genetic variation in this specific G protein is causally linked to the observed differences in BMI and weight retention or is merely a marker for the responsible mutation, as well as what the mechanism might be, are both questions that require further investigation (Feldman and Hegele, 2000).

GENETIC DETERMINANTS

The understanding of the genetic influences on overweight and obesity in humans has increased dramatically. Individuals show significant heterogeneity in their body weight and body fatness responses to altered energy balance, dietary components, and changing activity levels. It is now well-established that overweight and obesity have a significant genetic component, with estimates of the contribution of genetic variation to observed variation in obesity-related phenotypes (such as BMI, fat mass, and leptin levels) ranging from 30 to 70 percent (Comuzzie et al., 1993, 1994, 1996). However, little is yet known about the specific causes of heterogeneity (Pérusse and Bouchard, 1999). It seems clear that energy metabolism and neural control of appetite are involved in regulating body weight and may contribute to the etiology of obesity. Studies of resting metabolic rate show that the variation within families is less than the variation among families (Bogardus et al., 1986).

Several studies have evaluated the potential mechanisms by which genetic factors may contribute to obesity. One of the mechanisms by which differences in energy metabolism may contribute to obesity may involve defects in uncoupling proteins (UCP). Several types of uncoupling proteins have been identified. Fleury and colleagues (1997) first described human uncoupling protein 2 (UCP-2) and its links to obesity and hyperinsulinemia. Bouchard (1997) noted that markers near the UCP-2 gene in humans are linked to differences in resting metabolic rate. Thus, genetic differences in UCP-2, and perhaps other UCPs, may contribute to human obesity.

There is a group of at least 20 Mendelian syndromes in which obesity is a component, including Prader-Willi, Bardet-Biedl, Borjeson, Cohen, and Wilson-Turner (Gunay-Aygun et al., 1997; Reed et al., 1995). These genetic disorders are rare, and family studies do not suggest that the genes responsible for these syndromes are involved in the common forms of human obesity. For more than 99 percent of obese humans, the genetic basis of their obesity is unknown.

Animal Models of Genetic Obesity

The strongest evidence for genetic weight-regulating mechanisms is the recent elucidation of single gene defects that are associated with excessive weight gain in animals. Single gene mutations can indisputably cause obesity in both rodent models and in humans. In rodents, such mutations have been identified in at least five genes: the *obese* gene for the circulating adipose tissue-secreted factor leptin; the *db* gene for the receptor of leptin; the *agouti yellow* mutation, which controls hair color in mice through the production of melanin pigments (with its human equivalent, agouti signaling protein gene); the *fat* mutation in the carboxipeptidase E gene, which is a prohormone processing enzyme; and the *tub* mutation, the function of which has yet to be determined. Of the five gene products that currently have been associated with weight regulation, leptin is the best characterized. Genetic defects in leptin are associated with extreme obesity in both humans and laboratory animals. In addition, serum concentrations of leptin are elevated in close proportion to body fat in obese people with no defect in the leptin gene. Recent studies show that administration of recombinant leptin to lean and obese individuals results in dose-dependent weight loss (Heymsfield et al., 1999). Further research is needed to assess the potential role of leptin in obesity treatment.

Familial Aggregation of Risk for Obesity

Using the comprehensive Danish adoption registry, Stunkard and colleagues (1986) found that adopted children who were raised separately from their biological parents had body weights closer to those of their biological parents than to those of their adoptive parents. The children in this study were separated from their parents at a very early age, generally before 3 months, so the opportunity for the biological parents to instill eating and activity habits was very limited. Another study of adoptees showed a significant genetic influence on obesity, but none of the environmental indicators evaluated were found to contribute, although a number of the conditions considered have previously been associated with obesity (Sorensen et al., 1998). Stunkard and colleagues (1986) estimated that as much as 70 percent of the variance in the occurrence of obesity could be attributed to genetic factors, but other authors have postulated that as little as 20 percent of the variance is due to genetic factors. The general consensus is that genetic factors account for about 30 to 50 percent of the variance in the occurrence of obesity (Bouchard, 1997).

Twin studies provide the most impressive clinical evidence that genetic factors play an important role in the etiology of obesity in humans. Stunkard and colleagues (1990) studied identical and nonidentical twins who were reared together and others who were reared apart. They found a high correlation of body weight among identical twins, even if they were reared apart. Bouchard and colleagues (1990) studied twins who were isolated in the Canadian wilderness with no access to foods other than those provided by the investigators. Identical twins were overfed for a period of 100 days, and their gains in body weight and adipose tissue were evaluated. There was a closer association of both body weight and intra-abdominal adipose tissue (visceral fat) within twin pairs than among twin pairs.

The maximal heritability of obesity has been estimated to range from 30 to 50 percent, based on a review of family studies (Chagnon et al., 2000). Although extensive efforts have been made to identify mutations in the genes identified as obesity-associated in rodents and in other candidate genes for obesity in humans, to date only a handful of individuals have been identified with mutations in any of the genes that have produced obesity in rodents. Specifically, several humans have been identified with mutations in the leptin gene or its receptor, but no individuals have yet been found with mutations in the other genes identified in rodents.

In total, single gene mutations have been identified as responsible for obesity in 25 persons, with these mutations appearing in 7 genes (12 different mutations) (Pérusse et al., 1999) or in 5 genes (Chagnon et al., 2000). Studies of quantitative trait loci (QTL) in rodents have suggested at least 98 different QTLs associated with obesity (Chagnon et al., 2000).

Currently, the major effort in the search for specific genes that contribute to human overweight and obesity is based on the use of genome scanning. In genome scanning, linkage analysis is conducted to identify QTLs that affect the specific phenotype under study. The use of genome scanning has provided evidence of QTLs that influence body weight and the number of fat cells (Chagnon et al., 2000).

Comparison of the risks of obesity in spouses and in first-degree relatives has suggested that genetic factors may be of greater prominence in more severe obesity (Katzmarzyk et al., 2000). Among the members of families that contain at least one morbidly obese person, a major gene effect was transmitted in a codominant fashion, suggesting a gene-environment interaction (Rice et al., 1999). Both multifactorial and major gene effects have been suggested. Efforts are ongoing to identify the genetic and molecular basis of overweight and obesity, and it is likely that many genes (and within these genes and their promoters, many different mutations or variants) that are responsible for the genetic variation of obesity in humans will be identified.

The development of obesity likely involves a combination of shared environment and shared genetic propensities. The rapid increase in prevalence of obesity in the United States, as well as in many other countries, across all age groups may reflect a removal of environmental constraints (e.g., high levels of daily activity and food availability) on the expression of obesity genotypes. Knowledge of the genetic components of obesity is not likely to be useful to the military in the near term, but identification of markers of potential risk of obesity may well have implications for future screening.

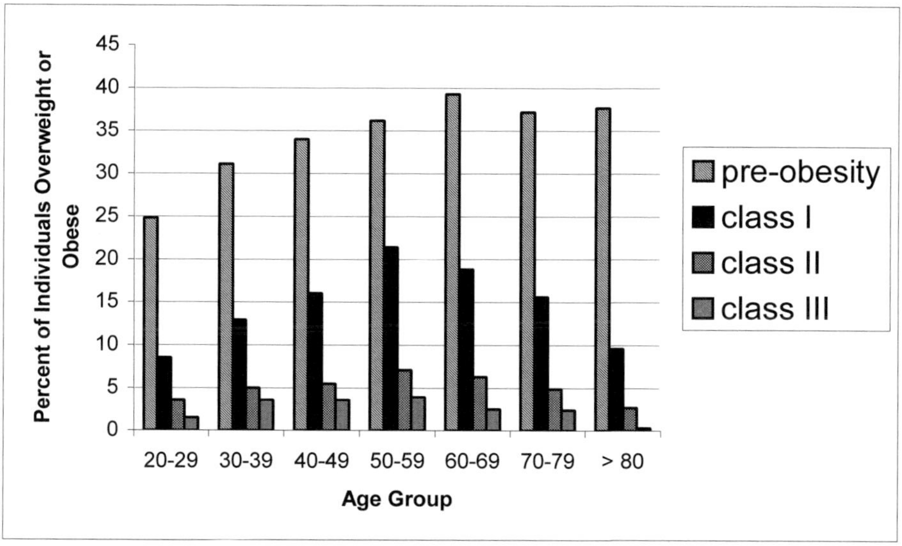

FIGURE 3-1 The prevalence (%) of overweight and obesity of men and women by age in the U.S. population. Preobesity = body mass index (BMI) of 25–29.9, class I obesity = BMI of 30–34.9, class II obesity = BMI of 35–39.9, and class III obesity = BMI ≥ 40. SOURCE: Third National Health and Nutrition Examination Survey, 1988–1994, Must et al. (1999).

AGE

Cross-sectional and longitudinal studies indicate a gradual increase in the average BMI of Americans up to the ages of 50 to 60 years (IOM, 1995). This trend is similar, with some variation, across males and females and across all evaluated ethnic groups. Population studies also indicate a decline in body weight and BMI among the elderly, usually in the seventh and eighth decades (IOM, 1995; Kuczmarski et al., 1994; NHLBI, 1998). The same trends have been identified in changes in total body fat and percent body fat (Chumlea et al., 2002). Overweight and obesity thus reach maximal rates among middle-aged adults. This pattern is shown in Figure 3-1.

The age-related body mass increase up to the fifth and sixth decades is accompanied by additional anatomical, structural, and body compositional changes. Stature declines from about age 30 onward, with rates in women faster than those in men and for postmenopausal women faster than their premenopausal counterparts. Declining stature accounts for a small portion of the age-related increase in BMI (Gallagher et al., 1996).

Many weight-management experts agree that body weight becomes progressively more difficult to maintain with age, but there appears to be little rationale for increasing the upper BMI range consistent with good health as individuals become older. Williams (1997) indicated that body weight and associated circumferences would increase with advancing age unless food intake is reduced and physical activity is substantially increased.

A large number of cross-sectional studies, however, do demonstrate that body fat increases with age, even after controlling for changes in body weight and physical activity levels (Baumgartner et al., 1995; Flynn et al., 1989; Forbes, 1987; Forbes and Reina, 1970; Gallagher et al., 1996, 1997; Noppa et al., 1980; Novak, 1972; Steen et al., 1979). Gallagher and colleagues (1996) demonstrated that the mean body-fat content in nonexercising civilian women with a BMI of 25 increased from 30 percent for those between the ages of 17 and 20 years to 36 percent for those ages 40 years and older. The implication of this is that lean body mass and, frequently, skeletal mass, decrease with age. Additionally, partitioning of adipose tissue between the subcutaneous and visceral compartments is also moderated by age (Borkan et al., 1983). Men have more visceral adipose tissue than do women at all ages, and the rate of visceral adipose tissue increase with age is greater in men than in women (Blaak, 2001).

In contrast to body fat, skeletal muscle mass declines with age beginning around the third decade of life (Dutta and Hadley, 1995). This observation is true not only for the general population, but it is also evident in military personnel (USAF, 1975). The rates of decline may accelerate after the onset of menopause in women (Aloia et al., 1991) and for both genders in the seventh and eighth decades (Flynn et al., 1989). Losses of skeletal muscle parallel changes in skeletal minerals with advancing age and are present even after controlling for loss in body weight (Gallagher et al., 2000). The mechanisms of body composition change with aging are multifactorial and include physical inactivity, diet, and hormonal and cytokine alterations. The loss of lean mass and gain in fat mass occur even with no apparent change in body weight. Since lean mass contributes the larger share of metabolic activity, total energy expenditure during rest or low activity will also decrease proportionally with the loss of lean mass.

Total energy expenditure and thus, energy requirements, decrease with advancing age (Tzankoff and Norris, 1978). Physical activity levels are lower in older individuals, which account for a portion of the energy expenditure reduction that comes with aging. Resting energy requirements are also lower in the elderly, due largely to decreases in all metabolically active tissues, including skeletal muscle, brain, and visceral organs. In laboratory animals, the heat produced by tissues per unit of mass decreases with age (a decrease in the specific resting energy expenditure of organs), but it remains uncertain whether this observation also applies to humans. The practice of resistance training by people over the age of 50 years may enhance fat-free mass, primarily skeletal muscle, and thereby help offset the age-related decline in resting metabolic rate (Hill and Saris, 1998; Tzankoff and Norris, 1977). In women, loss of ovarian function accounts for a lower rate of overall heat production compared with that observed in premenopausal women (Poehlman and Tchernof, 1998). Thus, both older men and women have lower rates of energy expenditure and, unless counterbalanced by increased physical activity and reduced food intake, older individuals, in general, will gain weight over time.

RACE/ETHNICITY

Whether there are racial/ethnic differences in response to the various components of weight management is a legitimate research question that has been explored to only a moderate extent. Data from National Health and Nutrition Examination Surveys (NHANES) clearly indicate that there are racial/ethnic differences in the prevalence of overweight and obesity. Flegal and coworkers (2002), reporting on 1999–2000 NHANES data, determined that in men 20 years of age and older, the prevalence of overweight (BMI $\geq$ 25) was 67.4 percent for non-Hispanic whites, 60.7 percent for non-Hispanic blacks, and 74.7 percent for Mexican Americans. The differences were not statistically significant, but sample sizes were relatively small. However, for women ages 20 years and older, the prevalence of overweight was 57.3 percent in non-Hispanic whites, 77.3 percent in non-Hispanic blacks, and 71.9 percent in Mexican Americans. The difference in prevalence between non-Hispanic white and non-Hispanic black women was statistically significant (Flegal et al., 2002). The causes of these differences in the prevalence of overweight have not been clearly identified, but are likely to be a combination of physiology, culture, and behavior.

The relationship of BMI to percent body fat is also affected by race/ethnicity. Fernandez and colleagues (2003) recently reported the results of an analysis of 11 cross-sectional studies involving body composition assessments of African-American men and women, Hispanic-American men and women, and European-American men and women. The average age ranged from 42.6 to 50.8 years, and the average BMI ranged from 25.1 (European-American women) to 29.8 (African-American women). Total body fat was measured using dual-energy X-ray absorptiometry. There were no differences in the estimation of percent body fat from BMI for men across ethnic groups. However, for women with BMIs less than 30, Hispanic-American women had a significantly higher percent of body fat at a given BMI than did African-American or European-American women. However, at BMIs greater than 35, European-American women had a higher percent body fat than either of the other two groups of women. Some earlier studies have reported greater fat free mass in African-American women compared with Caucasian women with the same

BMI, primarily due to the greater skeletal mass in African-American women (Gallagher et al., 1996; Ortiz et al., 1992).

A number of studies have examined possible physiological reasons for these race/ethnic differences. Foster and colleagues (1997) explored differences in resting energy expenditure (REE) between obese African-American women and Caucasian-American women. They found that REE was most closely correlated to body weight and that African-American women had lower REE than Caucasian-American women. Melby and coworkers (2000) examined behavioral and physiological characteristics related to obesity risk in young, sedentary, nonobese African-American and Caucasian-American women. The two groups were similar in age and anthropometric characteristics. Parameters examined included REE, respiratory exchange rates (RER), insulin sensitivity, and maximal oxygen consumption. REE was 3 to 4 percent lower in African-American women, but the difference was not statistically significant. However, the resting RER was significantly lower in African-American women. The African-American women also had significantly lower insulin sensitivity values that resulted in higher acute phase insulin response to glucose. Total daily energy expenditure and physical activity energy expenditure were significantly lower in the African-American women.

Tanner and coworkers (2002) recently identified a relationship between muscle fiber type and obesity. In a study of lean and obese African-American and Caucasian women, type I muscle fibers (slow twitch, oxidative muscle fibers) were significantly reduced in obese women compared with the lean women, and type IIb fibers (fast twitch, glycolytic muscle fibers) were significantly increased. These differences between lean and obese women were greater in African-Americans than in Caucasians. The type IIb phenotype is insulin resistant and deficient with regard to lipid disposal. The authors speculated that the prevalence of the type II fibers might result in partitioning lipid toward storage in skeletal muscle or adipose tissue rather than oxidation within the skeletal muscle, resulting in a positive fat balance.

A number of studies have also examined social and behavioral factors that may contribute to the difference in the prevalence of overweight between African-American and Caucasian women (Kumanyika et al., 1993; Stevens et al., 1994). Attitudinal and behavioral factors that limit the ability of some African-American women to lose weight or maintain weight loss have been identified. Regardless of whether or not they were overweight, African-American women were half as likely as Caucasian women to consider themselves overweight. There is a much greater cultural tolerance of overweight among African-Americans, and they have different body image perceptions. Although African-American women responded physiologically to a weight-reduction program in the same manner as Caucasian women, their drop-out rate from the program was double that of Caucasian women (Glass et al., 2002).

PHYSICAL ACTIVITY

While recent studies point to the importance of genetic factors in the etiology of obesity (Bouchard, 1997; Chagnon et al., 2000), the rapid rise in the prevalence of overweight and obesity in the last 20 years likely reflects major environmental shifts in exercise habits and food availability, which can be controlled.

Physical activity represents an important component of volitional energy expenditure. Modern transportation and other conveniences have reduced the need for energy expenditure in the form of physical exertion. Reductions in physical activity over the past several decades likely contribute to the evolution of the positive energy balance and weight-gain characteristics of all industrialized societies. Lack of physical activity begins in youth, with television watching time correlated with BMI, as well as with both prevalence and severity of overweight (Dietz and Gortmaker, 1985; Katzmarzyk et al., 1998; Tanasescu et al., 2000). A reduced emphasis on school physical education classes has been accompanied by a gradual decline in childhood fitness (Luepker, 1999). Indeed, physical inactivity is a major risk factor for development of obesity in children and adults (Astrup, 1999; Goran, 2001). Among adults who have maintained weight loss over time, a common factor is increased physical activity (Klem et al., 1997).

The effects of physical activity on weight and health may be influenced by age. Owens and coworkers (1992) evaluated the effects of physical activity on both weight change and the risk factors for cardiovascular disease during the perimenopausal period. Women who increased their activity levels during the 3-year study period (as measured using the Paffenbarger Physical Activity Questionnaire) had the smallest increases in body weight and the smallest decrement in high-density lipoprotein cholesterol.

Flatt (1987) has pointed out that to avoid increased fat deposition, both energy balance and macronutrient balance (especially fat balance) are necessary. When dietary fat is elevated, there is limited capacity to reduce total body fat by fat oxidation. Exercise, especially in bouts of 30 minutes of activity or more (Pate et al., 1995), can promote fat oxidation because the substrate that is preferentially oxidized switches from carbohydrate to fat. Thus, chronic extended bouts of exercise may, in effect, substitute for expansion of the adipose tissue, allowing the physically active individual to achieve fat balance while maintaining a lower body-fat mass than the sedentary individual (Flatt, 1987). Jakicic and coworkers (1995) initially demonstrated that over the short term, four 10-minute bouts of exercise per day, four times per week is more effective in reducing body weight than a single 30 to 40 minute period of exercise. However, the long-term data indicated that the short-term bouts of exercise were not as effective as the long bouts in reducing weight and maintaining weight loss (Jakicic et al., 1999).

Most fatty-acid oxidation in the human body occurs in muscle (Calles-Escandon and Poehlman, 1997). The intrinsic capacity of muscle to oxidize fat can be impaired by physical inactivity and possibly by loss of estrogen in women, but it is amenable to partial correction by exercise training (Calles-Escandon and Poehlman, 1997). A decrease in aerobic capacity and fat-free mass, rather than aging per se, is responsible for the decrease in fat oxidation seen in elderly women (Calles-Escandon and Poehlman, 1997). Exercise training increases oxidative disposal of fatty acids and improves muscle metabolism in both young and old individuals. However, the elderly do not increase fat utilization in response to exercise to the same extent as the young, despite performing exercise to the same intensity and for the same duration (Blaak, 2000; Calles-Escandon and Poehlman, 1997).

In a study of 970 healthy, female twins with a wide range of percent body fat, both total body fat and central adiposity were associated with physical activity (Samaras et al., 1999). Moderate-intensity sports of 1 and 2 hour durations accounted for within-pair differences of 1.0 kg and 1.4 kg, respectively, of total body fat. Among participants in whom one of a pair of twins was overweight, higher levels of physical activity were still associated with 3.96 kg lower total body fat and 0.53 kg lower central abdominal fat. In other words, even persons with an apparent genetic predisposition to adiposity showed an effect of physical activity on body-fat mass (Samaras et al., 1999). Studies of energy expenditure in individuals and families show that differences are greater between families than within families (Bogardus et al., 1986). Some differences in energy expenditure between families are due to genetic factors and some are due to differences in activity patterns.

Hormones affect the relationship of physical activity, body fat, and fat-free mass. Guo and coworkers (1999) found that associations between physical activity and fat-free mass were more pronounced in postmenopausal women than in premenopausal women, and that hormone replacement therapy had beneficial effects on body composition. Monozygotic twin pairs who were concordant for smoking and hormone replacement therapy status, but discordant for moderate-intensity activity, showed greater within-pair differences in total body fat than those who were concordant for activity level (Samaras et al., 1999), suggesting that the effect of physical activity is greater than that of hormonal status.

Habitual physical activity also affects other physical characteristics. Gilliat-Wimberly and coworkers (2001) found that an association exists between habitual physical activity and maintenance of resting metabolic rate in middle-aged women. Physical activity also may reduce the incidence of chronic diseases by favorably altering blood lipid profiles, reducing body fat, and improving lean body mass (Eliakim et al., 1997; Schwartz et al., 1991; Wei et al., 1997; Wilbur et al., 1999).

FOOD

Intake

In conjunction with the importance of physical activity levels, energy intake must be matched to energy expenditure. Positive energy balance results if energy intake is greater than energy expenditure. Increased energy consumption, decreased energy expenditure, or both can result in positive energy balance.

While the etiology of obesity is multifactoral, the common characteristic of all obese people is excessive energy storage in the form of body fat. Whether obese people consume more energy than do lean people has been a major source of controversy. Studies in modern respiratory chambers using doubly-labeled water have shown that weight-stable obese people have a higher resting metabolic rate and total 24-hour energy expenditure than do lean people (Jequier and Schutz, 1983; Ravussin et al., 1982; Zed and James, 1986), which demonstrates that average energy intake must indeed be higher in the obese. Some differences in energy expenditure, and consequently in energy intake, among families are due to genetic factors and differences in activity patterns. Social and cultural factors also contribute to individual food intake differences (de Castro, 1999).

Since the energy in food is derived from the macronutrients protein, fat, and carbohydrate (CHO), plus the optional energy source, alcohol, diets that are high in fat tend to be low in complex CHOs such as fiber. There is still considerable controversy over whether the role of diet composition or simply total energy intake is important in maintaining a healthy body weight.

Composition

A high energy intake or an energy intake that is not adjusted downward with declining physical activity or age-related decreases in lean body mass is associated with the development of overweight or obesity in susceptible individuals. In addition to total energy intake, the character of the diet may play a role in the etiology of obesity. High-fat diets may promote increased energy intake or may be associated with metabolic changes that promote the deposition of adipose tissue.

Dietary Fat

Research in both animals and humans suggests that high-fat (low in complex CHOs) diets promote obesity (Astrup et al., 2000; Bahceci et al., 1999; Blundell and Cooling, 2000; Cheverud et al., 1999; Maffeis et al., 2001). Because fat is more energy dense than other foods (9 kcal/g versus 4 kcal/g for protein and CHO), eating high-fat foods results in a greater energy intake than would eating a similar quantity of lower-fat foods. Fat modifies the taste of food and, in some people, promotes excess intake. Fatty foods tend to be easier to chew or may not require chewing, thus making larger quantities easier to eat in a shorter time than foods that require more mastication. Dietary fat also has a weaker satiation effect than CHOs, which results in the over consumption of fat (Rolls and Hammer, 1995; Rolls et al., 1999).

Some of the difference in weight gain on a high-fat versus a low-fat diet may be explained by differences in the metabolic processing of fat. Compared with dietary fat, CHOs require additional energy expenditure for digestion, assimilation, and conversion to fat. When energy intake exceeds expenditure, 23 percent of energy consumed is required to convert and store CHO as fat, compared with only 3 percent to store fat. Two studies in laboratory animals have demonstrated this effect of dietary fat on body weight and body composition (Donato and Hegsted, 1985; Lin et al., 1979).

The link between dietary fat and obesity in humans is not conclusive because of difficulties in accurately measuring or controlling the food intake and energy expenditure of individuals and the need to rely on estimates of body composition. Nonetheless, increasing evidence from clinical studies suggests that dietary fat promotes weight gain in humans as well as in animals. Studies in which people were overfed diets varying in the proportion of energy from fat (40 to 53 percent of kcal as fat) showed that high-fat diets promoted weight gain more efficiently than did lower-fat diets (Sims et al., 1973).

A positive correlation between the proportion of fat in the diet and the incidence of obesity has been noted among various cultures, as well as within ethnic groups that have migrated to the United States and adopted American dietary patterns (Curb and Marcus, 1991; Kushi et al., 1985). While these correlations all point to a causal role for dietary fat in obesity, they are subject to confounding variables such as differences in energy intake and expenditure, health status, and genetic and environmental influences. However, based on information such as that described above, Danforth (1985) recommended shifting to a higher-CHO and lower-fat diet to reduce the high prevalence of obesity in affluent societies such as the United States.

Obesity is more closely correlated with the level of dietary fat than with total energy intake (Dreon et al., 1988; Romieu et al., 1988). A low incidence of obesity has been observed among vegetarians who typically consume low-fat, high-CHO diets (Knuiman and West, 1982; Sacks et al., 1975). However, those who adhere to vegetarian diets for religious rather than nutritional reasons probably have a higher-fat diet (Dhurandhar and Kulkarni, 1993), and the prevalence of obesity among these types of vegetarians is high compared with that of omnivores (Dhurandhar and Kulkarni, 1992).

Some studies have failed to demonstrate an association between fat intake and body weight in free-living populations. On the basis of food frequency questionnaires, Macdiarmid and colleagues (1994) stratified 1,800 people by their fat consumption (high was considered to be 45 percent or more kcal as fat and low was considered to be 35 percent or less kcal as fat) and found no statistically significant difference in age, BMI, or social class between the two groups. However, the high-fat group rated their general diet and health as poorer. The high-fat group also consumed significantly more protein and total energy, but less CHO and fiber; consumed meat and high-fat dairy products more frequently; and consumed fewer fruits, vegetables, and cereals.

Results of a small study suggest that the amount of energy required to maintain body weight may be related to the proportion of fat in the diet, regardless of an individual's weight status (Prewitt et al., 1991). These findings suggest that dietary fat may promote greater weight gain and body-fat accumulation than expected on the basis of energy intake alone. In contrast, Leibel and colleagues (1992) found no relationship between the ratio of dietary fat/CHO and the total energy required to maintain body weight. CHO ranged from 15 to 85 percent of total intake, and kcal from fat ranged from 0 to 70 percent of total intake. The disparity between findings of these two studies may be due to the shorter duration of the second study (33 days average and ranging from 15 to 56 days compared with 140 days in the Prewitt study). Differences among the normal-weight patients in the study of Prewitt and colleagues (1991) were not seen consistently before 13 to 16 weeks. Also, body composition was not assessed in the Leibel study, and results of animal studies suggest that isocaloric diets of varying fat content may produce differences in percent of body fat without changing body weight (Boozer et al., 1990, 1993).

The arguments for whether dietary fat promotes obesity were summarized in two recent, competing editorials. Willett (1998a, 1998b) argues that obesity has increased in the United States despite reductions in intake of dietary fat and that ecological studies have found no relationship between fat intake and obesity. In contrast, Bray and Popkin (1998) argue that individuals who gained weight may not have decreased (or may have increased) their intake of dietary fat. They also argue that ecological studies may not be appropriate to study the relationship between fat intake and obesity, that body weight is a poor measure of body fatness, and that most of the previous studies focused on outcomes other than obesity. Although the literature is not clear, results of studies on laboratory animals and the small number of human studies suggest that dietary fat does promote obesity. Recently, Astrup and colleagues (2002) reviewed evidence on the effects of low-fat diets. Four meta-analyses of weight change occurring on low-fat diets in intervention trials with overweight subjects were reviewed. These analyses consistently demonstrated significant weight loss in both normal-weight and overweight subjects.

Carbohydrates

Several rationales have been postulated for the use of high-protein, low-CHO diets: (1) intake of a high proportion of kcal as CHO has adverse physiological consequences, such as increasing insulin secretion, promoting fat deposition, and increasing serum triglycerides levels; (2) low-CHO diets can lead to a "ketogenic" state, which has been hypothesized to suppress appetite; (3) a high-protein diet preserves lean body mass during weight loss; and (4) the thermogenic effect of protein is the highest of the three macronutrients, resulting in increased energy expenditure for a similar intake.

There is at least some scientific rationale for the above hypotheses (Skov et al., 1999a, 1999b). A high-protein diet has been found to: stabilize blood glucose during nonabsorptive periods and reduce insulin response following test meals (Layman et al., 2003b), improve glucose oxidation (Piatti et al., 1994), decrease lipid oxidation (Piatti et al., 1994), produce positive changes in blood lipids (Layman et al., 2003b), and provide greater satiety than diets higher in CHO (Layman et al., 2003a). Although more research is needed on the subject of amino acid flux measurements and how it relates to blood glucose levels, data from Layman and colleagues (2003b) support the idea that the ratio of dietary protein and CHO can have a significant effect on metabolic balance and specifically on glucose homeostasis during weight loss.

The role of CHO in soft drinks in producing obesity is controversial. Some studies suggest that an increase in the consumption of soft drinks may have contributed to the increased prevalence of obesity (French et al., 2000; Troiano et al., 2000), whereas others do not support this hypothesis (Gibson, 2000; Macdiarmid et al., 1998; O'Brien et al., 1982).

Portion Size

There is little research available on the role of portion size in the increasing prevalence of overweight in the United States. However, common sense dictates that it is a contributing factor. For example, a single serving of meat is considered to be 3 to 4 oz based on the Dietary Guidelines and the U.S. Food Guide Pyramid. However, in restaurants (where Americans are spending a greater portion of their food dollars), an 8-oz portion of red meat would be considered a "petite" serving; the standard serving would be 12 to 16 oz. Thus, an individual consuming a 16-oz steak in a restaurant would be likely to report (if asked in a dietary survey) consuming a single serving of red meat, when in reality 4 to 5 servings were consumed.

The intake of soft drinks has increased dramatically in the last 40 years, as has the trend towards larger portion sizes (Hill and Peters, 1998). While a standard serving of a soft drink in 1960 consisted of one 6-oz serving, the standard size serving today is 12 oz, and many vendors sell 20-oz bottles almost exclusively. Fountain drinks have also increased to the "super-jumbo" 32- to 64-oz sizes. It is not unusual for individuals to consume some 500 to 1,000 kcal per day from soft drinks in addition to their usual solid-food diet.

The change to larger portion sizes has been particularly apparent in fast-food restaurants where portion size has been used as a competitive tool. Full-service restaurants also have adopted the practice of serving larger meals. Similar to the increase in soft drink portions sizes, fast-food restaurants now offer "super-size" portions for a minimal increase in cost. For example, a "jumbo super-size" order of a large hamburger, french fries, and soft drink at a fast-food restaurant may now contain more than 1,500 kcal for a single meal (Nielsen and Popkin, 2003; Young and Nestle, 2002, 2003). One of the distinguishing features of dining out in Europe compared with the United States is the difference in restaurant portion sizes, a factor that may contribute to the lower prevalence of obesity in Europe.

A recent trend analysis of portion size was conducted by Nielsen and Popkin (2003). Data were taken from four national food-consumption surveys covering the period 1977 to 1996. Food consumption was estimated as energy intake in kcal and as average portion sizes using food models to assist respondents in identifying portion size. Results demonstrated that for foods eaten both inside and outside the home, portions sizes have increased for salty snacks, desserts, soft drinks, fruit drinks, french fries, hamburgers, cheese-burgers, and Mexican food.

Meal Patterns and Eating Habits

Eating patterns that are appropriate for an active lifestyle may continue after the individual changes to a more sedentary lifestyle. Individuals for whom this observation has been made include athletes and a large percentage of people with increasing age and changing occupational responsibilities. Athletes who are in training expend large amounts of energy each day and, for many organized sports, are encouraged to eat large quantities to maintain their weight at an artificially high level. When activity declines, the eating pattern established during training may not be adjusted to meet the new lower energy needs. The same is true of military personnel. During initial entry training, advanced individual training, and special forces training, large amounts of energy are expended on a daily basis. By the time training is completed, individuals have been habituated to consume large amounts of food over a very short period of time.

In many occupations, tasks that require more physical activity are assigned to younger workers. As these workers age and acquire more responsibility, their work may become more sedentary, but eating patterns may not change. This pattern of decreased occupational energy expenditure with job promotion may be common in the military as well. Privates, airmen, and junior noncom-missioned officers are more active than senior officers and noncommissioned officers. Despite strong commitments to engage in daily physical fitness, which may be unchanged or even increased in more senior individuals, the decrease in activities of daily living and job performance can lead to a positive energy balance unless particular care is taken to reduce energy intake.

The ubiquitousness of vending machines and fast-food outlets ensures constant access to foods at work—usually foods with a high caloric content largely in the form of fat or refined CHO. A major contributing factor to the epidemic of obesity in recent years is likely the rise in the proportion of meals eaten away from home (eating out), along with the increase in access to foods in virtually all locations. These changes have contributed in several ways to promoting obesity. Because more families include two-wage earners, adults spend more time out of the home and do not have time to prepare meals as they customarily did in the past. Meals consumed at restaurants tend to be larger and have a higher caloric content than those consumed at home, mainly because of higher fat content and larger portion sizes (Young and Nestle, 2003). In addition, a high percentage of meals eaten away from home are eaten in fast-food restaurants or consist of fast-food take-out. The presence of food in virtually every circumstance of daily life, from fast-food outlets to vending machines, encourages and allows individuals to consume multiple calorically dense meals and snacks per day (Bell et al., 1998; Rolls, 2000).

PHYSIOLOGICAL FACTORS

A number of phenotypic characteristics have been associated with the risk of weight gain, notably alterations in nonvolitional components of energy expenditure. Energy expenditure can be divided into three main components:

- *Resting metabolic rate (RMR),* the rate of energy expended at rest, under thermo-neutral conditions, and in a post-absorptive state.
- *Thermic effect of feeding*, the incremental increase in energy expenditure after a meal is consumed due to the energy costs of absorption and the transport of nutrients, as well as the synthesis and storage of protein, fat, and CHO. Some of the thermic effect of feeding may be mediated by sympathetic nervous system activity.
- *Energy expended for physical activity,* including involuntary movements associated with shivering, fidgeting, and postural control.

RMR accounts for 60 to 75 percent of total energy expended in most adults. RMR is primarily related to the maintenance of fat-free mass, reflecting such activities as protein synthesis and breakdown, temperature and cellular homeostasis, and cardiovascular, pulmonary, and central nervous system function. Metabolism associated with visceral organ mass makes the largest contribution to RMR, followed by that of skeletal muscle mass and adipose tissue (Gallagher et al., 1998). RMR is consistently greater in men than in women due to the greater lean tissue mass of males. A low RMR relative to body size was found to predict weight gain (Ravussin et al., 1988) in both men and women, although some studies have not confirmed this observation (Weinsier et al., 2000). RMR begins to decrease with age in the middle of the fourth decade. Gilliat-Wimberly and coworkers (2001) found that an association exists between physical activity and maintaining RMR in middle-aged women.

The thermic effect of feeding usually accounts for 5 to 10 percent of daily energy expenditure and varies between lean and obese individuals (Astrup, 1996). Extensive studies have been inconsistent in supporting the view that excessive weight gain is secondary to a reduced thermic effect of food (Tataranni et al., 1995).

Recent studies support the view that small, nonvolitional physical activities such as fidgeting may account for individual differences in energy expended with changes in energy balance (Levine et al., 1999; Zurlo et al., 1992). Although relatively small in caloric magnitude, these activities may account for some of the between-individual differences observed in the regulation of body weight.

These three phenotypic energy expenditure characteristics serve as markers for potential weight gain over the long term. Many factors may contribute to these individual energetic differences, and the origin of these differences is the basis of intensive study.

ENVIRONMENTAL FACTORS

Smoking and Alcohol

Cigarette smoking increases metabolic rate and may limit food intake, and weight gain is a common consequence of smoking cessation (Perkins, 1993; Russ et al., 2001). The use of alcoholic beverages may also have an impact on body weight. Energy consumed as alcohol that is in excess of need is converted to and stored as fat. Drinking alcohol has been shown to be associated with a greater energy intake than drinking nonalcoholic beverages, perhaps due to increased appetite (Tremblay and St-Pierre, 1996; Tremblay et al., 1995).

A recent, large prospective study of a cohort of men ages 40 to 59 with a 5-year follow-up found that mean BMI increased significantly from the light-to-moderate to the very-heavy alcohol intake group. The study concluded that heavy alcohol intake (defined as $\geq$ 30 g/day of alcohol) contributed directly to weight gain and obesity, regardless of the type of alcohol consumed (Wannamethee and Shaper, 2003).

Pharmacological Agents That Produce Weight Gain

Numerous drugs can produce weight gain and fat gain. These include glucocorticoids (e.g., prednisone), hypoglycemic agents (e.g., insulin, sulfonylureas), certain antihypertensive agents (e.g., prazocin), anti-allergens (e.g., cyproheptadine), and numerous drugs that affect the central nervous system (e.g., thorazine, tricyclic antidepressants, valproic acid, lithium). Most of these drugs are used for diseases that mandate separation from the military, but there are a number of drugs that may be taken by military personnel that are not deemed a rationale for separation.

SOCIAL FACTORS

Americans live in a culture in which food is abundant. A well-developed and efficient food transportation and storage system assures a readily available and affordable food supply throughout the entire year.

The relative affluence of Americans has led to an increase in consumption of snack foods (Morgan and Goungetas, 1986) and an increase in the proportion of foods of animal origin compared with that of foods of plant origin (Senauer, 1986). Foods of animal origin are likely to be higher in energy and fat than comparable quantities of foods of plant origin.

The availability and abundance of food in the U.S. marketplace has accelerated dramatically in the past 30 years. The per capita energy content of food entering the American marketplace increased about 500 calories on a daily basis during this time period. In addition, fat intake has also increased steadily, although the relative intake of fat has been decreasing since the 1970s (Putnam and Allshouse, 1999). This decrease in fat intake has been associated with an increase in average total energy intake (Bray and Popkin, 1998). Food-supply studies indicate that the increase in the number of calories consumed is accompanied by a shift in macronutrient consumption that reflects an increase in refined CHO consumption and a decrease in consumption of fruits and vegetables (Putnam and Allshouse, 1999).

Family and Ethnicity

Eating is an intensely social activity, and many eating habits are acquired in a familial or ethnic setting. People tend to imitate the eating habits of their parents, so quantity and quality of foods eaten and meal patterns tends to be established early. Traditions that arise around eating patterns in a more agrarian or active society may favor excess consumption. Ethnic groups differ in their perceptions about appropriate body size and what constitutes overweight (Bhadrinath, 1990; Root, 1990).

Studies of changes in diet with immigration and acculturation show, for example, that Japanese who migrated to California and Hawaii have tended to abandon the traditional low-fat Japanese diet for American food patterns (Burchfiel et al., 1995; Curb and Marcus, 1991; Goodman et al., 1992; Hara et al., 1996; Ziegler et al., 1996). The result has been a marked increase in weight among these immigrants. Similarly, Japanese children who remain in Japan, but whose diet is increasingly western, are also getting heavier (Murata, 2000; Takada et al., 1998). Thus, dietary change is strongly associated with increased weight in both of these carefully studied population groups. The same phenomenon is observed in studies of South Asians who have migrated to the United Kingdom and who have modified their diet and physical activity patterns (McKeigue et al., 1992).

Socioeconomic Status

Social class and socioeconomic status (SES) influence the prevalence of overweight. In many countries of the world, lower SES is linked to increased body weight (Molarius et al., 2000). In contrast, in some developing countries and primitive societies, obesity is considered a sign of affluence or fertility (Molarius et al., 2000). However, some researchers who contend that obesity decreases economic status have disputed the belief that lower SES causes obesity in the United States. For example, one study reported that women who were overweight in late adolescence or early adult life were more likely to have lower income, greater levels of poverty, and decreased rates of marriage than were normal-weight women with comparable degrees of disability (Gortmaker et al., 1993).

The Potential Role of Viruses in the Etiology of Obesity

The possibility exists that at least some cases of human obesity are due to viral infection. Five viruses and scrapie agents cause obesity in animals (Bernard et al., 1988, 1993; Carp et al., 1998; Carter et al., 1983a, 1983b; Dhurandhar et al., 1990, 1992, 1997, 2000; Gosztonyi and Ludwig, 1995; Lyons et al., 1982; Nagashima et al., 1992). One of these viruses is a human adenovirus, Ad-36, which has been shown to produce a syndrome of increased body fat and paradoxically decreased serum cholesterol and triglycerides in chickens and mice (Dhurandhar et al., 2000). Preliminary data have been reported that demonstrated similar results in monkeys (Atkinson et al., 2000). Other preliminary studies suggest that humans with serum antibodies to Ad-36 have a higher BMI and lower serum lipids than do Ad-36 antibody-negative individuals (Atkinson et al., 1998).

Humans in Bombay, India, who had serum antibodies to SMAM-1, an avian adenovirus, were noted to be significantly heavier and to have lower serum lipids compared with antibody-negative individuals. Viral antigen was found in the serum of two of the individuals with SMAM-1 antibodies (Dhurandhar et al., 1997).

More research is needed to confirm the hypothesis generated from the above data that some cases of human obesity might be due to a viral infection.

Since adenoviruses are common cold viruses, the possibility of the spread of Ad-36 and perhaps other obesity-producing viruses in the military community may be of significant concern.

SUMMARY

The brief review of factors influencing body weight presented in this chapter demonstrate that maintaining a healthy body weight is an extremely complex issue. Maintenance of fitness and appropriate body-fat standards by military personnel is affected by each individual's genetics, developmental history, physiology, age, physical activity level, environment, diet, ethnicity, and social background.

4

Weight-Loss and Maintenance Strategies

The most important component of an effective weight-management program must be the *prevention* of unwanted weight gain from excess body fat. The military is in a unique position to address prevention from the first day of an individual's military career. Because the military population is selected from a pool of individuals who meet specific criteria for body mass index (BMI) and percent body fat, the primary goal should be to foster an environment that promotes maintenance of a healthy body weight and body composition throughout an individual's military career. There is significant evidence that losing excess body fat is difficult for most individuals and the risk of regaining lost weight is high. From the first day of initial entry training, an understanding of the fundamental causes of excess weight gain must be communicated to each individual, along with a strategy for maintaining a healthy body weight as a way of life.

INTRODUCTION

The principle of weight gain is simple: energy intake exceeds energy expenditure. However, as discussed in Chapter 3, overweight and obesity are clearly the result of a complex set of interactions among genetic, behavioral, and environmental factors. While hundreds, if not thousands, of weight-loss strategies, diets, potions, and devices have been offered to the overweight public, the multi-factorial etiology of overweight challenges practitioners, researchers, and the overweight themselves to identify permanent, effective strategies for weight loss and maintenance. The percentage of individuals who lose weight and successfully maintain the loss has been estimated to be as small as 1 to 3 percent (Andersen et al., 1988; Wadden et al., 1989).

Evidence shows that genetics plays a role in the etiology of overweight and obesity. However, genetics cannot account for the increase in overweight observed in the U.S. population over the past two decades. Rather, the behavioral and environmental factors that conspire to induce individuals to engage in

TABLE 4-1 Benefits of Physical Activity

Benefit	Reference
Improved maintenance of lost weight	Pavlou et al., 1989a, 1989b; Phinney, 1992; Skender et al., 1996; Wadden, 1993; Wing, 1992; Wing and Greeno, 1994
Preservation of lean body mass	Calles-Escandon and Horton, 1992; Wadden, 1993
Improved cardiovascular, respiratory, and musculoskeletal fitness	Calles-Escandon and Horton, 1992
Improved psychological profile and self-esteem	ACSM, 2000
Improved mood	Wadden, 1993
Improved plasma blood glucose levels, blood pressure, and blood lipid and lipoprotein values	Calles-Escandon and Horton, 1992; Pate et al., 1995; Pavlou et al., 1989a, 1989b
Reduced risk for morbidity and mortality	Blair, 1993; Dyer, 1994; Pate et al., 1995

too little physical activity and eat too much relative to their energy expenditure must take most of the blame. It is these factors that are the target of weight-management strategies. This chapter reviews the efficacy and safety of strategies for weight loss, as well as the combinations of strategies that appear to be associated with successful loss. In addition, the elements of successful weight maintenance also will be reviewed since the difficulty in maintaining weight loss may contribute to the overweight problem. A brief discussion of public policy measures that may help prevent overweight and assist those who are trying to lose weight or maintain weight loss is also included.

PHYSICAL ACTIVITY

Increased physical activity is an essential component of a comprehensive weight-reduction strategy for overweight adults who are otherwise healthy. One of the best predictors of success in the long-term management of overweight and obesity is the ability to develop and sustain an exercise program (Jakicic et al., 1995, 1999; Klem et al., 1997; McGuire et al., 1998, 1999; Schoeller et al., 1997). The availability of exercise facilities at military bases can reinforce exercise and fitness programs that are necessary to meet the services' physical readiness needs generally, and for weight management specifically. For a given individual, the intensity, duration, frequency, and type of physical activity will depend on existing medical conditions, degree of previous activity, physical limitations, and individual preferences. Referral for additional professional evaluation may be appropriate, especially for individuals with more than one of the above extenuating factors. The benefits of physical activity (see Table 4-1) are significant and occur even in the absence of weight loss (Blair, 1993; Kesaniemi et al., 2001). It has been shown that one of the benefits, an increase in high-density lipoproteins, can be achieved with a threshold level of aerobic exercise of 10 to 11 hours per month.

For previously sedentary individuals, a slow progression in physical activity has been recommended so that 30 minutes of exercise daily is achieved after several weeks of gradual build-up. This may also apply to some military personnel, especially new recruits or reservists recalled to active duty who may be entering service from previously very sedentary lifestyles. The activity goal has been expressed as an increase in energy expenditure of 1,000 kcal/wk (Jakicic et al., 1999; Pate et al., 1995), although this quantity may be insufficient to prevent weight regain. For that purpose, a weekly goal of 2,000 to 3,000 kcal of added activity may be necessary (Klem et al., 1997; Schoeller et al., 1997). Thus, mental preparation for the amount of activity necessary to maintain weight loss must begin while losing weight (Brownell, 1999).

For many individuals, changing activity levels is perceived as more unpleasant than changing dietary habits. Breaking up a 30-minute daily exercise "prescription" into 10-minute bouts has been shown to increase compliance over that of longer bouts (Jakicic et al., 1995, Pate et al., 1995). However, over an 18-month period, individuals who performed short bouts of physical activity did not experience improvements in long-term weight loss, cardiorespiratory fitness, or physical activity participation in comparison with those who performed longer bouts of exercise. Some evidence suggests that home exercise equipment (e.g., a treadmill) increases the likelihood of regular exercise and is associated with greater long-term weight loss (Jakicic et al., 1999). In addition, individual preferences are paramount considerations in choices of activity.

When strength training or resistance exercise is combined with aerobic activity, long-term results may be better than those with aerobics alone (Poirier and Despres, 2001; Sothern et al., 1999). Because strength training tends to build muscle, loss of lean body mass may be minimized and the relative loss of body fat may be increased. An added benefit is the attenuation of the decrease in resting metabolic rate associated with weight loss, possibly as a consequence of preserving or enhancing lean body mass.

As valuable as exercise is, the existing research literature on overweight individuals indicates that exercise programs alone do not produce significant weight loss in the populations studied. It should be emphasized, however, that a large number of such studies have been conducted with middle-aged Caucasian women leading sedentary lifestyles. The failure of exercise alone to produce significant weight loss may be because the neurochemical mechanisms that regulate eating behavior cause individuals to compensate for the calories expended in exercise by increasing food (calorie) intake. While exercise programs can result in an average weight loss of 2 to 3 kg in the short-term (Blair, 1993; Pavlou et al., 1989a; Skender et al., 1996; Wadden and Sarwer, 1999), outcome improves significantly when physical activity is combined with dietary intervention. For example, when physical activity was combined with a reduced-calorie diet and lifestyle change, a weight loss of 7.2 kg was achieved after 6 months to 3 years of follow-up (Blair, 1993). Physical activity plus diet produces better results than either diet or physical activity alone (Blair, 1993; Dyer, 1994; Pavlou et al., 1989a, 1989b; Perri et al., 1993). In addition, weight regain is significantly less likely when physical activity is combined with any other weight-reduction regimen (Blair, 1993; Klem et al., 1997). Continued follow-up after weight loss is associated with improved outcome if the activity plan is monitored and modified as part of this follow-up (Kayman et al., 1990).

While studies have shown that military recruits were able to lose significant amounts of weight during initial entry training through exercise alone, the restricted time available to consume meals during training probably contributed to this weight loss (Lee et al., 1994).

BEHAVIOR AND LIFESTYLE MODIFICATION

The use of behavior and lifestyle modification in weight management is based on a body of evidence that people become or remain overweight as the result of modifiable habits or behaviors (see Chapter 3), and that by changing those behaviors, weight can be lost and the loss can be maintained. The primary goals of behavioral strategies for weight control are to increase physical activity and to reduce caloric intake by altering eating habits (Brownell and Kramer, 1994; Wilson, 1995). A subcategory of behavior modification, environmental management, is discussed in the next section. Behavioral treatment, which was introduced in the 1960s, may be provided to a single individual or to groups of clients. Typically, individuals participate in 12 to 20 weekly sessions that last from 1 to 2 hours each (Brownell and Kramer, 1994), with a goal of weight loss in the range of 1 to 2 lb/wk (Brownell and Kramer, 1994). In the past, behavioral approaches were applied as stand-alone treatments to simply modify eating habits and reduce caloric intake. However, more recently, these treatments have been used in combination with low-calorie diets, medical nutrition therapy, nutrition education, exercise programs, monitoring, pharmacological agents, and social support to promote weight loss, and as a component of maintenance programs.

Self-Monitoring and Feedback

Self-monitoring of dietary intake and physical activity, which enables the individual to develop a sense of accountability, is one of the cornerstones of behavioral treatment. Patients are asked to keep a daily food diary in which they record what and how much they have eaten, when and where the food was consumed, and the context in which the food was consumed (e.g., what else they were doing at the time, what they were feeling, and who else was there). Additionally, patients may be asked to keep a record of their daily physical activities. Self-monitoring of food intake is often associated with a relatively immediate reduction in food intake and consequent weight loss (Blundell, 2000; Goris et al., 2000). This reduction in food intake is believed to result from increased awareness of food intake and/or concern about what the dietitian or nutrition therapist will think about the patient's eating behavior. The information obtained from the food diaries also is used to identify personal and environmental factors that contribute to overeating and to select and implement appropriate weight-loss strategies for the individual (Wilson, 1995). The same may be true of physical activity monitoring, although little research has been conducted in this area. Self-monitoring also provides a way for therapists and patients to evaluate which techniques are working and how changes in eating behavior or activity are contributing to weight loss. Recent work has suggested that regular self-monitoring of body weight is a useful adjunct to behavior modification programs (Jeffery and French, 1999).

Other Behavioral Techniques

Some additional techniques included in behavioral treatment programs include eating only regularly scheduled meals; doing nothing else while eating; consuming meals only in one place (usually the dining room) and leaving the table after eating; shopping only from a list; and shopping on a full stomach (Brownell and Kramer, 1994).

Reinforcement techniques are also an integral part of the behavioral treatment of overweight and obesity. For example, subjects may select a positively reinforcing event, such as participating in a particularly enjoyable activity or purchasing a special item when a goal is met (Brownell and Kramer, 1994).

Another important component of behavioral treatment programs may be cognitive restructuring of erroneous or dysfunctional beliefs about weight regulation (Wing, 1998). Techniques developed by cognitive behavior therapists can be used to help the individual identify specific triggers for overeating, deal with negative attitudes towards obesity in society, and realize that a minor dietary infraction does not mean failure. Nutrition education and social support, discussed later in this chapter, are also components of behavioral programs.

Behavioral treatments of obesity are frequently successful in the short-term. However, the long-term effectiveness of these treatments is more controversial, with data suggesting that many individuals return to their initial body weight within 3 to 5 years after treatment has ended (Brownell and Kramer, 1994; Klem et al., 1997). Techniques for improving the long-term benefits of behavioral treatments include: (1) developing criteria to match patients to treatments, (2) increasing initial weight loss, (3) increasing the length of treatment, (4) emphasizing the role of exercise, and (5) combining behavioral programs with other treatments such as pharmacotherapy, surgery, or stringent diets (Brownell and Kramer, 1994).

Recent studies of individuals who have achieved success at long-term weight loss may offer other insights into ways to improve behavioral treatment strategies. In their analysis of data from the National Weight Control Registry, Klem and coworkers (1997) found that weight loss achieved through exercise, sensible dieting, reduced fat consumption, and individual behavior changes could be maintained for long periods of time. However, this population was self-selected so it does not represent the experience of the average person in a civilian population. Because they have achieved and maintained a significant amount of weight loss (at least 30 lb for 2 or more years), there is reason to believe that the population enrolled in the Registry may be especially disciplined. As such, the experience of people in the Registry may provide insight into the military population, although evidence to assert this with authority is lacking. In any case, the majority of participants in the Registry report they have made significant permanent changes in their behavior, including portion control, low-fat food selection, 60 or more minutes of daily exercise, self-monitoring, and well-honed problem-solving skills.

Eating Environments

A significant part of weight loss and management may involve restructuring the environment that promotes overeating and underactivity. The environment includes the home, the workplace, and the community (e.g., places of worship, eating places, stores, movie theaters). Environmental factors include the availability of foods such as fruits, vegetables, nonfat dairy products, and other foods of low energy density and high nutritional value. Environmental restructuring empha-sizes frequenting dining facilities that produce appealing foods of lower energy density and providing ample time for eating a wholesome meal rather than grabbing a candy bar or bag of chips and a soda from a vending machine. Busy lifestyles and hectic work schedules create eating habits that may contribute to a less than desirable eating environment, but simple changes can help to counter-act these habits.

Commanders of military bases should examine their facilities to identify and eliminate conditions that encourage one or more of the eating habits that promote overweight. Some nonmilitary employers have increased healthy eating options at worksite dining facilities and vending machines. Although multiple publications suggest that worksite weight-loss programs are not very effective in reducing body weight (Cohen et al., 1987; Forster et al., 1988; Frankle et al., 1986; Kneip et al., 1985; Loper and Barrows, 1985), this may not be the case for the military due to the greater controls the military has over its "employees" than do nonmilitary employers.

Eating habits that may promote overweight:

1. Eating few or no meals at home
2. Opting for high-fat, calorie-dense foods
3. Opting for high-fat snack foods from strategically placed vending machines or snack shops combined with allowing insufficient time to prepare affordable, healthier alternatives.
4. Consuming meals at sit-down restaurants that feature excessive portion sizes or "all-you-can-eat" buffets

Simple changes that can modify the eating environment:

1. Prepare meals at home and carry bag lunches
2. Learn to estimate or measure portion sizes in restaurants
3. Learn to recognize fat content of menu items and dishes on buffet tables
4. Eliminate smoking and reduce alcohol consumption
5. Substitute low-calorie for high-calorie foods
6. Modify the route to work to avoid a favorite food shop

Physical Activity Environment

Major obstacles to exercise, even in highly motivated people, include the time it takes to complete the task and the inaccessibility of facilities or safe places to exercise. Environmental interventions emphasize the many ways that physical activity can be fit into a busy lifestyle and seek to make use of whatever opportunities are available (HHS, 1996). Environmental changes may be needed to encourage female participation in exercise programs, such as accommodation of the need for more after-exercise "repair time" by women and worksite facilities that are more "user friendly," such as measured indoor walking routes and lunchtime low-level aerobics classes (Wasserman et al., 2000). The availability of safe sidewalks and parks and alternative methods of transportation to work, such as walking or bicycling, also enhance the physical activity environment. Establishing "car-free" zones is an example of an environmental change that could promote increased physical activity.

Nutrition Education

Management of overweight and obesity requires the active participation of the individual. Nutrition professionals can provide individuals with a base of information that allows them to make knowledgeable food choices.

Nutrition education is distinct from nutrition counseling, although the contents overlap considerably. Nutrition counseling and dietary management tend to focus more directly on the motivational, emotional, and psychological issues associated with the current task of weight loss and weight management. It addresses the *how* of behavioral changes in the dietary arena. Nutrition education on the other hand, provides basic information about the scientific foundation of nutrition that enables people to make informed decisions about food, cooking methods, eating out, and estimating portion sizes. Nutrition education programs also may provide information on the role of nutrition in health promotion and disease prevention, sports nutrition, and nutrition for pregnant and lactating women. Effective nutrition education imparts nutrition knowledge and its use in healthy living. For example, it explains the concept of energy balance in weight management in an accessible, practical way that has meaning to the individual's lifestyle, including that in the military setting.

Written materials prepared by various government agencies or by nonprofit health organizations can be used effectively to provide nutrition education. However, written materials are most effective when used to reinforce informal classroom or counseling sessions and to provide specific information, such as a table of the calorie content of foods. The format of education programs varies considerably, and can include formal classes, informal group meetings, or teleconferencing. A common background among group members is helpful (but seldom possible).

Educational formats that provide practical and relevant nutrition information for program participants are the most successful. For example, some military weight-management programs include field trips to post exchanges, restaurants (fast-food and others), movies, and other places where food is purchased or consumed (Vorachek, 1999).

The involvement of spouses and other family members in an education program increases the likelihood that other members of the household will make permanent changes, which in turn enhances the likelihood that the program participants will continue to lose weight or maintain weight loss (Hart et al., 1990; Hertzler and Schulman, 1983; Sperry, 1985). Particular attention must be directed to involvement of those in the household who are most likely to shop for and prepare food. Unless the program participant lives alone, nutrition management is rarely effective without the involvement of family members.

DIET

Weight-management programs may be divided into two phases: weight loss and weight maintenance. While exercise may be the most important element of a weight-maintenance program, it is clear that dietary restriction is the critical component of a weight-loss program that influences the rate of weight loss.

Activity accounts for only about 15 to 30 percent of daily energy expenditure, but food intake accounts for 100 percent of energy intake. Thus, the energy balance equation may be affected most significantly by reducing energy intake. The number of diets that have been proposed is almost innumerable, but whatever the name, all diets consist of reductions of some proportions of protein, carbohydrate (CHO) and fat. The following sections examine a number of arrangements of the proportions of these three energy-containing macronutrients.

Nutritionally Balanced, Hypocaloric Diets

A nutritionally balanced, hypocaloric diet has been the recommendation of most dietitians who are counseling patients who wish to lose weight. This type of diet is composed of the types of foods a patient usually eats, but in lower quantities. There are a number of reasons such diets are appealing, but the main reason is that the recommendation is simple—individuals need only to follow the U.S. Department of Agriculture's Food Guide Pyramid. The Pyramid recommends that individuals eat a variety of foods, with the majority being grain products (e.g., bread, pasta, cereal, rice), eat at least five servings per day of fruits and vegetables; eat only moderate amounts of dairy and meat products; and limit the consumption of foods that are high in fat or sugar or contain few nutrients. In using the Pyramid, however, it is important to emphasize the portion sizes used to establish the recommended number of servings. For example, a majority of consumers do not realize that a portion of bread is a single slice or that a portion of meat is only 3 oz.

A diet based on the Pyramid is easily adapted from the foods served in group settings, including military bases, since all that is required is to eat smaller portions. Even with smaller portions, it is not difficult to obtain adequate quantities of the other essential nutrients. Many of the studies published in the medical literature are based on a balanced hypocaloric diet with a reduction of energy intake by 500 to 1,000 kcal from the patient's usual caloric intake. The U.S. Food and Drug Administration (FDA) recommends such diets as the "standard treatment" for clinical trials of new weight-loss drugs, to be used by both the active agent group and the placebo group (FDA, 1996).

Meal Replacement

Meal replacement programs are commercially available to consumers for a reasonably low cost. The meal replacement industry suggests replacing one or two of the three daily meals with their products, while the third meal should be sensibly balanced. In addition, two snacks consisting of fruits, vegetables, or diet snack bars are recommended each day. Using this plan, individuals consume approximately 1,200 to 1,500 kcal/day.

A number of studies have evaluated long-term weight maintenance using meal replacement, either self-managed (Flechtner-Mors et al., 2000; Heber et al., 1994; Rothacker, 2000), with active dietary counseling, or with behavior modification programs (Ashley et al., 2001; Ditschuneit and Flechtner-Mors, 2001; Ditschuneit et al., 1999) compared with traditional calorie-restricted diet plans. The largest amount of weight loss occurred early in the studies (about the first 3 months of the plan) (Ditschuneit et al., 1999; Heber et al., 1994). One study found that women lost more weight between the third and sixth months of the plan, but men lost most of their weight by the third month (Heber et al., 1994). All of the studies resulted in maintenance of significant weight loss after 2 to 5 years of follow-up. Hill's (2000) review of Rothacker (2000) pointed out that the group receiving meal replacements maintained a small, yet significant, weight loss over the 5-year program, whereas the control group gained a significant amount of weight. Active intervention, which included dietary counseling and behavior modification, was more effective in weight maintenance when meal replacements were part of the diet (Ashley et al., 2001). Meal replacements were also found to improve food patterns, including nutrient distribution, intake of micronutrients, and maintenance of fruit and vegetable intake.

Long-term maintenance of weight loss with meal replacements improves biomarkers of disease risk, including improvements in levels of blood glucose (Ditschuneit and Fletchner-Mors, 2001), insulin, and triacylglycerol; improved systolic blood pressure (Ditschuneit and Fletchner-Mors, 2001; Ditschuneit et al., 1999); and reductions in plasma cholesterol (Heber et al., 1994).

Winick and coworkers (2002) evaluated employees in high-stress jobs (e.g., police, firefighters, and hospital and aviation personnel) who participated in worksite weight-reduction and maintenance programs that used meal replacements. The meal replacements were found to be effective in reducing weight and maintaining weight loss at a 1-year follow-up. In contrast, Bendixen and coworkers (2002) reported from Denmark that meal replacements were associated with negative outcomes on weight loss and weight maintenance. However, this was not an intervention study; participants were followed for 6 years by phone interview and data were self-reported.

Unbalanced, Hypocaloric Diets

Unbalanced, hypocaloric diets restrict one or more of the calorie-containing macronutrients (protein, fat, and CHO). The rationale given for these diets by their advocates is that the restriction of one particular macronutrient facilitates weight loss, while restriction of the others does not. Many of these diets are published in books aimed at the lay public and are often not written by health professionals and often are not based on sound scientific nutrition principles. For some of the dietary regimens of this type, there are few or no research publications and virtually none have been studied long term. Therefore, few conclusions can be drawn about the safety, and even about the efficacy, of such diets. The major types of unbalanced, hypocaloric diets are discussed below.

High-Protein, Low-Carbohydrate Diets

There has been considerable debate on the optimal ratio of macronutrient intake for adults. This research usually compares the amount of fat and CHO; however, there has been increasing interest in the role of protein in the diet (Hu et al., 1999; Wolfe and Giovannetti, 1991). Studies have looked for the effects of a higher protein diet (CHO/protein ratio ~1.0) compared with a higher CHO diet (CHO/protein ratio ~3.0). Although the high-protein diet does not produce significantly different weight loss compared with the high-CHO diet (Layman et al., 2003a, 2003b; Piatti et al., 1994), the high-protein diet has been reported to stimulate greater improvements in body composition by sparing lean body mass (Layman et al., 2003a; Piatti et al., 1994).

High-protein, low-CHO diets were introduced to the American public during the 1970s and 1980s by Stillman and Baker (1978) and by Atkins (Atkins, 1988; Atkins and Linde, 1978), and more recently, by Sears and Lawren (1998). Some of these diets are high in fat (> 35 percent of kcal), while others have moderate levels of fat (25–35 percent of kcal). While most of these diets have been promoted by nonscientists who have done little or no serious scientific research, some of the regimens have been subjected to rigorous studies (Skov et al., 1999a, 1999b). There remains, however, a lack of randomized clinical trials of 2 or more years' duration, which are needed to evaluate the potent beneficial effect of weight loss (accomplished using virtually any dietary regimen, no matter how unbalanced) on blood lipids. In addition, longer studies are needed to separate the beneficial effects of weight loss from the long-term effects of consuming an unbalanced diet.

Authors of books aimed at the lay public have proposed advantages of high protein diets, including that eating a high-protein, low-CHO diet produces a "near-euphoric" state of maximal physical and mental performance (Sears and Lawren, 1998). These claims are unsupported by scientific data.

Although these diets are prescribed to be eaten ad libitum, total daily energy intake tends to be reduced as a result of the monotony of the food choices, other prescripts of the diet, and an increased satiety effect of protein. In addition, the restriction of CHO intake leads to the loss of glycogen and marked diuresis (Coulston and Rock, 1994; Miller and Lindeman, 1997; Pi-Sunyer, 1988). Thus, the relatively rapid initial weight loss that occurs on these diets predominantly reflects the loss of body water rather than stored fat. This can be a significant concern for military personnel, where even mild dehydration can have detrimental effects on physical and cognitive performance. For example, small changes in hydration status can affect a military pilot's ability to sense changes in equilibrium.

Results of several recent studies suggest that high-protein, low-CHO diets may have their benefits. In addition to sparing fat-free mass (Piatti et al., 1994) and producing greater weight and fat losses than high-CHO diets (Skov et al., 1999b), high-protein diets have been associated with decreases in fasting triglycerides and free fatty acids in healthy subjects and with the normalization of fasting insulin levels in hyperinsulinemic, normoglycemic obese subjects (Baba et al., 1999; Skov et al., 1999b). Furthermore, a 45-percent protein diet reduced resting energy expenditure to a significantly lesser extent than did a 12-percent protein diet (Baba et al., 1999). The length of these studies that examined high-protein diets only lasted 1 year or less; the long-term safety of these diets is not known.

Low-Fat Diets

Low-fat diets have been one of the most commonly used treatments for obesity for many years (Astrup, 1999; Astrup et al., 1997; Blundell, 2000; Castellanos and Rolls, 1997; Flatt, 1997; Kendall et al., 1991; Pritikin, 1982). The most extreme forms of these diets, such as those proposed by Ornish (1993) and Pritikin (1982), recommend fat intakes of no more than 10 percent of total caloric intake. Although these stringent diets can lead to weight loss, the limited array of food choices make them difficult to maintain for extended periods of time by individuals who wish to follow a normal lifestyle.

More modest reductions in fat intake, which make a dietary regimen easier to follow and more acceptable to many individuals, can also promote weight loss (Astrup, 1999; Astrup et al., 1997, 2000; Blundell, 2000; Castellanos and Rolls, 1997; Flatt, 1997; Kendall et al., 1991; Shah and Garg, 1996). For example, Sheppard and colleagues (1991) reported that after 1 year, obese women who reduced their fat intake from approximately 39 percent to 22 percent of total caloric intake lost 3.1 kg of body weight, while women who reduced their fat intake from 38 percent to 36 percent of total calories lost only 0.4 kg.

Results of recent studies suggest that fat restriction is also valuable for weight maintenance in those who have lost weight (Flatt 1997; Miller and Lindeman, 1997). Dietary fat reduction can be achieved by counting and limiting the number of grams (or calories) consumed as fat, by limiting the intake of certain foods (for example, fattier cuts of meat), and by substituting reduced-fat or nonfat versions of foods for their higher fat counterparts (e.g., skim milk for whole milk, nonfat frozen yogurt for full-fat ice cream, baked potato chips for fried chips) (Dywer, 1995; Miller and Lindeman, 1997). Over the past decade, pursuit of this latter strategy has been simplified by the burgeoning availability of low-fat or fat-free products, which have been marketed in response to evidence that decreasing fat intake can aid in weight control.

The mechanisms for weight loss on a low-fat diet are not clear. Weight loss may be solely the result of a reduction in total energy intake, but another possibility is that a low-fat diet may alter metabolism (Astrup, 1999; Astrup et al., 2000; Castellanos and Rolls, 1997; Shah and Garg, 1996). Support for the latter possibility has come from studies showing that the short-term adherence to a diet containing 20 or 30 percent of calories from fat increased 24-hour energy expenditure in formerly obese women, relative to an isocaloric diet with 40 percent of calories from fat (Astrup et al., 1994).

Over the past two decades, fat consumption as a percent of total caloric intake has declined in the United States (Anand and Basiotis, 1998), while average body weight and the proportion of the American population suffering from obesity have increased significantly (Mokdad et al., 1999). Several factors may contribute to this seeming contradiction. First, all individuals appear to selectively underestimate their intake of dietary fat and to decrease normal fat intake when asked to record it (Goris et al., 2000; Macdiarmid et al., 1998). If these results reflect the general tendencies of individuals completing dietary surveys, then the amount of fat being consumed by obese and, possibly, nonobese people, is greater than routinely reported. Second, although the proportion of total calories consumed as fat has decreased over the past 20 years, grams of fat intake per day have remained steady or increased (Anand and Basiotis, 1998), indicating that total energy intake increased at a faster rate than did fat intake. Coupled with these findings is the fact that since the early 1990s, the availability of low-fat and nonfat, but calorie-rich snack foods (e.g., crackers, candy, cookies, cake, frozen desserts) has grown dramatically. However, total energy intake still matters, and overconsumption of these low-fat snacks could as easily lead to weight gain as intake of their high-fat counterparts (Allred, 1995).

Two recent, comprehensive reviews have reported on the overall impact of low-fat diets. Astrup and coworkers (2002) examined four meta-analyses of weight change that occurred on intervention trials with ad libitum low-fat diets. They found that low-fat diets consistently demonstrated significant weight loss, both in normal-weight and overweight individuals. A dose-response relationship was also observed in that a 10 percent reduction in dietary fat was predicted to produce a 4- to 5-kg weight loss in an individual with a BMI of 30. Kris-Etherton and colleagues (2002) found that a moderate-fat diet (20 to 30 percent of energy from fat) was more likely to promote weight loss because it was easier for patients to adhere to this type of diet than to one that was severely restricted in fat (< 20 percent of energy).

High-Fiber Diets

Most low-fat diets are also high in dietary fiber, and some investigators attribute the beneficial effects of low-fat diets to the high content of vegetables and fruits that contain large amounts of dietary fiber. The rationale for using high-fiber diets is that they may reduce energy intake and may alter metabolism (Raben et al., 1994). The beneficial effects of dietary fiber might be accomplished by the following mechanisms: (1) caloric dilution (most high-fiber foods are low in calories and low in fat); (2) longer chewing and swallowing time reduces total intake; (3) improved gastric and intestinal motility and emptying and less absorption (French and Read, 1994; Leeds, 1987; McIntyre et al., 1997; Rigaud et al., 1998; Schonfeld et al., 1997; Vincent et al., 1995); and (4) decreased hunger and enhanced satiety (Pasman et al., 1997a, 1997b, 1997c). Dietary fiber is not a panacea, and the vast majority of controlled studies of the effects of dietary fiber on weight loss show minimal or no reduction in body weight (LSRO, 1987; Pasman et al., 1997b, 1997c).

Many individuals and companies promote the use of dietary fiber supplements for weight loss and reductions in cardiovascular and cancer risks. Numerous studies, usually short-term and using purified or partially purified dietary fiber, have shown reductions in serum lipids, glucose, or insulin (Jenkins et al., 2000). Long-term studies have usually not confirmed these findings (LSRO, 1987; Pasman et al., 1997b). Current recommendations suggest that instead of eating dietary fiber supplements, a diet of foods high in whole fruits and vegetables may have favorable effects on cardiovascular and cancer risk factors (Bruce et al., 2000). Such diets are often lower in fat and higher in CHOs.

Very-Low-Calorie Diets

Very-low-calorie diets (VLCDs) were used extensively for weight loss in the 1970s and 1980s, but have fallen into disfavor in recent years (Atkinson, 1989; Bray, 1992a; Fisler and Drenick, 1987). FDA and the National Institutes of Health define a VLCD as a diet that provides 800 kcal/day or less. Since this does not take into account body size, a more scientific definition is a diet that provides 10 to 12 kcal/kg of "desirable" body weight/day (Atkinson, 1989). The VLCDs used most frequently consist of powdered formulas or limited-calorie servings of foods that contain a high-quality protein source, CHO, a small percentage of calories as fat, and the daily recommendations of vitamins and minerals (Kanders and Blackburn, 1994; Wadden, 1995). The servings are eaten three to five times per day. The primary goal of VLCDs is to produce relatively rapid weight loss without substantial loss in lean body mass. To achieve this goal, VLCDs usually provide 1.2 to 1.5 g of protein/kg of desirable body weight in the formula or as fish, lean meat, or fowl. Fisler and Drenick (1987) reviewed the literature and concluded that about 70 g/day of protein is needed to ensure that nitrogen balance is achieved within a short period of time on a VLCD.

VLCDs are not appropriate for all overweight individuals, and they are usually limited to patients with a BMI of greater than 25 (some guidelines suggest a BMI of 27 or even 30) who have medical complications associated

TABLE 4-2 One through Five-Year Maintenance of Initial Weight Loss of Individuals (%) Placed on Either Very-Low-Calorie Diets or Hypocaloric-Balanced Diets

Diet	1 year	2 years	3 years	4 years	5 years
Very-low-calorie diet	16.1	9.7	7.8	7	6.2
Hypocaloric-balanced diet	7.2	4.2	3.5	2.8	2

SOURCE: Adapted from Anderson et al. (2001).

with being overweight and have already tried more conservative treatment programs. Additionally, because of the potential detrimental side effects of these diets (e.g., gallstone formation, nutritional deficiencies, cardiac arrhythmias), medical and nutritional monitoring is important while individuals are on the diet.

On a short-term basis, VLCDs are relatively effective, with weight losses of approximately 15 to 30 kg over 12 to 20 weeks being reported in a number of studies (Anderson et al., 1992, 1999; Apfelbaum et al., 1987; Atkinson, 1989; Fisler and Drenick, 1987; Kanders and Blackburn, 1994). However, the long-term effectiveness of these diets is somewhat limited. Approximately 40 to 50 percent of patients drop out of the program before achieving their weight-loss goals. In addition, relatively few people who lose large amounts of weight using VLCDs are able to sustain the weight loss when they resume normal eating. In two studies, only 30 percent of patients who reached their goal were able to maintain their weight loss for at least 18 months. Within 1 year, the majority of patients regained approximately two-thirds of the lost weight (Apfelbaum et al., 1987; Kanders and Blackburn, 1994). In a more recent study with longer follow-up, the average regain over the first 3 years of follow-up was 73 percent. However, weight tended to stabilize over the fourth year. At 5 years, the dieters had maintained an average of 23 percent of their initial weight loss. At 7 years, 25 percent of the dieters were maintaining a weight loss of 10 percent of their initial body weight (Anderson et al., 1999, 2001).

It appears that VLCDs are more effective for long-term weight loss than hypocaloric-balanced diets. In a meta-analysis of 29 studies, Anderson and colleagues (2001) examined the long-term weight-loss maintenance of individuals put on a VLCD diet with behavioral modification as compared with individuals put on a hypocaloric-balanced diet. They found that VLCD participants lost significantly more weight initially and maintained significantly more weight loss than participants on the hypocaloric-balanced diet (see Table 4-2).

SUPPORT SYSTEMS

Almost any kind of assistance provided to participants in a weight-management program can be characterized as support services. These can include emotional support, dietary support, and support services for physical activity. The support services used most often are structured in a standard way. Other services are developed to meet the specific needs of a site, program, or the individual involved. With few exceptions, almost any weight-management program is likely to be more successful if it is accompanied by support services (Heshka et al., 2000). However, not all services will be productively applicable to all patients, and not all can be made available in all settings. Furthermore, some weight-loss program participants will be reluctant to use any support services.

Counseling and Psychotherapy Services

Psychological and emotional factors play a significant role in weight management. Counseling services are those that consider psychological issues associated with inappropriate eating and that are structured to inform the patient about the nature of these issues, their implications, and the possibilities available for their ongoing management. This intervention is less elaborate, intense, and sustaining than psychotherapy services. For example, it should be useful to help patients understand the existence and nature of a sabotaging household or the phenomenon of stress-related eating without undertaking continuing psychotherapy. A counselor or therapist can provide this service either in individual or group sessions. These counselors should, however, be sufficiently familiar with the issues that arise with weight-management programs, such as binge eating and purging. Short-term, individual case management can be helpful, as can group sessions because patients can hear the perspective of other individuals with similar weight-management concerns while addressing their individual concerns (Hughes et al., 1999; Perri et al., 2001; Wadden and Sarwer, 1999).

Psychotherapy services, both individual and group, can also be useful. However, the costs of this type of service limits its applicability to many patients. Nevertheless, the value for individual patients can be substantial, and the option should not be dismissed simply because of cost. Concerns about childhood abuse, emotional linkages to sustaining obesity (fat-dependent personality), and the management of coexisting mental health problems are the kinds of issues that might be addressed with this type of support service. The individual therapist can structure the format of the therapy but, as with counseling services, the therapist should be familiar with weight-management issues.

Patient-Led Groups

Nonprofessional patient-led groups and counseling, such as those available with organized programs like Take Off Pounds Sensibly and Overeaters Anonymous, can be useful adjuncts to weight-loss efforts. These programs have the advantages of low cost, continuing support and encouragement, and a semi-structured approach to the issues that arise among weight-management patients. Their disadvantage is that, since the counseling is nonprofessional in nature, the programs are only as good as the people who are involved. These peer-support programs are more likely to be productive when they are used as a supplement to a program with professional therapists and counselors. In Overeaters Anonymous, a variant of these groups is a sponsor-system program that pairs individuals who can help one another.

Commercial Groups

Certain commercial programs like Weight Watchers and Jenny Craig can also be helpful. Since commercial groups have their own agenda, caution must be exercised to avoid contradictions between the advice of professional counselors and that of the supportive commercial program. Since the counselors in commercial programs are not likely to be professionals, the quality of counseling offered by these programs varies with the training of the counselors.

Other Community Resources

Many communities offer supplemental weight-management services. Educational services, particularly in nutrition, may be provided through community adult education using teaching materials from nonprofit organizations such as the American Heart Association, the American Diabetes Association, and government agencies (FDA, National Institutes of Health, and U.S. Department of Agriculture). Many community hospitals have staff dietitians who are available for out-patient individual counseling (Pavlou et al., 1989a). However, the military's TRICARE health services contracts would need to be modified to include dietitian services from community hospitals or other community services since these contracts do not currently include medical nutrition therapy (and therefore dietitian counseling).

Family Support

The family unit can be a source of significant assistance to an individual in a weight-management program. For example, program dropout rates tend to be lower when a participant's spouse is involved in the program (Jeffery et al., 1984). With simple guidance and direction, the involvement of the spouse as a form of reinforcement (rather than as a source of discipline and monitoring) can become a resource to assist in supporting the participant. However, individual family members (or the family as a group) can become an obstacle when they express reluctance to make changes in food and eating patterns within the household. Issues of family conflict become more complex when the participants are children or adolescents or when spouses are reluctant to relinquish status quo positions of control.

Internet Services

A variety of Internet- and web-related services are available to individuals who are trying to manage their weight (Davison, 1997; Gray and Raab, 1999; Riva et al., 2000). As with any other Internet service, the quality of these sites varies substantially (Miles et al., 2000). An important role for weight-management professionals is to review such sites so they can recommend those that are the most useful. The use of e-mail counseling services by military personnel who travel frequently or who are stationed in remote locations has been tested at one facility; initial results are promising (James et al., 1999a). The use of web-based modalities by qualified counselors or facilitators located at large military installations would extend the accessibility of such services to personnel located at small bases or stationed in remote locations.

Physical Activity Support Services

Support is also required for military personnel who need to enhance their levels of physical fitness and physical activity. All branches of the services have remedial physical fitness training programs for personnel who fail their fitness test, but support is also needed for those who need to lose weight and for all personnel to aid in maintaining proper weight. Support services should include personnel, facilities, and equipment, and should provide practical advice on how to begin and progress through physical training routines (including proper use of training equipment and how to prevent musculoskeletal injuries), as well as advice on when and how to eat in conjunction with physical activity demands.

PRESCRIPTION AND OVER-THE-COUNTER DRUGS AND SUPPLEMENTS

Success in the promotion of weight loss can sometimes be achieved with the use of drugs. Almost all prescription drugs in current use cause weight loss by suppressing appetite or enhancing satiety. One drug, however, promotes weight loss by inhibiting fat digestion. To sustain weight loss, these drugs must be taken on a continuing basis; when their use is discontinued, some or all of the lost weight is typically regained. Therefore, when drugs are effective, it is expected that their use will continue indefinitely. For maximum benefit and safety, the use of weight-loss drugs should occur only in the context of a comprehensive weight-loss program. In general, these drugs can induce a 5- to 10-percent mean drop in body weight within 6 months of treatment initiation, but the effect can be larger or smaller depending on the individual. As with any drug, the occurrence of side effects may exclude their use in certain occupational contexts. Current convention recommends the use of weight-loss drugs in otherwise healthy individuals who have a BMI ≥ 30, or in individuals with a BMI between

27 and 30 with an existing comorbid condition (e.g., hypertension, diabetes, heart disease). Recognition that weight-related diseases, such as diabetes and hypertension, occur in individuals with BMI levels below 25, and that weight loss improves these conditions in these individuals, suggests that indications for weight-loss drugs need to be individualized to the specific patient.

A number of hormonal and metabolic differences distinguish obese people from lean people (Leibel et al., 1995; Pi-Sunyer, 1993), suggesting that genetic factors play a role in weight. Weight loss alters metabolism in obese individuals, limiting energy expenditure and reducing protein synthesis. This alteration suggests that the body may attempt to maintain an elevated body weight.

The facts that genetics might play a role in hormonal and metabolic differences between people and that weight loss alters metabolism imply that obesity is not a simple psychological problem or a failure of self-discipline. Instead, it is a chronic metabolic disease similar to other chronic diseases and it involves alterations of the body's biochemistry. Like most other chronic diseases that require ongoing pharmacotherapy to prevent the recurrence of symptoms, obesity management and relapse prevention may someday be accomplished through this form of treatment. The following sections provide a brief review of the mechanisms of action, efficacy, and safety of prescription agents that have been approved for weight loss and the various over-the-counter substances that are promoted for weight loss.

Mechanisms of Action of Obesity Drugs

Obesity drugs act by a variety of mechanisms (see Box 4-1), but all must either reduce energy intake and/or increase energy output (Arch, 1981; Aronne, 1998; Astrup et al., 1998; Bray et al., 1996; Bross and Hoffer, 1995; Cole et al., 1998; Hanotin et al., 1998a, 1998b; Heal et al., 1998; Hollander et al., 1998; Jonderko and Kucio, 1989; Kogon et al., 1994; McNeely and Benfield, 1998; Rolls et al., 1998; Scalfi et al., 1993; Sjostrom et al., 1998; Tonstad et al., 1994; Troiano et al., 1990; van Gaal et al., 1998). Energy intake may be curbed by reducing hunger or appetite or by enhancing satiety.

Some obesity drugs may reduce the preference for dietary fat or refined CHOs (Blundell et al., 1995; Bray, 1992b; Foltin et al., 1995; Leibowitz, 1995; Wurtman et al., 1987). For example, the drug orlistat reduces the absorption of fat, which results in energy loss in the feces; other drugs not approved for obesity treatment reduce CHO absorption (Heal et al., 1998; McNeely and Benfield, 1998; Sjostrom et al., 1998; van Gaal et al., 1998). These drugs may produce sufficiently adverse effects, such as oily stools or increased flatus, so that patients reduce consumption of high-fat foods in favor of less energy-dense foods (McNeely and Benfield, 1998; Sjostrom et al., 1998; van Gaal et al., 1998).

BOX 4-1 Summary of Potential Mechanisms of Action of Obesity Drugs

1. Reductions in food intake
   a. Reduction in hunger and/or appetite
   b. Enhanced satiety
   c. Reduction of fat and/or carbohydrate preference
   d. Reduction of nutrient absorption
2. Increases in energy expenditure
   a. Increased physical activity
      i. Tremor
      ii. Spontaneous physical activity (fidgeting)
      iii. Increased willingness to exercise
   b. Increased metabolic rate
      i. Increased resting metabolic rate
      ii. Increased thermogenesis with food intake, cold, activity
   c. Altered nutrient partitioning: increased fat oxidation

Obesity drugs also may increase activity levels or stimulate metabolic rate. Drugs such as fenfluramine or sibutramine were reported to increase energy expenditure in some studies (Arch, 1981; Astrup et al., 1998; Bross and Hoffer, 1995; Heal et al., 1998; Scalfi et al., 1993; Troiano et al., 1990), but not in others (Schutz et al., 1992; Seagle et al., 1998). Fluoxetine, although not approved for obesity treatment, has been shown to increase resting metabolic rate (Bross and Hoffer, 1995). Ephedrine and caffeine, which act on adenosine receptors, may increase metabolic rate, reduce body-fat storage, and increase lean mass (Liu et al., 1995; Stock, 1996; Toubro et al., 1993). With one exception (orlistat), all currently available prescription obesity drugs act on either the adrenergic or serotonergic systems in the central nervous system to regulate energy intake or expenditure (Bray, 1992b). These adrenergic and serotonergic agonists increase secretion of norepinephrine, serotonin, and/or dopamine, or inhibit neuronal reuptake. Table 4-3 summarizes the mechanism of action of pharmacological agents used for treating obesity, which are discussed in detail below.

Efficacy and Safety of Currently Available Prescription Obesity Drugs

Adrenergic and Serotonergic Agents

Efficacy. Phentermine, an adrenergic agent, is the most commonly used prescription drug for obesity and has one of the lowest costs of all prescription agents. Weight loss is comparable with that of other single agents (Silverstone,

1992). Diethylpropion, phendimetrazine, and benzphetamine are other adrenergic agents that stimulate central norepinephrine secretion and produce weight loss similar to that of phentermine (Griffiths et al., 1979; Silverstone, 1992). The categorization of phendimetrazine and benzphetamine as Drug Enforcement Agency Schedule III drugs may have limited their use, although little evidence exists to suggest that they have a higher abuse potential than does phentermine. Diethylpropion was reported to have a higher reinforcement potential in nonhuman primates than that of the other Schedule III and IV adrenergic drugs (Griffiths et al., 1979).

No currently available agents for treating obesity are exclusively serotonergic. Fluoxetine and sertraline are selective serotonin reuptake inhibitors that produce weight loss (Bross and Hoffer, 1995; Goldstein et al., 1993, 1995; Ricca et al., 1997; Wadden et al., 1995), but they do not have FDA approval for use in obesity treatment. Fluoxetine produced good weight loss after 6 months, but 1-year results were not different from those of placebo treatment (Goldstein et al., 1993). Sertraline also produced short-term weight loss (Ricca et al., 1997; Wadden et al., 1995).

Sibutramine inhibits reuptake of both norepinephrine and serotonin in central nervous system neurons. At doses of 15 mg/day, the drug produced a 1-year weight loss of 6 to 10 percent (Astrup et al., 1998; Bray et al., 1996; Hanotin et al., 1998b; Seagle et al., 1998). Blood pressure rose slightly in normotensive subjects, but fell in hypertensive subjects (Heal et al., 1998). Decreases in fasting blood glucose, insulin, waist circumference, waist-hip ratio, and computerized tomography-estimated abdominal fat were greater with sibutramine than with placebo (Heal et al., 1998). The greater weight losses observed in the sibutramine group compared with the placebo group may be responsible for the greater improvements in other parameters.

Safety. Common complaints with the use of centrally active adrenergic and serotonergic obesity drugs include dry mouth, fatigue, hair loss, constipation, sweating, sleep disturbances, and sexual dysfunction (Atkinson et al., 1997; Bray, 1998). Sibutramine can increase blood pressure and pulse rate in occasional patients and may cause dizziness and increased food intake (Cole et al., 1998; Hanotin et al., 1998a, 1998b). Mazindol may cause penile discharge (van Puijenbroek and Meyboom, 1998).

Drugs Affecting Absorption: Lipase and Amylase Inhibitors

Efficacy. Orlistat binds to lipase in the gastrointestinal tract and inhibits absorption of about one-third of dietary fat (Hollander et al., 1998; James WP et al., 1997; McNeely and Benfield, 1998; Sjostrom et al., 1998; Tonstad et al., 1994; van Gaal et al., 1998; Zhi et al., 1994). Thus, consumption of over 100 g of fat/day should result in about 30 g or more of fat reaching the colon. Average

TABLE 4-3 Prescription Pharmacological Agents for Weight-Loss Treatment and Mechanisms of Action

Drug Class	Drug
Adrenergic (DEA[a] II)	Amphetamine[b,d]
	Methamphetamine[b,d]
Adrenergic (DEA[a] III)	Benzphetamine
	Phedimetrazine
Adrenergic (DEA[a] IV)	Diethylpropion[b]
	Mazindol[c]
	Phentermine
Adrenergic over-the-counter	Phenylpropanolamine[c]
Serotonergic	d,1-fenfluramine[c]
	d-norfenfluramine[c]
	SSRI anti-depressants[d]
Combined adrenergic and serotonergic (DEA[a] IV)	Sibutramine
Drugs affecting absorption	Orlistat
	Acarbose[d]

[a] DEA = Drug Enforcement Agency
[b] High abuse potential – measured by the ratio of anorexiant dose to reinforcing dose.

weight loss on orlistat is about 8 to 11 percent of initial body weight at 1 year (James WP et al., 1997; Sjostrom et al., 1998).

Compared with the effects of a placebo, orlistat treatment resulted in greater improvements in total cholesterol, low-density lipoprotein (LDL) cholesterol, LDL/high-density lipoprotein ratio, and concentrations of glucose and insulin (Hollander et al., 1998; James WP et al., 1997; McNeely and Benfield, 1998; Sjostrom et al., 1998; Tonstad et al., 1994; van Gaal et al., 1998). Although weight loss may be responsible for some of the observed improvements, orlistat lowered LDL independently of its effect on weight loss.

Acarbose is an alpha glucosidase inhibitor that inhibits or delays absorption of complex CHOs (Wolever et al., 1997). This drug is approved by FDA for the treatment of diabetes mellitus, but not for weight loss. Although it produces modest weight loss in animals, it has minimal or no effect on humans.

Safety. Adverse side effects of orlistat include abdominal cramping, increased flatus formation, diarrhea, oily spotting, and fecal incontinence (Hollander et al., 1998; James WP et al., 1997; McNeely and Benfield, 1998; Sjostrom et al., 1998; Tonstad et al., 1994; van Gaal et al., 1998; Zhi et al., 1994). These adverse effects may serve as a behavior modification tool to reduce the level of fat in the diet and presumably to reduce energy intake. Orlistat has been shown to produce small reductions in serum levels of fat-

Mechanism of Action	Efficacy/Safety
	DEA[a] II drugs rarely used for obesity treatment due to high abuse potential
Stimulates norepinephrine release	Weight loss varies but significant compared with placebo; insomnia and dry mouth
Stimulates norepinephrine release	
Stimulates norepinephrine release	Weight loss varies but significant compared with placebo; insomnia and dry mouth
Blocks norepinephrine reuptake	
Stimulates norepinephrine release	
α_1 Agonist	Significant weight loss compared with placebo but less than class III and IV adrenergics
Acts to block serotonin reuptake	Significant weight loss compared with placebo; plateau at 6 months; dry mouth and insomnia; pulmonary hypertension
Acts to enhance serotonin release	
Acts to block serotonin reuptake	
Stimulates norepinephrine and serotonin release or blocks uptake	Significant weight loss compared with placebo; dry mouth and insomnia; raises blood pressure in some individuals
Inhibits lipase activity	Significant weight loss compared with placebo; abdominal cramps and diarrhea

[c] Removed from market by manufacturers.
[d] Not approved by the Food and Drug Administration for weight-loss treatment
SOURCE: Bray (1998); James et al. (1997).

soluble vitamins. The manufacturer recommends that a vitamin supplement containing vitamins A, D, E, and K be prescribed for patients taking orlistat.

Drugs Approved for Other Conditions

A variety of drugs currently on the market for other conditions, but not approved by FDA for obesity treatment, have been evaluated for their ability to induce weight loss. Metformin (Lee and Morley, 1998), cimetidine (Rasmussen et al., 1993; Stoa-Birketvedt, 1993), diazoxide (Alemzadeh et al., 1998), bromocriptine (Cincotta and Meier, 1996), nicotine (Grant et al., 1997; Jensen et al., 1995; Nides et al., 1994), bupropion (Croft et al., 2000; Gadde et al., 1999), and topiramate (Rosenfeld et al., 1997) have produced modest weight loss. Additional studies are needed to support these findings.

Drugs Used in Combination

Efficacy. Although chronic diseases often require treatment with more than one drug, few studies have evaluated combination therapy for obesity. Private practitioners have used various combinations in an off-label fashion. The available data suggest that combination therapy is somewhat more effective than therapy with single agents. Combinations such as phentermine and fenfluramine or ephedrine and caffeine produce weight losses of about 15 percent or more of initial body weight compared with about 10 percent or less with single drug use. However, due to reported side-effects of cardiac valve lesions and pulmonary hypertension, fenfluramine and dexfenfluramine are no longer available.

Results of tests using combinations of phentermine with selective serotonin reuptake inhibitors (mainly fluoxetine or sertraline) have been reported in abstracts or preliminary reports (Dhurandhar and Atkinson, 1996; Griffen and Anchors, 1998). These combinations produced weight losses somewhat less than that of the combination treatment of ephedrine-caffeine, but greater than that of treatment with single agents (Dhurandhar and Atkinson, 1996).

Safety. Anchors (1997) used the combination of phentermine and fluoxetine in a large series of patients and suggested that this combination is safe and effective. Griffen and Anchors (1998) reported that the combination of phentermine-fluoxetine was not associated with the cardiac valve lesions that were reported for fenfluramine and dexfenfluramine.

Alternative Medicines, Herbs, and Diet Supplements

In 1994, Congress passed the Dietary Supplement Health and Education Act, which exempted dietary supplements (including those promoted for weight loss) from the requirement to demonstrate safety and efficacy. As a result, the variety of over-the-counter preparations touted to promote weight loss has exploded. Dietary supplements include compounds such as herbal preparations (often of unknown composition), chemicals (e.g., hydroxycitrate, chromium), vitamin preparations, and protein powder preparations. With the exception of herbal preparations of ephedrine and caffeine, none of these compounds have produced more than a minimal weight loss and most are ineffective or have been insufficiently studied to determine their efficacy. Furthermore, while little is known about the safety of many of these compounds, there are a growing number of adverse event reports for several of them. Table 4-4 summarizes the current safety and efficacy profile of a number of alternative compounds promoted for the purpose of weight loss.

The combination of ephedrine and caffeine to treat obesity has been reported to produce weight losses of 15 percent or more of initial body weight (Daly et al., 1993; Toubro et al., 1993). Both drugs are the active ingredients in a number of herbal weight-loss preparations. Weight loss is maximal at about 4 to 6 months on this combination, but body-fat levels may continue to decrease through 9 to 12 months, with increases in lean body mass (Toubro et al., 1993). This observation suggests that the combination may be a beta-3 adrenergic agonist (Liu et al., 1995; Toubro et al., 1993).

Reports of cardiovascular and cerebrovascular events following use of ephedrine and caffeine to treat obesity have reached sufficient frequency that FDA and the Federal Trade Commission have begun to investigate the safety of this combination and have issued warnings to consumers. In addition, FDA has proposed new regulations for the labeling of products containing ephedrine, which would require warning statements for potential adverse health effects. Use of ephedrine alone or in combination with caffeine has been associated with a wide range of cardiovascular, cerebrovascular, neurological, psychological, gastrointestinal, and other symptoms in adverse events reports (Haller and Benowitz, 2000; Shekelle et al., 2003). Some prospective studies do not support the concept that there are major adverse events with ephedrine and caffeine (Boozer et al., 2001, 2002; Greenway, 2001; Kalman et al., 2002), but these studies were conducted using healthy individuals selected using careful exclusion criteria.

FUTURE DRUGS FOR THE TREATMENT OF OBESITY

Body weight, body fat, energy metabolism, and fat oxidation are regulated by numerous hormones, peptides, neurotransmitters, and other substances in the body. Drug companies are devoting a large amount of resources to find new agents to treat obesity. Potential candidates include cholecystokinin, corticotropin-releasing hormone, glucagon-like peptide 1, growth hormone and other growth factors, enterostatin, neurotensin, vasopressin, anorectin, ciliary neurotrophic factor, and bombesin, all of which potentially either inhibit food intake or reduce body weight in humans or animals (Bray, 1992b, 1998; Ettinger et al., 2003; Okada et al., 1991; Rudman et al., 1990; Smith and Gibbs, 1984). Neuropeptide Y and galanin are central nervous system neurotransmitters that stimulate food intake (Bray, 1998; Leibowitz, 1995), so antagonists to these substances might be expected to reduce food intake. Beta-3 adrenergic receptor agonists reduce body fat and increase lean body mass in animals (Stock, 1996; Yen, 1995), but human analogs have not been identified that are effective and safe in humans. Several types of uncoupling proteins have been identified as being involved with the regulation of energy metabolism and body fat (Bao et al., 1998; Bouchard et al., 1998; Chagnon et al., 2000; Pérusse et al., 1999), but no agents based on these proteins have yet been produced to treat obesity.

As discussed in Chapter 3, seven single gene defects have been reported to produce obesity in humans (Pérusse et al., 1999). The leptin gene is defective in ob/ob mice, and leptin administration has been shown to be highly effective in reducing body weight in these mice (Campfield et al., 1995; Halaas et al., 1995; Pelleymounter et al., 1995). A very small number of humans with this gene defect have been identified, and at least one responded to leptin (Clement et al., 1998; Pérusse et al., 1999). Leptin levels are high in most obese individuals (Considine et al., 1996; Phillips, 1998), and preliminary trials of administration of leptin to these individuals show modest effects. Defects in the genes for

TABLE 4-4 Alternative Medicines, Herbs, and Supplements Used for Weight Loss

Name/Compound	Description
Bladderwrack	Fucus vesiculosus
Chitosan	Polymer of glucosamine derived from chitin
Chromium	Cr—an essential element
CLA	Conjugated linoleic acid
DHEA	Dehydroepiandrosterone
Ephedrine fat-burning stack	Ephedrine with caffeine and aspirin, ma huang with guarana and willow bark
Garcinia cambogia	Contains hydroxycitrate (HCA)
Germander	Teucrium chamaedrys
HMB	β-Hydroxy-β-methylbutryrate
Olestra (Lawson et al., 1997)	Mixture of hexa-, hepta-, and octa-esters of sucrose formed from long-chain fatty acids isolated from edible oils
Plantago	Plantain leaf or psyllium seed
Pyruvate	A 3-carbon compound
Sunflower	Helianthus annuus
St. John's Wort	Hypericum perforatum

SOURCE: Allison et al. (2001).

protein convertase subtilisin/kexin type 1, PPAR-gamma, and pro-opiomelanocortin and in the genes for the receptors for leptin, thyroid hormone, and melanocortin-4R (Bouchard et al., 1998; Chagnon et al., 2000; Pérusse et al., 1999) have been identified in humans. It may be possible in the future to develop gene therapy or products that correct these defects in order to treat obesity.

Summary

Although obesity drugs have been available for more than 50 years, the concept of long-term treatment of obesity with drugs has been seriously advanced only in the last 10 years. The evidence that obesity, as opposed to overweight, is a pathophysiological process of multiple etiologies and not simply a problem of self-discipline is gradually being recognized—obesity is

Safety	Efficacy for Weight/Fat Loss
No, increases risk of hyperthyroidism	Insufficient data
Insufficient data	No (Pittler et al., 1999; Wuolijoki et al., 1999)
Yes, when used in recommended doses	Likely ineffective (Hallmark et al., 1996; Lukaski et al., 1996; Trent and Thieding-Cencel, 1995)
Yes, preliminary report	Yes, preliminary report (Blankson et al., 2000)
No	Yes, but studies are limited
Adverse effects have been reported (Haller and Benowitz, 2000; HHS/FDA, 1997; Shekelle et al., 2003)	Yes, appropriate dose and in combination with caffeine (Astrup et al., 1992a, 1992b; Boozer et al., 2001)
Insufficient data	Insufficient data, possibly ineffective at dose of 1,500 mg/d in obese adults (Heymsfield et al., 1998)
No	Insufficient data
Yes, short-term	Yes
Yes	Insufficient data
Unknown, may cause gastrointestinal distress and affect absorption of medications	Insufficient data
Insufficient data	No
Yes	Insufficient data
Insufficient data	Insufficient data

similar to other chronic diseases associated with alterations in the biochemistry of the body. Most other chronic diseases are treated with drugs, and it is likely that the primary treatment for obesity in the future will be the long-term administration of drugs. Unfortunately, current drug treatment of obesity produces only moderately better success than does diet, exercise, and behavioral modification over the intermediate term. Newer drugs need to be developed, and combinations of current drugs need to be tested for short- and long-term effectiveness and safety. As drugs are proven to be safe and effective, their use in less severe obesity and overweight may be justified.

The appropriateness of using weight-loss drugs in the military population requires careful consideration. On average, a 5 to 10 percent weight loss can improve comorbid conditions associated with obesity, but it is not known if this degree of weight reduction by itself would improve fitness or if it could be expected to improve performance in all military contexts. The side effects that are sometimes encountered might also restrict the use of weight-loss drugs in some military contexts. On the other hand, the military is losing or is in danger of losing otherwise qualified individuals who cannot "make weight." Such people might be able to keep their weight within regulation if they are allowed to take weight-loss drugs for the remainder of their term in the military. The frequency of known side effects of current weight-loss drugs is sufficiently low that the potential for adverse events would not seem to be a reason to avoid the use of these drugs by military personnel.

The use of available dietary supplements and herbal preparations to control body weight is generally not recommended because of a lack of demonstrated efficacy of such preparations, the absence of control on their purity, and evidence that at least some of these agents have significant side effects and safety problems. The occurrence of potential adverse effects (e.g., dehydration, mood alterations) would be of particular concern for military personnel.

SURGERY

Although it would be expected that very few active duty military personnel would qualify for consideration for obesity surgery, a review of weight-management programs would not be complete without a discussion of this option.

For massively obese individuals (those with a BMI above 35 or 40), the modest weight losses from behavioral treatments and/or drugs do not alter their obese status. For these individuals, obesity surgery may produce massive, long-term weight loss. Recent studies have shown dramatic improvements in the morbidity and mortality of those who are massively obese, and surgery is being recommended with increasing frequency for these individuals (Hubbard and Hall, 1991). Table 4-5 presents the rationale and results of all forms of obesity surgery.

Individuals who are candidates for obesity surgery are those who (1) exhibit any of the complications of obesity such as diabetes, hypertension, dyslipidemia, sleep disorders, pulmonary dysfunction, or increased intracranial pressure and have a BMI above 35, or (2) have a BMI above 40.

Gastric bypass is currently the most commonly used procedure for obesity surgery. Following this procedure, patients lose about 62 to 70 percent of excess weight and maintain this loss for more than 5 years (Kral, 1998; MacDonald et al., 1997; Pories et al., 1992, 1995; Sugerman et al., 1989). Biliopancreatic bypass, another type of obesity surgery, and its variations produce weight losses comparable or superior to gastric bypass (Kral, 1998). In addition to massive weight loss, individuals who undergo obesity surgery experience improvements in health status relative to hypertension, dyslipidemia, sleep apnea, pulmonary function (oxygen saturation and oxyhemoglobin levels and decreased carbon dioxide saturation) (Sugerman, 1987; Sugerman et al., 1986, 1988), obesity-hypoventilation syndrome, and pseudotumor cerebri, urinary incontinence, and pulmonary dysfunction possibly due to increased intra-abdominal pressure (Sugerman et al., 1995, 1999).

Obesity surgery is, however, considered the treatment of last resort because of the short- and long-term complications associated with the surgery. Perioperative mortality is small but significant (about 0.3 to 2 percent) and appears to vary inversely with the experience of the surgeon (Kral, 1998). Other potential side effects include vomiting, diarrhea, electrolyte abnormalities, liver failure, renal stones, pseudo-obstruction syndrome, arthritis syndrome, and bacterial overgrowth syndromes.

THE USE OF STRUCTURED MAINTENANCE PROGRAMS

When to Use a Maintenance Program

The long-term success of weight management appears to depend on the individual participating in a specific and deliberate follow-up program. Programs to aid personnel in weight maintenance or prevention of weight gain are appropriate when:

- An individual has successfully achieved his or her weight-loss goal and now seeks to maintain the new weight,
- An individual who is gaining weight has taken a weight-loss readiness assessment and has determined that he or she is not ready for weight loss at this time, or
- An overweight individual is temporarily excluded from a weight-reduction program until a medical, physical, or psychological problem stabilizes.

Components of a Maintenance Program

A comprehensive weight-maintenance strategy has five fundamental components:

1. It helps the patient select a weight range within which he or she can realistically stay and, if possible, minimize health risks.
2. It provides an opportunity for continued monitoring of weight, food intake, and physical activity.
3. It helps the patient understand and implement the principle of balancing the energy consumed from food with routine physical activity.
4. It helps the patient establish and maintain lifestyle change strategies for a sufficiently long period of time to make the new behaviors into permanent habits (a minimum of 6 months has been suggested [Wing, 1998]).
5. It considers the long-term use of drugs.

TABLE 4-5 Surgical Procedures Used for Treatment of Obesity in Humans

Procedure	Proposed Mechanism
Intestinal resection (Kral, 1989)	Small intestine malabsorption
Intestinal bypass (Kral, 1998)	Small intestine malabsorption
Jujuno-ileal bypass (Hallberg et al., 1975; Kral, 1998; Payne and DeWind, 1969)	
End-to-end, end-to-side (Bray et al., 1977)	
Biblio-pancreatic bypass (Kral, 1998; Scopinaro et al., 1979, 1998)	Small intestine malabsorption
Stomach to ileum (Kral, 1998)	Small intestine malabsorption
Gastric stapling (MacLean et al., 1993)	Partial gastric outlet obstruction, limited food intake
Gastric bypass (Benotti et al., 1989; Linner, 1982; Yale, 1989)	Reduced food intake secondary to very small stomach size and restricted flow rate into small intestine, reduced intestinal absorption
Vertical banded gastroplasty (Benotti et al., 1989; Linner, 1982; Mason, 1982; Yale, 1989)	Reduced food intake secondary to very small stomach size and restricted flow rate into small intestine, reduced intestinal absorption
Gastric wrapping (Kral, 1998)	Reduced food intake secondary to very small stomach size and restricted flow rate into small intestine, reduced intestinal absorption
Jaw wiring	Prevents solid food consumption
Subdiaphragmatic truncal vagotomy ± pyloroplasty (Holle and Bauer, 1978)	Loss of motor function leads to stomach distension which causes a feeling of fullness that may signal the central nervous system
Liposuction (Kral, 1998)	Removal of subcutaneous fat

[a] Humoral or neural effects of exposure of ileum to nutrients may lead to increased effects.

Helping Patients Learn How to Balance Energy

Individuals who have achieved a weight-loss goal generally fall into one of two groups: those who see no point in participating in a maintenance program since they believe they know how to keep the weight off and those who remain open to change and improving their skills in weight management.

The critical role of the health care provider is to motivate the former group to learn the skills necessary for weight management. The skills necessary to:

Results	Notes
	80% Decrease in energy intake in immediate postoperative period Gradual weight increase over 2 years
High failure rate	
	Considered more effective than vertical banded gastroplasty and gastric wrapping, causes dumping, laparoscopic (leads to decrease in perioperative complications)[a] Rarely used due to large number of complications
100% Failure	
Average weight loss ≈ 20 kg	Procedure abandoned
Effects minimal	Cosmetic use only

- Maintain regular exercise for at least 60 min/day or an expenditure of 2,000 to 3,000 kcal/wk (8,368 kJ) (Klem et al., 1997; Schoeller et al., 1997).
- Decrease the amount of energy-dense foods eaten (especially those that are low in nutrients).
- Practice healthy eating by including fruits, vegetables, and whole grains in the diet.
- Understand portion control.
- Access the services of nutrition counselors or other forms of guidance.

Helping Patients Establish Permanent Lifestyle Change Strategies

As mentioned above, individuals who have lost weight need to make permanent lifestyle changes in order to maintain their loss. To assist patients in making these changes, successful maintenance programs will include education on and assistance with the following factors (Foreyt and Goodrick, 1993, 1994; Kayman et al., 1990):

- *Self-monitoring*. Regular weighing and recording of daily food intake and physical activity for the first month or two of the maintenance period and during periods of increased exposure to food (e.g., during the holidays). If weight gain occurs, reinstitution of this practice may help bring weight back into control. Frequent follow-up contact with counselors is also crucial (Perri et al., 1993). Effective follow-up consists of a schedule of regular weekly to monthly contacts by mail, phone, or in person. Support groups may substitute for some of this follow-up with a health care provider, but should not replace it.
- *Physical activity*. Daily physical activity is key to successful weight maintenance; it is the factor cited as the most important in maintaining weight loss by the majority of individuals in the National Weight Loss Registry (Klem et al., 1997). An average of 80 min/day of moderate activity or 35 min/day of vigorous activity is needed to maintain weight (Schoeller et al., 1997).
- *Problem solving*. Learning to identify and anticipate problems that threaten to undermine success is necessary. Problem solving skills allow the individual to craft strategies that will resolve problems as they emerge.
- *Stress management*. Exercise, relaxation, and social support can help reduce stress. Techniques to reduce stress can be critical for some individuals who overeat in response to stress.
- *Relapse prevention*. Relapse, temporary loss of control, and return to old behaviors is common. The key to relapse prevention is learning to anticipate high-risk situations and to devise plans to reduce the damages. Patients need to learn to forgive themselves for a lapse and view it as a "learning experience." Reestablishing control is crucial.
- *Social influence/support*. Sabotage by family or friends is seen often and may be stressful for the individual who is trying to maintain weight. The skills to recognize intentional or unintentional sabotage may be learned. In extreme cases, a choice may need to be made between the weight-maintenance program or the relationship. Identifying a fresh circle of supporters or starting a support group may be useful.

PUBLIC POLICY MEASURES

To the extent that the epidemic of obesity can be attributed to changes in our living and working environments (the increased availability of calorie-dense foods and decreased opportunity to expend energy), public policy efforts may help prevent overweight and may assist those who are trying to lose weight or maintain weight loss (Koplan and Dietz, 1999). Some measures that have been suggested and/or tried include the following:

- Increasing choices and decreasing prices of low-calorie (and low-fat) foods (e.g., fruits and vegetables) offered at worksite eating places and in vending machines (French et al., 1997; Hoerr and Louden, 1993)
- Instituting workplace and community programs that include regular monitoring, nutrition and health promotion, overweight prevention education, and exercise classes or groups
- Renovating community spaces to provide more and safer spaces for physical activity
- Modifying work environments or schedules to encourage greater physical activity on and off the job
- Mandating regular physical activity during the workday (IOM, 1998).

SUMMARY

Apart from the obvious need to increase energy expenditure relative to intake, none of the strategies that have been proposed to promote weight loss or maintenance of weight loss are universally recognized as having any utility in weight management. The efficacy of individual interventions is poor, and evidence regarding the efficacy of combinations of strategies is sparse, with results varying from one study to another and with the individual. Recent studies that have focused on identifying and studying individuals who have been successful at weight management have identified some common techniques. These include self-monitoring, contact with and support from others, regular physical activity, development of problem-solving skills (to deal with difficult environments and situations), and relapse-prevention/limitation skills. However, an additional factor identified among successful weight managers, and one not generally included in discussing weight-management techniques, is individual readiness, that is, strong personal motivation to succeed in weight management.

5

Response to the Military's Questions

Based on a thorough review of the scientific literature, the material presented at the workshop, and current military data and discussions with workshop speakers and others, the subcommittee provides the following responses to the questions posed by the military. It should be noted, however, that prevention of weight and fat gain throughout an individual's military career would be preferable to even the most comprehensive weight-loss program.

QUESTION 1

What are the essential components of an effective weight/fat loss program, and the most effective strategies for sustaining weight loss?

Years of research have demonstrated that a program for weight/fat loss can only be effective when it is closely integrated with a program for sustaining weight loss. The rate of failure to maintain weight loss for those individuals who have successfully completed weight-loss programs has been disappointingly high. Successful cases clearly demonstrate that permanent major lifestyle changes must be adopted during the weight-loss phase of the program in order to prevent regain of the weight lost. Even in the most successful programs, the majority of patients regain some of their lost weight over time. **The greatest likelihood of success requires an integrated program, both during and after the weight-loss phase, in which assessment, increased energy expenditure through exercise and other daily activities, energy intake reduction, nutrition education, lifestyle change, environmental change, and psychological support are all components.**

Essential Components of an Effective Weight/Fat Loss Program

The first component of an effective weight/fat loss program is an appropriate assessment. In most cases, body weight and height measurements should be taken and the individual's body mass index (BMI) calculated from this data. If the BMI is within the acceptable range as defined by the Department of Defense (DOD), no further measurement is necessary. However, if the height and weight measurements indicate that the individual exceeds the service's standards or that the calculated BMI exceeds the newly adopted DOD maximum of 27.5, then additional anthropometric measures should be taken to assess body-fat content. DOD has extensively validated the circumference equations used to estimate percent body fat, and a single equation for men and one for women has now been mandated across all service branches (DOD, 2002). Care should be taken to assure that the standard procedures for measuring body circumferences are followed. Proper training and adequate criteria for assessing technician skill in conducting accurate circumference measurements should be standardized across DOD. Considering the seriousness of the consequences of overweight for military personnel, validation of technician skill and availability of the data demonstrating the reliability and repeatability of a technician's circumference measures is warranted. Once there are clear indications that an individual's body-fat mass exceeds desired standards, a medical evaluation should be conducted to determine if a medical condition exists that might be the underlying cause of body-fat accumulation. In the absence of any apparent medical condition, the individual can enter a weight-reduction program.

The essential components of a weight/fat loss program include:

- *Exercise.* For overweight adults who are otherwise healthy, increased physical activity is an essential component of a comprehensive weight-reduction strategy. There is compelling evidence that habitual physical activity is associated not only with weight/fat loss, but also with desirable health outcomes (Angotti and Levine, 1994; IOM, 2002; Kesaniemi et al., 2001), and there is evidence from industrial research that workers are more productive and lose fewer days due to health problems when provisions are made for regular exercise. Retrospective analyses of weight regain as a function of energy expended in physical activity indicated a threshold for weight maintenance of 11.23 kcal (47 kJ)/kg of body weight/day. This corresponds to an average of 80 min/day of moderate activity or 35 min/day of vigorous activity added to a sedentary lifestyle (Schoeller et al., 1997). As indicated, this would be considered the threshold level and would likely need to be higher (either longer time periods or greater intensity) to effect weight loss. There is good evidence that peak rates of lipid oxidation are achieved at exercise intensities of approximately 45 percent of VO_{2max} (Bergman and Brooks, 1999; Brooks, 1998; Wolfe, 1998).
- *Behavioral modification.* The use of behavior and lifestyle modification in weight management is based on a body of evidence that people become or remain overweight as a result of modifiable habits or behaviors and that by changing these behaviors, weight can be lost and weight loss can be maintained. The modifications that need to be made are: increased activity, decreased energy

intake, and improved diet quality. In addition, the individual needs to learn to effectively deal with stress and identify situations that may trigger excessive intake or inactivity.

- *Net dietary energy deficit.* Energy expended must exceed energy consumed on a consistent basis over an extended period of time, the length of which depends on the degree of overweight. While balanced macronutrient diets are usually recommended, the composition of the diet may vary to suit individual preferences and health concerns that may need to be addressed. There is no scientific consensus on the ideal dietary composition, but extremes of individual macronutrients should be avoided. For military personnel who stand to lose their livelihood if they cannot reduce their weight, options such as high-protein diets should not be precluded. Recent data suggest that these types of diets may better preserve lean body mass, lower insulin levels, and enhance energy expenditure (protein has the highest thermal effect of feeding).

A potential downside to high-protein diets, particularly if they are quite low in carbohydrate, is that there may be changes in levels of potassium and other cations. Evidence suggests that the initial weight that is lost on high-protein diets is mostly fluid and thus, dehydration is a risk, particularly for military pilots.

- *Education.* Information on nutrition principles, food-portion control, and the need for energy balance is essential for individuals to develop appropriate eating behaviors.
- *Psychological Support.* Any weight-management program is likely to be more successful if it is accompanied by structured support mechanisms (e.g., from professional counselors, commanders, coworkers, and family).
- *Environmental changes*. The services should take measures to change the environments that foster underactivity and overconsumption of energy. Examples of environmental changes include putting low-fat, healthy snacks in vending machines; increasing the variety of low-fat, low-calorie entrees in base dining facilities; selecting commercial food establishments for base contracts that provide a variety of low-fat, healthy menu items; and encouraging the consumption of low-fat, low-calorie snacks during working hours. Environmental changes that promote greater activity are also essential (e.g., using stairs rather than elevators and escalators). The environment includes the home, the workplace, and the community.
- *Structured monitoring.* The long-term success of weight-loss programs appears to depend on a specific and deliberate follow-up program. This structured follow-up should include monitoring body weight with weigh-ins at least weekly during weight loss and monthly during maintenance, monitoring food intake, and monitoring physical activity. Keeping a diary or record that includes this information, along with notations on feelings and challenges, can also be useful. The frequency of monitoring is usually weekly until new habits and be-

haviors are well established. After that, less frequent monitoring is needed unless the individual encounters difficulties and needs to get back on track.

Sustaining Weight Loss

Most studies in which patients are not provided weight-maintenance assistance following achievement of weight-loss goals show that complete weight regain will occur in a majority of the patients within 5 years (Stalonas et al., 1984; Wadden et al., 1989). A recent review of studies on the effectiveness of weight-maintenance strategies show that programs that incorporate continued professional guidance, skills training for coping with challenges, enhanced social support, enhanced aerobic exercise, and techniques for sustaining behavior change lower the rate of relapse (Perri et al., 1993). Although such strategies do not ensure success, the outcome is much more favorable. Considering that these studies were conducted with patients in the general population where relapse is undesirable, but often not punitive, makes the results even more compelling for the military where failure to maintain weight loss can have serious consequences for career progression.

A successful program for sustaining weight loss should include the following components:

- *Physical activity* is an essential component for long-term, sustained weight loss. Studies suggest that expenditure of at least 2,000 kcal (8,368 kJ) to 3,000 kcal (12,558 kJ) per week from exercise is necessary to prevent regain of lost weight (Klem et al., 1997; Schoeller et al., 1997). This is in addition to the normal daily activities of sedentary individuals.
- *Permanent lifestyle and behavioral modifications* are important for maintaining energy balance. The individual needs practice in problem solving and coping skills that are essential to balance daily energy intake and habitual levels of physical activity. This includes portion control, selecting foods lower in fat and calories, and consistently sustaining higher levels of daily physical activity. Sustained professional guidance, support, and feedback are essential for the maintenance of these skills.
- *Self-monitoring* is important to success in weight maintenance. Individuals who have been overweight need to weigh themselves at least once a week and record their weight. They should also be encouraged to periodically (about every 3 months) keep a 3-day diary of the type and amounts of foods consumed and the type and amounts of physical activity performed. The diary information can provide counselors with important clues on problem areas and highlight necessary changes in the diet and activity level needed to support weight maintenance.
- *Continuous structured support* is necessary for weight maintenance. At a minimum, an individual embarking on a weight-maintenance program, in addi-

tion to self-monitoring, should have follow-up visits or counseling via phone or the Internet every 2 to 4 weeks for the first 3 months, depending on the difficulty in maintaining a stable healthy weight, and every 1 to 2 months thereafter.

QUESTION 2

How do age and gender influence success in weight-management programs? Should age be considered in weight/fat standards and in weight-management programs and interventions?

Age

Research indicates that percent body fat increases with age even if weight has not changed. The current upper limits of DOD standards of 26 percent fat in men and 36 percent fat in women, however, are well within the limits of the healthy percent body-fat range even for men and women as old as 60 to 79 years of age. However, since the individual services all have body-fat limits more stringent than the DOD upper limits, increases with age up to the DOD limit appear to be appropriate.

Weight loss is more difficult with age due to decreases in physical activity, strength, and endurance without concomitant decreases in energy intake, coupled with decreases in lean body mass and increases (either absolute or relative) in percent body fat. Energy requirements may be reduced due to decreased lean body mass; therefore, energy intake must be carefully controlled. If the goal of the military is to maintain health, there should not be age-related BMI increases. However, increases in the allowable percent fat with increasing age are reasonable, but should not exceed the maximum of 36 percent in women and 26 percent in men. If the goal is performance, BMI and fat increases may not affect performance in some military occupations. (This is an area that needs further research.) In such occupational specialties, it may be reasonable to rely on performance-based physical training tests. If the goal is military appearance, there is little data to suggest that appearance standards are closely related to performance, health, fitness, or nutrition (IOM, 1998). However, from both an appearance and a health perspective, abdominal circumference should be used as an objective measure. Upper body adiposity as measured by abdominal circumference has been shown to be a separate risk factor for mortality and coronary heart disease. Current National Institutes of Health guidelines for maximum abdominal girths are 102 cm (approximately 40 in) for men and 89 cm (approximately 35 in) for women.

Gender

Women, because of their smaller body size, specific adipose tissue stores, and lower lean body mass, automatically have a higher percent body fat than men at the same BMI. In addition, excessive weight gain during pregnancy, as well as hormonal and metabolic changes after pregnancy and menopause, may be associated with higher body fat. This may make weight loss more difficult for women. Preventive measures would include counseling to keep pregnancy weight gain within the recommended range (IOM, 1990, 1992b).

QUESTION 3

Which strategies would be most and least effective in a military setting? Should military weight/fat loss programs involve direct participation interventions or only monitoring and guidance? Should military programs be more proactive in identifying and discouraging ineffective or dangerous weight-loss practices? Is a warning or cautionary zone prior to enrollment in a weight-control program an effective strategy? When should duty time be authorized for participation in intervention strategies for weight/fat loss?

Most and Least Effective Strategies

The effective strategies for a weight/fat loss program would be the same regardless of whether the setting is military or civilian. However, the implementation of some of these strategies could be facilitated in the military environment, particularly physical fitness, exercise, and behavior modification. The safest program designed for weight loss and maintenance is an increase of energy expenditure through exercise and daily activity coupled with control or reduction of energy intake, behavior modification, and lifestyle changes. A key factor in the control of energy intake is behavior modification—individuals who have an overweight problem have a pattern of food consumption and/or energy expenditure that contributes to positive energy balance.

The primary difficulty in the military setting would be in providing structured follow-up due to the mobility of the military population. When diet and exercise are insufficient, the addition of certain prescription drugs may be useful as an adjunct, but the use of drugs should be carefully monitored and controlled. A person whose overweight is severe enough to warrant drugs (BMI ≥ 30) is likely to require the drugs on a long-term basis. Such individuals may have genetic or other etiologies of obesity that make it difficult to adhere to lifestyle modification programs. In such cases, drug therapy may alter the biochemistry of the body sufficiently to allow them to adhere to a diet and exercise program that will bring them into compliance with weight regulations.

Direct Participation Interventions versus Monitoring and Guidance

Direct participation interventions have been demonstrated to improve compliance, increase the success rate of weight/fat loss, and support an improved level of weight maintenance. It is important that overweight individuals be counseled for individualized diet modification and exercise and be continually monitored. Do-it-yourself pamphlets may be useful to some people, but many individuals need one-on-one or group contact with competent counselors to address both diet and exercise. Weight loss and weight-loss maintenance programs have high rates of failure. The goal is to develop permanent behavior modification.

Long-term follow-up is clearly needed for individuals to maintain their weight loss. Innovative strategies, perhaps with centralized dietitians or other counselors who can follow military personnel via the Internet, might be developed. Since recidivism in overweight people is high, the military might consider mandating routine follow-up for anyone who has at any time exceeded the weight standards. While drastic, a focus on constant follow-up and feedback may prevent weight regain or identify a problem very early in its course, thus making it easier to rectify.

There is a correlation between frequency of monitoring and success in weight loss and maintenance of weight loss. A comprehensive program that individualizes the degree of direct participation intervention will increase the success rate of weight/fat loss and support an improved level of weight maintenance. If only monitoring and guidance are provided, individuals may seek help from unqualified nonmilitary weight-loss sources or pursue other unhealthy weight-loss approaches to meet their monitoring goals. Individuals' use of prescription drugs or nonprescription supplements unknown to their military health-care providers could have negative health consequences.

Identifying and Discouraging Ineffective or Dangerous Weight-Loss Practices

The military setting is unique in providing a strong disciplinary incentive to achieve and maintain a healthy body weight and body-fat content. Few employment environments have standards for weight and percent body fat and the authority to enforce them by affecting promotion and retention. In fact, the incentive is so strong that individuals in the military have been observed to practice high-risk crash dieting in order to pass weigh-ins.

It is appropriate for military weight programs to collect information and evaluate weight-loss practices of overweight (as well as normal-weight) individuals as a component of their medical evaluation. Research reports (McNulty, 1997a, 1997b, 2001; Peterson et al., 1995) demonstrate that unhealthy eating and purging behaviors are much more prevalent among military personnel compared with civilian populations. One method to reduce the incidence of dangerous practices is more frequent weigh-ins and an emphasis on appropriate diet and physical activity patterns at all times as part of a military lifestyle. Not only is this strategy in the individual's best interest, but also the military is responsible for the health and welfare of all uniformed personnel and must bear the cost of care for individuals who may be injured by unsafe weight-loss practices.

Is A Warning or Cautionary Zone Prior to Enrollment in a Weight-Control Program an Effective Strategy?

The use of a warning or cautionary zone in a military weight-control program, the Air Force has a 3-month warning period now in effect, appears to be an excellent strategy. A significant number of individuals are capable of correcting a marginal overweight condition with appropriate support. The restrictions associated with being assigned to a military weight/fat-loss program are very punitive to the individual and costly to the military service. Those who are able to solve their overweight/fat problems by themselves (or with minimal help) in a timely manner should be given the chance to accomplish this goal without being assigned to the military weight/fat-loss program with its attendant consequences. In addition, a strong, preventive weight-control effort should be added to military public health programs (beginning with initial entry training) to encourage young military personnel to monitor their body weight and seek help early if they find they are gaining weight.

Authorizing Duty Time for Participation in Intervention Strategies for Weight/Fat Loss

Certain tasks associated with the weight/fat loss program should be accomp-lished during duty time. They include any medical examination and tests that are appropriate before being assigned to the program, as well as counseling and monitoring. A weight-loss program should be viewed as treatment for a medical condition and, as such, be given the same priority as treatment for other medical conditions. Given the benefits of exercise for long-term obesity prevention, long-term health outcomes, and possibly for enhanced mental performance, the military might consider mandatory exercise at fixed times each day or other schemes to ensure that the vast majority of military personnel exercise several times per week.

Current DOD policy dictates regular exercise as a part of the duty day. This policy should be mandatory rather than at the unit commander's discretion. Unit commanders should provide (or require) regular exercise to ensure a high level of fitness and readiness. Allowing duty time for participation in associated activities of weight-management programs, such as exercise classes, support group sessions, and classes that teach appropriate dietary selection and new food preparation techniques, should be at the discretion of the unit commander. Such activities could be viewed as part of a healthy life style and the individual should be expected to do these tasks on their own time in the same manner as individuals who maintain a healthy weight.

QUESTION 4

To what extent should weight-control programs/policies be standardized across the services versus tailored to the individual service, installation, or unit? What are the advantages and disadvantages of standardization? Is the provision of state-of-the-art- techniques and knowledge a rationale for standardization?

Lower rates of recruitment, increased attrition of those who enter overweight, and reduced retention of skilled, highly trained older personnel threaten the long-term welfare and readiness of U.S. military forces. Therefore, the subcommittee provides the following responses regarding the standardization of weight-control policies.

Extent of Standardization Across the Services versus Tailored to an Individual Service

The specifics of implementation of weight-control policies and programs may need to be tailored for each service due to the different environments in which the programs will be carried out (e.g., aboard ships, on CONUS military bases, on overseas bases). However, they could be standardized across the services to a significant extent as indicated below. A limited number of military centers should be identified to provide scientifically-validated body composition evaluations (IOM, 1992a).

Body Composition Standards

The current DOD target for body fat, with a maximum body fat of 36 percent for women and 26 percent for men, seems appropriate based on considerations of health and chronic disease risk. This percentage of body fat should be acceptable if the fitness test is passed (IOM, 1998). Cut-off points for the maximum weight-for-height standards should reflect BMI categories that are consistent with the guidelines released by the National Heart, Lung and Blood Institute (NHLBI, 1998). A BMI < 18.5 constitutes underweight, a BMI of 18.5 to 24.9 constitutes healthy weight, a BMI of 25.0 to 29.9 constitutes overweight, and a BMI ≥ 30.0 constitutes obesity. **A BMI consistent with overweight does not by itself indicate that an individual is overfat.** Additional testing must be done to determine whether the excess weight in such individuals consists of fat or of lean mass. This is especially relevant because research has linked BMI to injury rates in initial entry training (Jones et al., 1992). In several small studies, an increased BMI was associated with reduced performance in 1- and 2-mile runs, sit-ups, and push-ups by men, and also was associated with an increased injury rate during initial entry training.

Body Composition Measurements

New technologies for measuring body composition should be adopted service-wide as they become available, once they are validated for accuracy and ease of use.

Appearance Standard

The DOD appearance standard is articulated in DOD Directive 1308.1, *DOD Physical Fitness and Body Fat Program* (DOD, 1995). This document states that ". . . maintaining desirable body composition is an integral part of physical fitness, general health, and military appearance" (p. 2). Further, Army Regulation 600-9 (U.S. Army, 1987) states that soldiers should present a physical appearance in uniform "that is trim and smart" and that enlarged waistlines detract from a good military appearance. The need to develop objective criteria has been highlighted previously (IOM, 1992a, 1998). The subcommittee commends the military for its recent adoption of waist circumference as a criteria for proper appearance (DOD, 2002), although research is needed to clarify whether the present appearance policy unfairly penalizes certain individuals (e.g., those of Hispanic heritage, female gender, older age) (Ellis et al., 1997; Thomas et al., 1997). The only objective health-based standard the subcommittee can offer that relates to appearance is that waist circumference should not exceed 40 inches in men and 35 inches in women.

Weight-Management Counselors

Those responsible for weight-control programs should be certified and their training should be standardized. The number of certified weight-management counselors should be increased in each of the military branches. These counselors should be experienced in weight management issues that are specific to gender, ethnic background, and age.

Internet-Based Weight-Management Programs

Web-based weight-management programs should be developed that are portable and consistent DOD-wide so that counseling, records, and support techniques move with military personnel when they are assigned to a permanent change of station.

What Are the Advantages and Disadvantages of Standardization?

The advantages of standardization are that all military personnel would have access to equivalent weight-management assistance and that the incorporation of new technologies for body composition assessment and the adoption of Internet-based services would be facilitated. In addition, the costs of producing education materials (e.g., portion size models, brochures) would be reduced.

The disadvantage of standardization is that it might limit autonomy within the branches of the armed forces. There is no scientific disadvantage.

Is the Provision of State-of-the-Art Techniques and Knowledge a Rationale for Standardization?

Standardization of weight-control program components would facilitate the incorporation of new technologies and provide a stronger base for program evaluation, which would in turn protect DOD investments in each soldier. Although programs would need to be tailored to some degree for the various military settings, all programs need to be multidisciplinary and comprehensive (e.g., all should incorporate the elements of successful programs as discussed earlier).

QUESTION 5

How can diet be effectively dealt with as a weight-management component in the military setting? Should pharmacological treatment (anorexiants) be considered for use in the military? In what cases? What factors bear on this decision?

Diet counseling needs to be administered by individuals fully trained in weight-management concepts and supported by appropriate professional personnel. For those military personnel who are on ships or are dependent on mess halls, more healthy, low-fat food choices and sufficient time for meal consumption are imperative. In any case, nutrition and lifestyle education are paramount and should be provided early in the initial entry training period and reinforced periodically. The development of distance-based education in nutrition and lifestyle modification may prove useful.

Pharmacological treatments should be considered for those who meet the standard criteria for the use of such compounds (i.e., BMI $\geq$ 30 or BMI $\geq$ 27 with comorbidities and who are in military operational specialties that do not preclude the use of central nervous system-active drugs. Current prescription weight-loss drugs appear to have minimal side effects; long-term use during an individual's military career may need to be considered.

QUESTION 6

How should resistiveness to weight/fat control be dealt with?

In the context of the military use of the term, resistiveness is a condition that generally refers to a genotype and/or a phenotype that is obesity-prone. An individual may have physiological factors that favor obesity (e.g., family history of obesity), thus making weight loss much more difficult. These individuals can lose weight, but usually have to work harder and may need additional assistance in the program and in the structured follow-up. Such individuals have a higher risk of being unresponsive to lifestyle modification; drug therapy may be the most efficient and effective long-term option for their treatment.

QUESTION 7

What are the knowledge gaps in weight-management programs relative to the military? What research is needed?

Chapter 6 has been partly dedicated to research needs from a health and weight-loss effectiveness perspective. This report does not address the fundamental issues of the relationship of body weight/fat standards to performance, nor does it consider the impact of military service policies on manpower needs. Additional research on the impact of modest overweight/overfat on performance in various military occupational specialties is recommended to address these issues.

6

Programmatic and Research Recommendations

Knowledge gaps concerning weight-management programs relative to the military are extensive. Much published research has been derived from studies on middle-class, middle-aged or perimenopausal, Caucasian women in clinical settings. This data may have little relevance to the military population where: (1) only about 25 percent of officers and warrant officers and about 6 percent of enlisted personnel are over the age of 40, (2) only 15 percent are women, and (3) approximately 40 percent are minorities. Considerable research is needed in the primary areas of prevention, treatment, and program evaluation. Research recommendations are focused on those areas that are of specific concern to the military community.

This chapter provides recommendations on the structure and content of military weight-management programs and highlights research needed under each of these areas. In addition, recommendations are provided for other potential areas of relevant research.

PREVENTION

National health survey data from the U.S. general population clearly demonstrate that a significant percentage of individuals are overweight or obese. This is true for both adolescents and adults. The existence of the Department of Defense's (DOD) weight-for-height and body-fat standards currently means that an estimated 13 to 18 percent of young men between the ages of 17 and 20 and 17 to 43 percent of young women in this age group would fail to meet military standards for accession (Nolte et al., 2002). While this situation will certainly have a negative impact on DOD's ability to meet recruitment goals, the fact that accession standards exist also offers an extremely unique opportunity to develop and study interventions to prevent weight gain.

Since the majority of military recruits will have met the DOD weight-for-height and body-composition standards at the time of entry into the service, the need for combat readiness (Robbins et al., 2001), optimal health, and economics (Robbins et al., 2002) dictate that the prevention of weight gain should be a major focus of military health programs and research.

Research is needed on interventions at the individual, group, worksite, and community levels to prevent overweight and obesity. Most of the studies that have evaluated prevention efforts in communities, in the workplace, or in schools have shown modest or no effect on body weight (Atkinson and Nitzke, 2001; Taylor et al., 1991). However, intervention studies in targeted individuals have been more positive (Angotti and Levine, 1994; Angotti et al., 2000; Latner et al., 2000; Perri et al., 2001). There is a general consensus that preventing the onset of obesity with appropriate interventions is likely to produce a better success rate than attempting to treat overweight or obesity after it develops; however, solid clinical research has not yet verified this assumption. Evidence from a large body of literature indicates that once an individual becomes overweight, loss of the excess weight is difficult to accomplish and the frequency of regain is high.

Early Education of Initial Entry Trainees

Almost uniquely in American society, the military has the ability to mold belief systems and behaviors of large groups of young people. This is apparent in the ability of the military to take people in their late teens and early twenties and instill in them character issues of discipline, honor, integrity, and hard work. If the military made a commitment to nutrition education and physical activity as part of the "military lifestyle," generations of young people would have a high possibility of adopting good nutrition and exercise habits as a part of expected behavior. The military currently expects and demands a commitment to physical fitness that far surpasses that which is customary in the civilian population, and recruits change behavior dramatically in regard to physical fitness. Initial entry training is a time of learning for individuals entering the military. Just as these individuals learn military tasks (e.g., how to fire a weapon), they could also learn nutritional principles and to adopt physically active lifestyles. It is recommended that classes be included in initial entry training that deal with appropriate nutrition behavior, eating patterns (such as consumption of ample quantities of fruits, vegetables, and whole grains and limiting portions of saturated fat), portion sizes, and the basic human biology of nutrition and energy balance. An early training effort can provide large benefits, including decreased loss of time from the job, reduced administration cost of weight-control programs, and improved morale.

Military mess halls have a long history of closer adherence to recommended dietary allowances than is usual in the civilian population. Educating recruits on why this is appropriate and expected may produce life-long eating habits that are healthier than that of the civilian population. The effectiveness of such a program, including its specific components, should be evaluated. Controlled studies of pilot programs could be conducted at selected bases to determine if behavior changes are observed in response to the nutrition and healthy lifestyle education and to identify the most appropriate methods of nutritional training. Large-scale, randomized trials with alternate classes of recruits, followed over time, could be highly useful in evaluating the efficacy of the preventive efforts and whether they prove to be helpful in preventing overweight and obesity later in military service. Positive results would encourage expansion of the program to the entire military.

Particular attention should be paid to the concept that, as daily physical activity declines with time in the service due to more administratively oriented duties, energy intake needs to decline in order to maintain energy balance, even if the level of fitness training remains unchanged.

Education of Families

Spouses and families of new military inductees should be included in instruction on nutrition and healthy lifestyle habits, just as they are in classes on military etiquette. Classes should also be set up for military spouses to learn appropriate nutrition, cooking skills, shopping skills, and the importance of a high level of exercise and activities of daily living. Evaluation of the effectiveness of these programs should be carried out as described above (for the initial entry trainees).

Exercise/Activity

As indicated in Chapters 3 and 4, there is much evidence to indicate that activity is an important factor in preventing excess adipose tissue gain. Activity may be divided into two categories: structured exercise and unstructured exercise (or activities of daily living). Both of these provide opportunities for research that could be of benefit to the military.

Structured Exercise

Current DOD policy dictates regular exercise as part of duty time, but this policy is routinely ignored due to time pressures. Enforcement of these policies by DOD or, for example, by holding commanders accountable for their units' achieving a minimum average level of performance on the physical fitness test, would engage commanders in the quest for routine exercise and attainment of physical fitness.

The use of exercise as entertainment, as competition, and as games can play an important role, especially among men. It is particularly valuable in military facilities in which personnel are often organized into units around which competition can be developed. Scheduling competitions that involve unit fitness could be tested as a method to improve overall fitness and activity. The competitions should require participation by the entire unit and could include activities such as comparisons of the unit-wide average performance on annual physical fitness tests. Competition among companies or battalions would necessitate that all individuals take part and would require nonmandated exercise to attain peak performance.

Activities of Daily Living

Structured exercise requires time and may impinge on the performance of other military duties. It usually is confined to a very limited period each day or to several times per week. Increasing the activities of daily living to increase unstructured exercise has been proposed as a way to help prevent overweight and obesity. This could be studied in the military environment in a number of ways, such as:

- *Comparisons of environmental changes that might promote increased activity*. Changes to the design of military facilities that encourage increased activity (a model that has been recommended but not tested in civilian life) include prohibiting the use of cars in the center of bases (or cities), thus increasing the likelihood of walking or biking, and designing (or renovating) buildings so that stairs are readily available and that elevators or escalators are not the first option for movement between a few floors. Such changes could only be introduced gradually, but would provide an opportunity for evaluating the effect on the prevalence of overweight or the average performance on physical fitness tests. The military setting provides a unique environment in which to examine the potential role of such features.
- *DOD-wide competitions for model activity programs*. A DOD-wide competition, held periodically, could stimulate innovative individuals to develop programs locally that could be tested and, if found to be effective, then applied on a broader scale. Awards for the most innovative, effective program locally, by region, by service, and throughout all services would bring attention to the possibilities, stimulate creative solutions, and take advantage of the huge range of talents of military personnel.

Diet and Nutrition

Recent research by the Air Force (Fiedler et al., 1999) showed that providing "heart-healthy" menus in base dining facilities was not only possible, but also that these menus improved body mass index (BMI) for women recruits with no detrimental effects on physical conditioning or visits to the doctor. Another study by the Army found that women consuming more than 14 reduced-energy foods per week had a lower BMI, exercised more, and had significantly higher intakes of dietary fiber, folate, calcium, and iron. (Arsenault and Cline, 2000).

Environmental Factors

Current theories to explain the epidemic of obesity point to an increased availability of foods, particularly energy-dense foods. Vending machines are a ubiquitous presence in both military and civilian life. The majority of foods in these machines are snack items containing high amounts of fat, calories, or both.

Careful studies could be undertaken to determine the roll of vending machines in promoting obesity or overweight. For example, studies could be conducted that compare the presence or absence of vending machines with the hypothesis that severely limiting their availability might reduce impulse eating. Also, offering alternatives such as fruit, low-calorie snacks, meal replacement bars and drinks, should be evaluated. It is possible that the availability of vending machines is important for morale on military bases, but the effect of removing these machines on the prevalence of overweight and on military morale are appropriate questions for well-designed studies. In addition, studies could be conducted to determine if increasing the price of high-energy and high-fat foods and reducing (or subsidizing) the price of fresh fruit and other low-calorie snacks encourages healthier eating behavior.

RECOMMENDATIONS ON PREVENTION

- Each service should provide its members training on diet and health, including the fundamentals of energy balance, the caloric content of common foods, portion sizes, and the importance of maintaining high levels of daily activity even after intensive training periods (e.g., initial entry training) to prevent weight gain.
- An education program on maintaining healthy weight should include components directed at the entire military family.
- Programs to reinforce the concept of exercise and activity as part of the military lifestyle should be developed, along with ones to encourage the reduction of alcohol consumption, which contributes to excess energy intake.
- Particular emphasis should be placed on providing or upgrading physical fitness facilities and equipment that encourage exercise. Creating bicycle paths and sidewalks, making community-owned bicycles available to personnel, discouraging the use of automobiles, and organizing competitions should be given high priority.

- The use of rewards for exercise achievement should be reinforced. More tangible and immediate benefits in recognition, awards, and personnel and performance ratings should be developed within military facilities.
- The military services should make the incorporation of "heart healthy" menus a standard for base dining facilities, with continued emphasis on training all military cooks in low-fat cooking techniques. In addition, low-calorie and low-fat food items should be offered in vending machines and at base exchange facilities. Lowering the costs of these items could be an incentive to increase their consumption.
- Priority consideration should be given to commercial eating establishments that routinely offer reasonable portion sizes and low-fat dining options when these establishments are competing for base contracts.

ASSESSMENT

The reissued instruction, *DOD Physical Fitness and Body Fat Program Procedures*, states that "service members shall maintain physical readiness through appropriate nutrition, health, and fitness habits," and that "aerobic capacity, muscular strength, muscle endurance and desirable body-fat composition" form the basis for the military's relevant programs (DOD, 2002). This policy also mandates that all service members, regardless of age, will be formally evaluated and tested for the record at least once annually unless under medical waiver. If the prevention of weight gain is an appropriate goal (as it should be), annual or semi-annual evaluations are clearly inadequate to aid in achievement of this goal. Individuals have ample opportunity to increase their weight and body composition to levels above standards over a 6- to 12-month period. They will have a much better chance of returning to standards if their problems are identified early. Thus, more frequent evaluations, while potentially costly, may be less costly than remedial programs. In addition, more frequent evaluations may decrease the number of disordered eating behaviors that have been documented to occur in military personnel within 3 months of their annual assessments (McNulty, 1997a, 1997b, 2001; Peterson et al., 1995). Ideally, evaluations (at least weigh-ins and body-fat assessments, if not physical fitness) should be performed quarterly.

Early Identification of Personnel at Risk

Many obesity experts believe that preventing obesity or treating it at the initial stages of overweight is more effective than individuals' attempting to lose significant amounts of weight. Inviting individuals at risk (e.g., those who have gained weight or body fat since their last assessment but are still within standards) and those who have only recently become overweight to enroll in weight-management programs may reduce the prevalence of personnel who later become significantly overweight. This deserves careful study. The Air Force has recently modified its weight-management program to include a 3-month cautionary zone prior to enrollment in the program itself (with its administrative consequences). Research is recommended on the impact of this program change on weight-management efforts before instituting such a change in the other services.

Identifying potential risk factors for weight gain (e.g., overweight at time of accession, family history of obesity, poor initial performance on physical fitness test, a weight gain of more than 5 percent over initial entry training weight) may help identify individuals who are at risk. Educating these individuals during initial entry training, or whenever risk factors are identified, about their risk of becoming overweight might allow self-directed preventive measures. An evaluation of the usefulness of these efforts should be undertaken as there is a potential for negative consequences: individuals identified as potentially at risk may be singled out for attention or suffer discrimination by their commanders.

The military appearance policy raises several concerns. Individuals differ anatomically and some accumulate adipose tissue in the abdomen (upper-body adiposity), while others tend to have a more even distribution of fat over several regions of the body. However, from an appearance perspective, an individual with abdominal fat may attract negative attention, while an individual with an even distribution of fat may not. Age, gender, and ethnic background (e.g., Hispanic, African-American) may exacerbate the disproportionate accumulation of abdominal adipose tissue, but the available data are insufficient to support these associations (IOM, 1998). Implementation of the appearance policy may unfairly penalize some individuals due to their demographics. In addition, an individual who has been accused of violating the appearance standard but is later found to be within the height and weight standards may suffer some loss of self-esteem. Also, the use of the appearance standard by unit commanders has frequently been criticized as being flawed because it is not uniformly applied to all personnel.

DOD is to be commended for the recent changes in procedure instructions relative to body fat that mandate the use of a single abdominal circumference-based equation for men and one for women to be used by all the services (DOD, 2002). The emphasis on abdominal circumference is appropriate as it is the site of human body-fat deposition most strongly associated with health risks and it corresponds most closely with military goals on appropriate appearance.

Underweight and Eating Disorders

One of the negative aspects of military enforcement of weight-for-height and body-fat standards is the possibility that such efforts may provoke the onset of eating disorders (e.g., bulimia, binge eating, anorexia nervosa). Questions that need research attention include:

1. What is the prevalence of bulimia, binge eating, and anorexia nervosa in military personnel? Some research has been conducted in this area, primarily by the Navy (McNulty, 1997a, 1997b, 2001). One study of Air Force weight-management program participants has been conducted (Peterson et al., 1995), but this information needs to be collected in both men and women across all the services.
2. Does the military lifestyle promote disordered eating behavior in military personnel?
3. Does the diagnosis of an eating disorder preclude retention in the military?
4. What are the effects of disordered eating on performance?

Performance

It is recognized that implementation of the new DOD policy requires that specific physical fitness standards for occupation specialties be established, and that once these standards are identified, physical fitness training and testing would be linked to occupational requirements. This should benefit personnel needs as performance can not always be linked to compliance with standards. For example, Sharp and colleagues (1994) found that in female Army recruits in initial entry training, women who exceeded the weight-for-height standards or the percent body-fat standards before initial entry training performed as well as or better than women who initially passed the standards. Thus, the standards at that time tended to eliminate stronger women. Implementation of the new DOD weight-for-height standards should alleviate this problem, but it merits investigation.

RECOMMENDATIONS ON ASSESSMENT

- Assessments for weight-for-height (BMI) and percent body fat should be conducted quarterly rather than annually or semi-annually to facilitate identifying personnel at risk of exceeding standards and to allow for early intervention. More frequent assessments should be evaluated to determine if they reduce disordered eating and other risky behaviors.

- Individuals at risk of increased weight gain or body fat (e.g., those entering the service over the standard or those with a family history of obesity) should be identified at the time of accession and their evaluations monitored so that interventions may be instituted as soon as adverse changes are identified.
- The incidence of disordered eating behaviors needs to be documented and addressed across all branches of the military.

TREATMENT

Military personnel who are identified as exceeding body composition standards are mandated to enter a military weight-management program for treatment. A good weight-management program must include two phases: weight loss and weight maintenance. Details of each are provided below. There are however, two overarching recommendations for military weight-management programs: (1) the critical components of the programs should be uniform across the services so that all personnel who are referred to such programs obtain equal assistance, and (2) the personnel administering these programs should have training in weight-management principles with respect to diet, physical activity, and counseling on behavior modification.

The particular problems of establishing these services for military personnel are immediately obvious. Treatment programs are based on the concept of long-term care. Military personnel are rarely stationed at one facility long enough to be able to take advantage of continuing services, even if they are available. The problem is compounded still further by the instability of the staff. Even if staff were available for a continuing care program, there would be no expectation that these personnel would be continuously assigned at one facility. These environmental factors make it more urgent that each service strive to have a uniform program that will allow the individual to continue to progress in weight control regardless of assigned duty station. Furthermore, where possible, the programs of all the services should be coordinated to the maximum extent to assist individuals who receive medical care from another service and to facilitate fairness across the services.

It may be possible to reorganize aspects of care to permit patients to maintain contact with individual service providers through e-mail, regardless of the location of patient or provider. This will only be useful, however, if computers are generally available to all service personnel and if resources are locally available for the patient to be able to follow-up on recommendations developed through this system.

Essential Components of Military Weight-Loss Programs

The key components of military weight-loss programs are diet, physical activity, behavior modification, and structured follow-up. Recommendations on each of these components are discussed in detail below.

Diet

General criteria for a diet that provides reasonable and steady weight loss are based on the principle of a hypocaloric-balanced diet. However, there is recent evidence that in obese individuals, use of very-low-calorie diets, coupled with behavior modification, may be more successful in initial weight loss and maintenance of weight loss than the hypocaloric-balanced diet.

Although there is still considerable controversy over the ideal macronutrient distribution of a hypocaloric-balanced diet, recent evidence suggests that there may be some benefits to diets with a higher ratio of protein to carbohydrate in terms of stabilization of blood glucose, maintenance of lean body mass during weight loss, and better satiety. In a recent comprehensive review, Astrup and coworkers (2002) examined four meta-analyses of weight change occurring on intervention trials with ad libitum low-fat diets and found that these diets consistently demonstrated significant weight loss both in normal-weight and overweight individuals. On the other hand, Kris-Etherton and colleagues (2002) found that a moderate-fat diet (20 to 30 percent of energy from fat) was more likely to promote weight loss because it was easier for patients to adhere to this type of diet than to one that was severely restricted in fat (< 20 percent of energy). Thus, the macronutrient distribution of a recommended diet could be tailored somewhat to individual preferences.

The most important dietary considerations are that:

- The diet must be deficient in energy, as determined by comparing its energy value with an estimate of the individual's energy expenditure. Energy intake should be sufficient, and the level of other essential nutrients adequate, to allow individuals to pursue their regularly scheduled activities and to maintain appropriate levels of fitness.
- The diet program should promote a new set of eating habits that can help to maintain weight loss over time and should emphasize changes in what, how much, and how often one eats.
- The diet should include at least five servings of fruits and vegetables a day and should be able to be readily incorporated into an individual's life style. It must be one that can be followed for a sufficient period of time to achieve desired weight loss.

- The diet should contain sufficient volume to promote feelings of satiety. It should also be palatable and familiar, with the foods reflecting the food preferences of the individual, if possible.
- The foods in the diet must be readily available and affordable. Additionally, given that personnel may be living in barracks or at home, married or single, in the United States or abroad, the diet must be easily adaptable to a variety of situations, including mess halls and other group feeding environments, restaurants, and home.

An appropriate weight-loss diet would be one that incorporates the points above and is energy deficient by 350 to 1,000 kcal/day (with intakes no lower than 800 kcal/day). For women, protein intake should be no less than 60 g/day, and for men, no less than 75 g/day. Fat content should be no greater than 30 percent of total calories and carbohydrate intake no less than 130 g/day. A daily multivitamin and mineral supplement may be useful.

Low-Carbohydrate Diets. Use of low-carbohydrate diets by military personnel should be discouraged. These diets have been associated with a number of potential side effects such as physiological dehydration, nausea, hyperuricemia, ketosis, and fatigue incidental to the depletion of glycogen stores, which could comprise performance (Phinney et al., 1980). Furthermore, the recently released Dietary Reference Intakes for macronutrients (IOM, 2002) concluded that the adult requirement for carbohydrate to supply adequate glucose for proper brain function is 100 g/day, with a recommended daily intake of 130 g/day. Thus, it is recommended that under no circumstances should weight-loss diets recommended for military personnel contain less than 130 g/day of carbohydrate.

Dietary Supplements. Little or no information is available to guide medical providers on possible interactions between weight-loss drugs and medications, herbals, or supplements taken for other purposes. Because military personnel must be combat-ready and side effects and interactions of supplements are largely unknown, personnel should be advised against the use of weight-loss supplements.

Physical Activity

A weight-reduction strategy based solely upon an increase in physical activity (in the absence of calorie restriction) is likely to yield only a modest weight loss of no more than 5 to 6 lb (Blair, 1993; Wadden and Sarwer, 1999). Weight-loss outcomes are optimized when physical activity is combined with dietary intervention (Dyer, 1994; Pavlou et al., 1989a, 1989b; Perri et al., 1993; Wing and Greeno, 1994). Finally, physically active dieters are far more likely to be successful in maintaining lost weight as compared with dieters who do not embrace physical activity (Kayman et al., 1990; Klem et al., 1997). It should be kept in mind that persons who include bouts of structured physical activity in their weight-reduction regimen may inadvertently reduce their activities of daily living.

It is difficult to develop specific physical activity recommendations for weight loss that may be appropriate for military programs. The amount of activity needed in conjunction with decreased energy intake will depend on whether the individual is genetically and phenotypically obesity-prone or obesity-resistant, and how much weight or body fat needs to be lost to bring them into compliance with military standards. There are few data available for physical activity requirements for predominantly young (< 50 y), male, overweight (as opposed to obese) individuals. Recent recommendations for normal-weight individuals are 60 min/day of moderately intense physical activity to maintain healthy weight (IOM, 2002). Data also indicate that the threshold of energy expenditure as physical activity needed to minimize weight regain in previously obese women is 47 kJ/kg body weight/day, which equates to an average of 80 min/day of moderate activity or 35 min/day of vigorous activity added to a sedentary lifestyle (Schoeller et al., 1997).

In a thorough review of the literature, Jakicic and colleagues (2001) developed a consensus statement for the American College of Sports Medicine that recommends an initial physical activity goal for overweight and obese individuals as a minimum of 150 min/wk of moderately intense exercise. To enhance weight loss and maintenance of this loss, exercise should be gradually increased to 200 to 300 min/wk (3.3–5 hr). Similar results may also be achieved through the expenditure of > 2,000 kcal/week through activities of daily living (Dunn et al., 1999). The physical activity component of a weight-loss program should include both structured and unstructured exercise (e.g., aerobics, strength training, increased activities of daily living).

Behavior Modification

The behavior modification component of a weight-loss program should include instructions on stimulus control, cognitive restructuring, relapse prevention, and self-monitoring, and it should provide mentoring.

The primary goals of behavioral strategies for weight control are to increase physical activity and to reduce energy intake by altering eating habits (Brownell and Kramer, 1994; Wilson, 1995). Self-monitoring of dietary intake and physical activity, which enables the individual to develop a sense of accountability, is one of the cornerstones of behavioral treatment (Jeffery and French, 1999). Patients are asked to keep a daily food/activity diary in which they record what and how much they have eaten, when and where the food was consumed, the context in which the food was consumed (e.g., what else they were doing at the time, what they were feeling, who else was there), and the types and amount of physical activity. The information obtained from the diary can also be used to identify personal and environmental factors that contribute to overeating and sedentary behavior, which helps in selecting and implementing appropriate weight-loss strategies for the individual (Wilson, 1995). Self-monitoring also provides a way for therapists and patients to evaluate which techniques are working and how changes in eating behavior and activity are contributing to weight loss.

The Use of Structured Follow-Up/Maintenance

Once individuals have achieved their weight-loss goals, systematic contact and follow-up from the weight-loss program staff is crucial to maintain the weight loss. This structured follow-up should include monitoring of body weight and weigh-ins weekly during the weight-loss phase and at least monthly during the weight-maintenance phase. Contact with program staff via phone or the Internet every 1 to 2 months, depending on the individual's difficulty in maintaining a stable weight, would facilitate continuity of care.

RECOMMENDATIONS ON THE SPECIFIC CONTENT OF WEIGHT-LOSS PROGRAMS

- *Diet.* A weight-loss diet should be energy deficient by 350 to 1,000 kcal/day, with a minimum intake of 800 kcal/day. It should provide a minimum of 60 g of protein/day for women and 75 g of protein/day for men. Fat should provide no more than 30 percent of total energy and carbohydrate content should be no less than 130 g/day. In addition, the daily use of a multivitamin-mineral supplement may help to ensure adequate micronutrient intake.
- *Exercise.* A combination of aerobic and strength training exercise, along with increased activities of daily living, is recommended. Energy expended in physical activity should be at least 200 to 300 min/wk of moderate intensity exercise (3.5–5 hr), or greater than 2,000 kcal/wk.
- *Behavior Modification.* Training and support in behavior modification should include stimulus control, relapse prevention, self-monitoring, cognitive restructuring, and mentoring.
- *Structured Follow-up.* Follow-up should include regular contact with weight management counselors, routine self-monitoring, and ongoing support that could be provided via the Internet.

PROGRAM EVALUATION

An important aspect of implementation of any weight-management program is an evaluation of the program results. The effectiveness of a weight-management program is determined by the success of the participants in losing the necessary amount of weight and being able to maintain that weight loss. This requires long-term tracking of these individuals. While this may be inherently more difficult in the military setting because of frequency of relocation and terms of enlistment, a minimum period of tracking would be 2 years. Because of the high rate of weight regain documented in many civilian settings, 5 and even 10 years of follow-up data would be optimal for program evaluation.

TRAINING

If one assumes a shortage of personnel trained to assist in weight management, it may be advantageous for the military services to establish weight-control training programs for professionals as a military occupational specialty. The development of a specialty skill in administering weight-management programs may be useful for personnel otherwise trained as nurses, dietitians, physician assistants, nurse practitioners, counselors, and psychologists and would aid in developing uniform quality of weight-loss programs across the services. Special efforts will be needed to develop these programs in an effective way and to recruit personnel with sufficient interest in, and understanding of, the problems in losing and maintaining weight loss, so that they can be effective in the delivery of services.

RECOMMENDATIONS ON A WEIGHT-MANAGEMENT MILITARY OCCUPATIONAL SPECIALTY

- Weight-control training programs should be established to train a multidisciplinary team of personnel associated with implementing weight-loss and weight-maintenance programs.
- Training standards for a weight-management military occupational specialty should include training in the principles of:
  - Nutrition
  - Physical activity/exercise
  - Behavior modification
  - Weight-loss aids (e.g., counseling, mentoring, psychological support).
- The program should include mandated continuing education requirements.

RESEARCH RECOMMENDATIONS

The modest success of weight-management endeavors in the civilian world sends a signal that losing weight and maintaining weight loss will not be easy and research on weight management in the military is sorely needed. Further suggestions for military research on overweight are presented in the following sections.

Use of the Internet

Internet-based programs could be developed using models already being used by the military (James et al., 1999a) in which participation may be completed during off-duty time. Emphasis should be given to the development of a number of options, testing their effectiveness overall, and identifying those with high response rates. Also, the range of individual responses of military personnel should be evaluated since there may be subpopulations that respond well to a given intervention even though overall response is not consistent.

The concept of web-based programs may be very fruitful. Also, with a few resources put into development, a program could be created that followed military personnel regardless of where they were stationed. Classes could be conducted on line and even live (with current technology, two-way video can be inexpensive). Individuals could do this on their own time at home. Since members of the military risk losing their job if they exceed standards, it may not be too much to expect them to spend some off-duty time working at a weight-loss or weight-management program. The military could develop its own program with its own personnel or it could contract to one or more of the outstanding civilian obesity-treatment programs (Brownell, 1999; Foreyt and Goodrick, 1994; Jakicic et al., 1995; McGuire et al., 1999; Wadden et al., 1989). These computerized weight-loss interventions optimize staff time (Wylie-Rosett et al., 2001) and could be used as a model for weight-reduction education in the military.

Evaluation of Existing Military Initiatives and Programs for Effectiveness

Evaluation of military weight-management programs is essential to determine their effectiveness. Recommendations provided in this report are based almost exclusively on data collected in civilian populations; effectiveness may be quite different in military populations. This type of evaluation research will require the identification and long-term monitoring of personnel who have completed military programs.

Computerized Follow-Up of Personnel at Risk

It is necessary to create an independent computerized database that can be used to identify individuals with risk factors for weight gain or overweight as described above, to maintain routine contact with these individuals to check on their weight and physical fitness status, and to identify problems early and intervene as needed. Such computerized information should be centrally maintained and used as a source of data for longitudinal studies on the effectiveness of prevention and treatment innovations. This data should *not* be available to unit commanders to avoid the possibility of discrimination against individuals at risk.

Evaluation of Pharmacological Treatments

Pharmacological treatments compatible with military performance need to be identified. Some military operational specialties preclude the use of central nervous system-active agents, but other types of Food And Drug Administration-approved drugs could be considered. For all other operational specialties, obesity drugs could be used on a long-term basis. Studies of individual weight-loss drugs and combinations of drugs to determine their effects on mental and physical performance of military duties, as well as on their success in reducing body weight, need to be carried out. Most current drugs have been evaluated as single agents, so research on the effects of drug combinations should receive special attention.

Evaluation of the Use of Dietary Supplements and Herbal Remedies

Many nonprescription preparations are being used for weight loss by the civilian population and are undoubtedly being used in the military population. Very little is known about their effects on body weight, body composition, overall health, and physical performance. It may be particularly important to assess their effects on military performance. Of particular importance is evaluation of the prevalence of the use of ephedrine/caffeine preparations and their effects. Although DOD has followed Food and Drug Administration warnings and removed this compound from post exchanges and base establishments, personnel may still obtain ephedrine/caffeine preparations from civilian establishments.

OTHER AREAS FOR RESEARCH

The military environment affords an excellent opportunity to conduct important research needed to fill gaps in knowledge about weight control and treatment for overweight. It is recognized that some of this research may not have a direct or apparent need in military operations and, therefore, may have lower priority in military research funding. However, in keeping with the current policy that encourages increased leveraging of resources for research in the federal government, the areas described below should be considered.

Body Weight and Aging

Little is known about developmental aspects of fat deposition or the effects of early attempts at weight control on later propensity for obesity. Because most personnel enter the military during late adolescence or young adulthood, and because the military has the capability to follow its personnel longitudinally, the military is in a unique position to follow a large population of young adults from the time of accession into retirement to examine the following questions:

- How do the mechanisms of fat deposition change with aging?
- Do individuals who remain in strenuous (heavy lifting or very physically active) occupations throughout their careers increase their proportion of body fat at a lower rate as they age than do those in low-activity occupations?
- Do they preserve lean body mass as they age?
- Do they remain healthier as they age?
- Do they cost the military less money as they age?
- Is bone mass/bone density better preserved as they age?

Gender

Information is needed on whether there are differences in gender responses to the various components of weight-management programs (e.g., do men and women respond differently to diet, physical activity, and behavioral change interventions). In addition, gestational weight gain is a major risk factor for overweight in women of childbearing age. Little is known about the factors responsible for postpartum weight retention or the effects of pregnancy and breastfeeding on military performance. Research is needed to answer the following questions:

- Does a program of regular physical activity throughout pregnancy (and/or beginning early in the postpartum period) reduce postpartum weight retention?
- Does weight loss at the rate that is required to return to within body composition standards in the recommended time frame (180 days) (IOM, 1998) permit adequate breastfeeding?
- Does competency in estimating portion sizes lead to less maternal weight gain and more rapid return to prepregnancy body weight and body composition?

- Is improved fitness when one becomes pregnant and throughout pregnancy associated with better outcomes (assessed by infant birth weight as well as by lower perinatal mortality and morbidity)?
- Does breastfeeding (which needs to be measured carefully and defined in terms of frequency and duration of feedings) lead to a more rapid return to prepregnancy body weight and body composition?

Genetic Screening

Currently, there are about 250 genes and gene markers that have been identified as associated with human obesity (Rankinen et al., 2002). As science progresses, common patterns of genes or gene markers may be identified that correlate with the development of obesity. While it would be an extremely sensitive area of research, the military could address the question of whether genetic screening for obesity-prone individuals is appropriate for its mission.

Role of Infectious Disease in Obesity

A provocative hypothesis that has been proposed as an explanation for at least some of the increase in the prevalence of obesity is that one or more viral infections may produce obesity. Several animal viruses produce obesity in animals, and both animal and human viruses have been associated with obesity in humans (Dhurandhar et al., 1997, 2000.).

Although the current committee was not constituted to evaluate this particular issue, it was presented at the committee's workshop and thus is mentioned here as an area where numerous research questions exist on the role of viruses in the etiology of obesity. Both basic and clinical studies are needed to identify whether human adenoviruses that have been demonstrated to produce obesity in animals are associated with obesity in humans.

References

Abenheim L, Moride Y, Brenot F, Rich S, Benichou J, Kurz X, Higenbottam T, Oakley C, Wouters E, Aubier M, Simonneau G, Begaud B. 1996. Appetite-suppressant drugs and the risk of primary pulmonary hypertension. International Primary Pulmonary Hypertension Study Group. *N Engl J Med* 335:609–616.

ACSM (American College of Sports Medicine). 2000. *ACSM's Guidelines for Exercise Testing and Prescription*. 6th ed. Philadelphia: Lippincott Williams & Wilkins. Pp. 3–21.

Alemzadeh R, Langley G, Upchurch L, Smith P, Slonim AE. 1998. Beneficial effect of diazoxide in obese hyperinsulinemic adults. *J Clin Endocrinol Metab* 83:1911–1915.

Allison DB, Fontaine KR, Manson JE, Stevens J, VanItallie TB. 1999. Annual deaths attributable to obesity in the United States. *J Am Med Assoc* 282:1530–1538.

Allison DB, Fontaine KR, Heshka S, Mentore JL, Heymsfield SB. 2001. Alternative treatments for weight loss: A critical review. *Crit Rev Food Sci Nutr* 41:1–28.

Allred JB. 1995. Too much of a good thing? An overemphasis on eating low-fat foods may be contributing to the alarming increase in overweight among U.S. adults. *J Am Diet Assoc* 95:417–418.

Aloia JF, McGowan DM, Vaswani AN, Ross P, Cohn SH. 1991. Relationship of menopause to skeletal and muscle mass. *Am J Clin Nutr* 53:1378–1383.

Altus WD. 1949. The height and weight of soldiers in association with scores earned on the Army general skills test. *J Soc Psychol* 29:201–210.

Anand RS, Basiotis PP. 1998. Is total fat consumption really decreasing? *Nutr Insights*. Online. Center for Nutrition Policy and Promotion, U.S. Department of Agriculture. Available at http://www.cnpp.usda.gov/insght5a.PDF. Accessed September 8, 2003.

Anchors M. 1997. *Safer Than Phen-Fen!* Rocklin, CA: Prima Publishing.

Andersen T, Stokholm KH, Backer OG, Quaade F. 1988. Long-term (5-year) results after either horizontal gastroplasty or very-low-calorie diet for morbid obesity. *Int J Obes* 12:277–284.

Anderson JW, Brinkman VL, Hamilton CC. 1992. Weight loss and 2-y follow-up for 80 morbidly obese patients treated with intensive very-low-calorie diet and an education program. *Am J Clin Nutr* 56:244S–246S.

Anderson JW, Vichitbandra S, Quian W, Kryscio RJ. 1999. Long-term weight maintenance after an intensive weight-loss program. *J Am Coll Nutr* 18:620–627.

Anderson JW, Konz EC, Frederich RC, Wood CL. 2001. Long-term weight-loss maintenance: A meta-analysis of U.S. studies. *Am J Clin Nutr* 74:579–584.

Angotti CM, Levine MS. 1994. Review of 5 years of a combined dietary and physical fitness intervention for control of serum cholesterol. *J Am Diet Assoc* 94:634–638.

Angotti CM, Chan WT, Sample CJ, Levine MS. 2000. Combined dietary and exercise intervention for control of serum cholesterol in the workplace. *Am J Health Promot* 15:9–16.

Apfelbaum M, Fricker J, Igoin-Apfelbaum L. 1987. Low- and very-low calorie diets. *Am J Clin Nutr* 45:1126–1134.

Arch JR. 1981. The contribution of increased thermogenesis to the effect of anorectic drugs on body composition in mice. *Am J Clin Nutr* 34:2763–2769.

Aronne LJ. 1998. Modern medical management of obesity: The role of pharmaceutical intervention. *J Am Diet Assoc* 98:S23–S26.

Arsenault JE, Cline AD. 2000. Nutrient intakes and characteristics of normal weight, female military personnel consuming foods reduced in fat or energy content. *Appetite* 34:227–233.

Ashley JM, St. Jeor ST, Perumean-Chaney S, Schrage J, Bovee V. 2001. Meal replacements in weight intervention. *Obes Res* 9:312S–320S.

Astrup A. 1996. Obesity and metabolic efficiency. *Ciba Found Symp* 201:159–168.

Astrup A. 1999. Macronutrient balances and obesity: The role of diet and physical activity. *Public Health Nutr* 2:341–347.

Astrup A, Breum L, Toubro S, Hein P, Quaade F. 1992a. The effect and safety of an ephedrine/caffeine compound compared to ephedrine, caffeine and placebo in obese subjects on an energy restricted diet. A double blind trial. *Int J Obes Relat Metab Disord* 16:269–277.

Astrup A, Buermann B, Christensen NJ, Toubro S, Thorbek G, Victor OJ, Quaade F. 1992b. The effect of ephedrine/caffeine mixture on energy expenditure and body composition in obese women. *Metabolism* 41:686–688.

Astrup A, Buemann B, Christensen NJ, Toubro S. 1994. Failure to increase lipid oxidation in response to increasing dietary fat content in formerly obese women. *Am J Physiol* 266:E592–E595.

Astrup A, Toubro S, Raben A, Skov AR. 1997. The role of low-fat diets and fat substitutes in body weight management: What have we learned from clinical studies? *J Am Diet Assoc* 97:S82–S87.

Astrup A, Hansen DL, Lundsgaard C, Toubro S. 1998. Sibutramine and energy balance. *Int J Obes Relat Metab Disord* 22:S30–S35.

Astrup A, Ryan L, Grunwald GK, Storgaard M, Saris W, Melanson E, Hill JO. 2000. The role of dietary fat in body fatness: Evidence from a preliminary meta-analysis of ad libitum low-fat dietary intervention studies. *Br J Nutr* 83:S25–S32.

Astrup A, Buemann B, Flint A, Raben A. 2002. Low-fat diets and energy balance: How does the evidence stand in 2002? *Proc Nutr Soc* 61:299–309.

Atkins RC. 1988. *Dr. Atkins Diet Revolution: The High Calorie Way to Stay Thin Forever*. New York: Bantam Books.

Atkins RC, Linde SM. 1978. *Dr. Atkins Super Energy Diet*. New York: Bantam Books.

Atkinson RL. 1989. Low and very low calorie diets. *Med Clin North Am* 73:203–215.

Atkinson RL, Nitzke SA. 2001. School based programmes on obesity. *Br Med J* 323:1018–1019.

Atkinson RL, Blank RC, Schumacher D, Dhurandhar NV, Ritch DL. 1997. Long term drug treatment of obesity in a private practice setting. *Obes Res* 5:578–586.

Atkinson RL, Dhurandhar NV, Allison DB, Bowen RL, Istael BA. 1998. Evidence for an association of an obesity virus with human obesity at three sites in the United States. *Int J Obes* 22:S57.

Atkinson RL, Dhurandhar NV, Abbott DH, Darken N. 2000. Weight gain and reduced serum lipids in non-human primates due to a human virus. *Int J Obes* 24:S39.

Baba NH, Sawaya S, Torbay N, Habbal Z, Azar S, Hashim SA. 1999. High protein vs high carbohydrate hypoenergetic diet for the treatment of obese hyperinsulinemic subjects. *Int J Obes Relat Metab Disord* 23:1202–1206.

Bahceci M, Tuzcu A, Akkus M, Yaldiz M, Ozbay A. 1999. The effect of high-fat diet on the development of obesity and serum leptin level in rats. *Eat Weight Disord* 4:128–132.

Bao S, Kennedy A, Wojciechowski B, Wallace P, Ganaway E, Garvey WT. 1998. Expression of mRNAs encoding uncoupling proteins in human skeletal muscle: Effects of obesity and diabetes. *Diabetes* 47:1935–1940.

Bauer RG, Stout RL, Holz RF. 1976. *Developing a Conceptual and Predictive Model of Discipline in the U.S. Army*. Alexandria, VA: Army Research Institute for Behavioral and Social Sciences.

Baumgartner RN, Stauber PM, McHugh D, Koehler KM, Garry PJ. 1995. Cross-sectional age differences in body composition in persons 60+ years of age. *J Gerontol* 50:M307–M316.

Bell EA, Castellanos VH, Pelkman CL, Thorwart ML, Rolls BJ. 1998. Energy density of foods affects energy intake in normal-weight women. *Am J Clin Nutr* 67:412–420.

Bendixen H, Madsen J, Bay-Hansen D, Boesen U, Ovesen LF, Bartels EM, Astrup A. 2002. An observational study of slimming behavior in Denmark in 1992 and 1998. *Obes Res* 10:911–922.

Benotti PN, Hollingshead J, Mascioli EA, Bothe A, Bistrian BR, Blackburn GL. 1989. Gastric restrictive operations for morbid obesity. *Am J Surg* 157:150–155.

Bergman BC, Brooks GA. 1999. Respiratory gas-exchange ratios during graded exercise in fed and fasted trained and untrained men. *J Appl Physiol* 86:479–487.

Bernard A, Zwingelstein G, Meister R, Wild TF. 1988. Hyperinsulinemia induced by canine distemper virus infection of mice and its correlation with the appearance of obesity. *Comp Biochem Physiol* 91B:691–696.

Bernard A, Fevre-Montange M, Bencsik A, Giraudon P, Wild TF, Confavreux C, Belin M-F. 1993. Brain structures selectively targeted by canine distemper virus in a mouse model infection. *J Neuropath Exp Neuro* 52:471–480.

Bhadrinath BR. 1990. Anorexia nervosa in adolescents of Asian extraction. *Br J Psychiatry* 156:565–568.

Bjorntorp P. 1992a. Abdominal fat distribution and the metabolic syndrome. *J Cardiovasc Pharmacol* 20:S26–S28.

Bjorntorp P. 1992b. Abdominal obesity and the metabolic syndrome. *Ann Med* 24:465–468.

Blaak EE. 2000. Adrenergically stimulated fat utilization and ageing. *Ann Med* 32:380–382.

Blaak E. 2001. Gender differences in fat metabolism. *Curr Opin Clin Nutr Metab Care* 4:499–502.

Blair SN. 1993. Evidence for success of exercise in weight loss and control. *Ann Intern Med* 119:702–706.

Blair SN, Kohl HW 3rd, Paffenbarger RS, Clark DG, Cooper KH, Gibbons LW. 1989. Physical fitness and all-cause mortality: A prospective study of healthy men and women. *J Am Med Assoc* 262:2395–2401.

Blair SN, Kohl HW 3rd, Barlow CE, Paffenbarger RS Jr, Gibbons LW, Macera CA. 1995. Changes in physical fitness and all-cause mortality: A prospective study of healthy and unhealthy men. *J Am Med Assoc* 273:1093–1098.

Blankson H, Stakkestad JA, Fagertun H, Thom E, Wadstein J, Gudmundsen O. 2000. Conjugated linoleic acid reduces body fat mass in overweight and obese humans. *J Nutr* 130:2943–2948.

Blundell JE. 2000. What foods do people habitually eat? A dilemma for nutrition, an enigma for psychology. *Am J Clin Nutr* 71:3–5.

Blundell JE, Cooling J. 2000. Routes to obesity: Phenotypes, food choices and activity. *Br J Nutr* 83:S25–S32.

Blundell JE, Lawton CL, Halford JCG. 1995. Serotonin, eating behavior, and fat intake. *Obes Res* 3:471S–476S.

Boardley DJ, Sargent RG, Coker AL, Hussey JR, Sharpe PA. 1995. The relationship between diet, activity, and other factors, and postpartum weight change by race. *Obstet Gynecol* 86:834–838.

Bogardus C, Lillioja S, Ravussin E, Abbot W, Zawadzki JK, Young A, Knowler WC, Jacobowitz R, Moll PP. 1986. Familial dependence of the resting metabolic rate. *N Eng J Med* 315:96–100.

Boozer CN, Choban PS, Atkinson RL. 1990. Ileal transposition surgery attenuates the increased efficiency of weight gain on a high fat diet. *Int J Obes* 14:869–878.

Boozer CN, Brasseur A, Atkinson RL. 1993. Dietary fat affects weight loss and adiposity during energy restriction in rats. *Am J Clin Nutr* 58:846–852.

Boozer CN, Nasser JA, Heymsfield SB, Wang V, Chen G, Solomon JL. 2001. An herbal supplement containing Ma Huang-Guarana for weight loss: A randomized, double-blind trial. *Int J Obes Relat Metab Disord* 25:316–324.

Boozer CN, Daly PA, Homel P, Solomon JL, Blanchard D, Nasser JA, Strauss R, Meredith T. 2002. Herbal ephedra/caffeine for weight loss: A 6-month randomized safety and efficacy trial. *Int J Obes Relat Metab Disord* 26:593–604.

Borkan GA, Hults DE, Gerzof DE, Robbins AH, Silbert CK. 1983. Age changes in body composition revealed by computed tomography. *J Gerontol* 38:673–677.

Bouchard C. 1997. Genetic factors and body weight regulation. In: Dalton S, ed. *Overweight and Weight Management. The Health Professional's Guide to Understanding and Practice*. Gaithersburg, MD: Aspen Publishers. Pp. 161–186.

Bouchard C, Tremblay A, Depres JP, Nadeau A, Lupien PJ, Theriault G, Dussault J, Moorjani S, Pinault S, Fournier G. 1990. The response to long-term overfeeding in identical twins. *N Engl J Med* 322:1477–1482.

Bouchard C, Pérusse L, Rice T, Rao DC. 1998. The genetics of human obesity. In: Bray GA, Bouchard C, James WPT, eds. *Handbook of Obesity*. New York: Marcel Dekker. Pp. 157–190.

Bray GA. 1992a. A retrospective view of obesity. *Int J Obes Relat Metab Disord* 16:S1–S4.

Bray GA. 1992b. Peptides affect the intake of specific nutrients in the sympathetic nervous system. *Am J Clin Nutr* 55:265S–271S.

Bray GA. 1996. Health hazards of obesity. *Endocrinol Metab Clin North Am* 25:907–919.

Bray GA. 1998. Pharmacological treatment of obesity. In: Bray GA, Bouchard C, James WPT, eds. *Handbook of Obesity*. New York: Marcel Dekker. Pp. 953–975.

Bray GA, Popkin BM. 1998. Dietary fat intake does affect obesity! *Am J Clin Nutr* 68:1157–1173.

Bray GA, Greenway FL, Barry RE, Benfield JR, Fiser RL, Dahms WT, Atkinson RL, Schwartz AA. 1977. Surgical treatment of obesity: A review of our experience and an analysis of published reports. *Int J Obes* 1:331–367.

Bray GA, Ryan DH, Gordon D, Heidingsfelder S, Cerise F, Wilson K. 1996. A double-blind randomized placebo-controlled trial of sibutramine. *Obesity Res* 4:263–270.

Bray RM, Sanchez RP, Ornstein ML, Lentine D, Vincus AA, Baird TU, Walker JA, Wheeless SC, Guess LL, Kroutil LA, Iannacchione VG. 1999. *Highlights 1998 Department of Defense Survey of Health Related Behaviors among Military Personnel*. Research Triangle Park, NC: Research Triangle Institute.

Brooks GA. 1997. Importance of the 'crossover' concept in exercise metabolism. *Clin Exp Pharmacol Physiol* 24:889–895.

Bross R, Hoffer LJ. 1995. Fluoxetine increases resting energy expenditure and basal body temperature in humans. *Am J Clin Nutr* 61:1020–1025.

Brownell KD. 1999. The central role of lifestyle change in long-term weight management. *Clin Cornerstone* 2:43–51.

Brownell KD, Kramer FM. 1994. Behavioral management of obesity. In: Blackburn GL, Kanders BS, eds. *Obesity: Pathophysiology, Psychology and Treatment*. New York: Chapman Hall. Pp. 231–252.

Bruce B, Spiller GA, Klevay LM, Gallagher SK. 2000. A diet high in whole and unrefined foods favorably alters lipids, antioxidant defenses, and colon function. *J Am Coll Nutr* 19:61–67.

Burchfiel CM, Curb JD, Sharp DS, Rodriguez BL, Arakaki R, Chyou PH, Yano K. 1995. Distribution and correlates of insulin in elderly men. The Honolulu heart program. *Arterioscler Thromb Vasc Biol* 15:2213–2221.

Calles-Escandon J, Horton ES. 1992. The thermogenic role of exercise in the treatment of morbid obesity: A critical evaluation. *Am J Clin Nutr* 55:533S–537S.

Calles-Escandon J, Poehlman ET. 1997. Aging, fat oxidation and exercise. *Aging Clin Exp Res* 9:57–63.

Cameron N, Demerath EW. 2002. Critical periods in human growth and their relationship to diseases of aging. *Yrbk Phys Anthropol* 45:159–184.

Campfield LA, Smith FJ, Guisez Y, Devos R, Burn P. 1995. Recombinant mouse OB protein: Evidence for a peripheral signal linking adiposity and central neural networks. *Science* 269:546–549.

Caprio S, Hyman LD, McCarthy S, Lange R, Bronson M, Tamborlane WV. 1996. Fat distribution and cardiovascular risk factors in obese adolescent girls: Importance of the intra-abdominal fat depot. *Am J Clin Nutr* 64:12–17.

Carlson DE, Burman KD. 1984. The effectiveness of carefully monitored modified fast as adjuvant therapy for exogenous obesity in active duty personnel. *Mil Med* 149:669–671.

Carp IR, Meeker H, Sersen E, Kozlowski P. 1998. Analysis of the incubation periods, induction of obesity and histopathological changes in senescence-prone and senescence-resistant mice infected with various scrapie strains. *J Gen Virol* 79:2863–2869.

Carter JK, Garlich JD, Donaldson WT, Smith RE. 1983a. Influence of diet on a retrovirus induced obesity and stunting syndrome. *Avian Dis* 27:317–322.

Carter JK, Ow CL, Smith RE. 1983b. Rous-associated virus type 7 induces a syndrome in chickens characterized by stunting and obesity. *Infect Immun* 39:410–422.

Castellanos VH, Rolls BJ. 1997. Diet composition and the regulation of food intake and body weight. In: Dalton S, ed. *Overweight and Weight Management. The Health Professional's Guide to Understanding and Practice.* Gaithersburg, MD: Aspen Publishers. Pp. 254–283.

Chagnon YC, Pérusse L, Weisnagel SJ, Rankinen T, Bouchard C. 2000. The human obesity gene map: The 1999 update. *Obes Res* 8:89–117.

Cheverud JM, Pletscher LS, Vaughn TT, Marshall B. 1999. Differential response to dietary fat in large (LG/J) and small (SM/J) inbred mouse strains. *Physiol Genomics* 1:33–39.

Choh AC, Gage TB, McGarvey ST, Comuzzie AG. 2001. Genetic and environmental correlations between anthropometric and blood pressure traits among adult Samoans. *Am J Phys Anthropol* 115:304–311.

Chumlea WC, Guo SS, Kuczmarski RJ, Flegal KM, Johnson CL, Heymsfield SB, Lukaski HC, Friedl K, Hubbard VS. 2002. Body composition estimates from NHANES III bioelectrical impedance data. *Int J Obes* 26:1596–1609.

Cincotta AH, Meier AH. 1996. Bromocriptine (Ergoset) reduces body weight and improves glucose tolerance in obese subjects. *Diabetes Care* 19:667–670.

Clement K, Vaisse C, Lahlu N, Cabrol S, Pelloux V, Cassuto D, Courmelen M, Dina C, Chambaz J, Lacorte JM, Basdevant A, Bougneres P, Lebouc Y, Froguel P, Guy-Grand B. 1998. A mutation in the human leptin receptor gene causes obesity and pituitary dysfunction. *Nature* 392:398–401.

Cohen RY, Stunkard AJ, Felix MRJ. 1987. Comparison of three worksite weight-loss competitions. *J Behav Med* 10:467–479.

Cole JO, Levin A, Beake B, Kaiser PE, Scheinbaum ML. 1998. Sibutramine: A new weight loss agent without evidence of the abuse potential associated with amphetamines. *J Clin Psychopharmacol* 18:231–236.

Comuzzie AG, Blangero J, Mahaney MC, Mitchell BD, Stern MP, MacCluer JW. 1994. Genetic and environmental correlations among skinfold measures. *Int J Obes Relat Metab Disord* 18:413–418.

Comuzzie AG, Blangero J, Mahaney MC, Haffner SM, Mitchell BD, Stern MP, MacCluer JW. 1996. Genetic and environmental correlations among hormone levels and measures of body fat accumulation and topography. *J Clin Endocrinol Metab* 81:597–600.

Connolly HM, Crary JL, McGoon MD, Hensrud DD, Edwards BS, Edwards WD, Schaff HV. 1997. Valvular heart disease associated with fenfluramine-phentermine. *N Engl J Med* 337:581–588.

Considine RV, Sinha MK, Heiman ML, Kriauciunas A, Stephens TW, Nyce MR, Ohannesian JP, Marco CC, McKee LJ, Bauer TL, Caro JF. 1996. Serum immunoreactive-leptin concentration in normal-weight and obese humans. *N Engl J Med* 334:292–295.

Coulston AM, Rock CL. 1994. Popular diets and use of moderate caloric restriction for the treatment of obesity. In: Blackburn GL, Kanders BS, eds. *Obesity: Pathophysiology, Psychology and Treatment*. New York: Chapman Hall. Pp. 185–196.

Croft H, Hauser T, Leadbetter R, Jamerson B, Metz A. 2000. Effect of bupropion SR on weight in the long-term treatment of depression. *Obes Res* 8:10S.

Curb JD, Marcus EB. 1991. Body fat and obesity in Japanese Americans. *Am J Clin Nutr* 53:1552S–1555S.

Daly PA, Krieger DR, Dulloo AG, Young JB, Landsberg L. 1993. Ephedrine, caffeine and aspirin: Safety and efficacy for treatment of human obesity. *Int J Obes* 17:S73–S78.

Danforth E. 1985. Diet and obesity. *Am J Clin Nutr* 41:1132–1145.

Davison K. 1997. The quality of dietary information on the World Wide Web. *Clin Perform Qual Health Care* 5:64–66.

de Castro JM. 1999. What are the major correlates of macronutrient selection in Western populations? *Proc Nutr Soc* 58:755–763.

Dennis KE, Pane KW, Adams BK, Qi BB. 1999. The impact of a shipboard weight control program. *Obes Res* 7:60–67.

Dhurandhar NV, Atkinson RL. 1996. Comparison of serotonin agonists in combination with phentermine for treatment of obesity. *FASEB J* 10:A561.

Dhurandhar NV, Atkinson RL. 1997. Correspondence. *N Engl J Med* 336:511; discussion 512–513.

Dhurandhar NV, Kulkarni PR. 1992. Prevalence of obesity in Bombay. *Int J Obes* 16:367–375.

Dhurandhar NV, Kulkarni PR. 1993. Outpatient weight management in India: A comparison with the west. *Int J Food Sci Nutr* 44:73–83.

Dhurandhar NV, Kulkarni PR, Ajinkya SM, Sherikar AA. 1990. Avian adenovirus leading to pathogenomic obesity in chickens. *J Bombay Vet College* 2:131–132.

Dhurandhar NV, Kulkarni PR, Ajinkya SM, Sherikar AA. 1992. Effect of adenovirus infection on adiposity in chickens. *Vet Microbiol* 31:101–107.

Dhurandhar NV, Kulkarni PR, Ajinkja SM, Sherikar AA, Atkinson RL. 1997. Association of adenovirus infection with human obesity. *Obes Res* 5:464–469.

Dhurandhar NV, Israel BA, Kolesar JM, Cook ME, Atkinson RL. 2000. Increased adiposity in animals due to a human virus. *Int J Obes* 24:989–996.

Dietz WH. 1994. Critical periods in childhood for the development of obesity. *Am J Clin Nutr* 59:955–959.

Dietz WH, Gortmaker SL. 1985. Do we fatten our children at the television set? Obesity and television viewing in children and adolescents. *Pediatrics* 75:807–812.

Ditschuneit HH, Flechtner-Mors M, Johnson TD, Adler G. 1999. Metabolic and weight-loss effects of a long-term dietary intervention in obese patients. *Am J Clin Nutr* 69:198–204.

Ditschuneit HH, Flechtner-Mors M. 2001. Value of structured meals for weight management: Risk factors and long-term weight maintenance. *Obes Res* 9:284S–289S.

DOD (U.S. Department of Defense). 1995. *DoD Physical Fitness and Body Fat Program Procedures*. DOD Directive 1308.1. July 20. Washington, DC: U.S. Government Printing Office.

DOD. 1999. *Active Duty Military Personnel Strength by Regional Area and by Country*. 309A. June 30. Washington, DC: U.S. Government Printing Office.

DOD. 2002. *DoD Physical Fitness and Body Fat Program Procedures*. Department of Defense Instruction 1308.3. November 5. Washington, DC: U.S. Government Printing Office.

DOD PEC (Pharmaco Economic Center). 1997. Pharmacoeconomic analysis of obesity treatment. *PEC Update* 05:1–17.

Donato KA, Hegsted DM. 1985. Efficiency of utilization of various sources of energy for growth. *Proc Natl Acad Sci (USA)* 82:4866–4870.

Dreon DM, Frey-Hewitt B, Ellsworth N, Williams P, Terry RB, Wood PD. 1988. Dietary fat:carbohydrate ratio and obesity in middle-aged men. *Am J Clin Nutr* 47:995–1000.

Dunn AL, Marcus BH, Kampert JB, Garcia ME, Kohl HW 3rd, Blair SN. 1999. Comparison of lifestyle and structured interventions to increase physical activity and cardiorespiratory fitness. A randomized trial. *J Am Med Assoc* 281:327–334.

Dutta C, Hadley EC. 1995. The significance of sarcopenia in old age. *J Gerontol* 50A:1–4.

Dwyer J. 1995. Popular diets. In: Brownell KD, Fairburn CG, eds. *Eating Disorders and Obesity: A Comprehensive Handbook*. New York: Guilford Press. Pp. 491–497.

Dyer RG. 1994. Traditional treatment of obesity: Does it work? *Baillieres Best Pract Res Clin Endocrinol Metab* 8:661–685.

Eliakim A, Burke GS, Cooper DM. 1997. Fitness, fatness, and the effect of training assessed by magnetic resonance imaging and skinfold-thickness measurements in healthy adolescent females. *Am J Clin Nutr* 66:223–231.

Ellis KJ, Abrams SA, Wong WW. 1997. Body composition of a young, multiethnic female population. *Am J Clin Nutr* 65:724–731.

Emery EM, Schmid TL, Kahn HS, Filozof PP. 1993. A review of the association between abdominal fat distribution, health outcome measures, and modifiable risk factors. *Am J Health Promot* 7:342–353.

Ettinger MP, Littlejohn TW, Schwartz SL, Weiss SR, McIlwain HH, Heymsfield SB, Bray GA, Roberts WG, Heyman ER, Stambler N, Heshka S, Vicary C, Guler H-P. 2003. Recombinant variant of ciliary neurotrophic factor for weight loss in obese adults. A randomized, dose-ranging study. *J Am Med Assoc* 289:1826–1832.

FDA (U.S. Food and Drug Administration). 1996. *Guidance for the Clinical Evaluation of Weight-Control Drugs.* Rockville, MD: FDA.

Feldman RD, Hegele RA. 2000. G-protein polymorphisms and maternal/neonatal metabolism: Still a weight for the answer. *Lancet* 355:1201–1202.

Fernandez JR, Heo M, Heymsfield SB, Pierson RN, Pi-Sunyer FX, Wang ZM, Wang J, Hayes M, Allison DB, Gallagher D. 2003. Is percentage body fat differentially related to body mass index in Hispanic Americans, African Americans, and European Americans? *Am J Clin Nutr* 77:71–75.

Fiedler ER, Cortner DM, Ktenidis H, Balch M. 1999. Healthy eating in practice: The U.S. Air Force demonstration at basic military training. *Appl Prev Psychol* 8:155–163.

Fisler JS, Drenick EJ. 1987. Starvation and semistarvation diets in the management of obesity. *Ann Rev Nutr* 7:465–484.

Flatt JP. 1987. Dietary fat, carbohydrate balance and weight maintenance: Effects of exercise. *Am J Clin Nutr* 45:296–306.

Flatt JP. 1997. Body fat content and the balance between fat and alcohol oxidation and consumption. In: Dalton S, ed. *Overweight and Weight Management. The Health Professional's Guide to Understanding and Practice.* Gaithersburg, MD: Aspen Publishers. Pp. 224–253.

Flechter-Mors M, Ditschuneit HH, Johnson TD, Suchard MA, Adler G. 2000. Metabolic and weight loss effects of long-term dietary intervention in obese patients: Four-year results. *Obes Res* 8:399–402.

Flegal KM, Carroll MD, Kuczmarski RJ, Johnson CL. 1998. Overweight and obesity in the United States: Prevalence and trends, 1960–1994. *Int J Obes Relat Metab Disord* 22:39–47.

Flegal KM, Carroll MD, Ogden CL, Johnson CL. 2002. Prevalence and trends in obesity among U.S. adults, 1999–2000. *J Am Med Assoc* 288:1723–1727.

Fleury C, Neverova M, Collins S, Raimbault S, Champigny O, Levi-Meyrueis C, Bouillaud F, Seldin MF, Surwit RS, Ricquier D, Warden CH. 1997. Uncoupling protein-2: A novel gene linked to obesity and hyperinsulinemia. *Nat Genet* 15:269–272.

Flynn MA, Nolph GB, Baker AS, Martin WM, Krause G. 1989. Total body potassium in aging humans: A longitudinal study. *Am J Clin Nutr* 50:713–717.

Foltin RW, Kelly TH, Fischman MW. 1995. Effect of amphetamine on human macronutrient intake. *Physiol Behav* 58:899–907.

Forbes GB. 1987. *Human Body Composition*. New York: Springer Verlag.

Forbes GB, Reina JC. 1970 Adult lean body mass declines with age: Some longitudinal observations. *Metabolism* 19:653–663.

Foreyt JP, Goodrick GK. 1993. National Institutes of Health Technology Assessment Conference: Evidence for success of behavior modification in weight loss and control. *Ann Intern Med* 119:698–701.

Foreyt JP, Goodrick GK. 1994. Attributes of successful approaches to weight loss and control. *Appl Prev Psychol* 3:209–215.

Forster JL, Jeffery RW, Snell MK. 1988. One-year follow-up study to a worksite weight control program. *Prev Med* 17:129–133.

Foster GD, Wadden TA, Vogt RA. 1997. Resting energy expenditure in obese African American and Caucasian women. *Obes Res* 5:1–8.

Frankle RT, McIntosh J, Bianchi M, Kane EJ. 1986. The Weight Watchers® at work program. *J Nutr Ed* 18:S44–S47.

Freedman DS, Khan LK, Serdula MK, Galuska DA, Dietz WH. 2002. Trends and correlates of class 3 obesity in the United States from 1990 through 2000. *J Am Med Assoc* 14:1758–1761.

French SA, Story M, Jeffery RW, Snyder P, Eisenberg M, Sidebottom A, Murray D. 1997. Pricing strategy to promote fruit and vegetable purchase in high school cafeterias. *J Am Diet Assoc* 97:1008–1010.

French SA, Harnack L, Jeffery RW. 2000. Fast food restaurants use among women in the Pound of Prevention study: Dietary behavioral and demographic correlates. *Int J Obes Relat Metab Disord* 24:1353–1359.

French SJ, Read NW. 1994. Effect of guar gum on hunger and satiety after meals of differing fat content: Relationship with gastric emptying. *Am J Clin Nutr* 59:87–91.

Friedl KE. 1992. Body composition and military performance: Origins of the Army standards. In: Marriott BM, Grumstrup-Scott J, eds. *Body Composition and Physical Performance.* Washington, DC: National Academy Press. Pp. 31–55.

Friedl KE, Vogel JA, Bovee MW, Jones BH. 1989. *Assessment of Body Weight Standards in Male and Female Army Recruits.* Technical Report No. T15–90. Natick, MA: U.S. Army Research Institute for Environmental Medicine.

Gadde KM, Ranga K, Krishnan K, Drezner MK. 1999. Bupropion SR shows promise as an effective obesity treatment. *Obes Res* 7:51S.

Gallagher D, Visser M, Sepulveda D, Pierson RN Jr, Harris T, Heymsfield SB. 1996. How useful is body mass index for comparison of body fatness across age, gender, and ethnic groups? *Am J Epidem* 143:228–239.

Gallagher D, Visser M, de Meersman RE, Sepulveda D, Baumgartner RN, Pierson RN, Harris TB, Heymsfield SB. 1997. Appendicular skeletal muscle mass: Effects of age, gender, and ethnicity. *J Appl Physiol* 83:229–239.

Gallagher D, Belmonte D, Deurenberg P, Wang Z, Krasnow N, Pi-Sunyer FX, Heymsfield SB. 1998. Organ-tissue mass measurement allows modeling of REE and metabolically active tissue mass. *Am J Physiol* 275:E249–E252.

Gallagher D, Ruts E, Visser M, Heshka S, Baumgartner RN, Wang J, Pierson RN, Pi-Sunyer FX, Heymsfield SB. 2000. Weight stability masks sarcopenia in elderly men and women. *Am J Physiol Endocrinol Metab* 279:E366–E375.

Gambera PJ, Schneeman BO, Davis PA. 1995. Use of the Food Guide Pyramid and U.S. Dietary Guidelines to improve dietary intake and reduce cardiovascular risk in active-duty Air Force members. *J Am Diet Assoc* 95:1268–1273.

GAO (U.S. General Accounting Office). 1998. *Gender Issues: Improved Guidance and Oversight are needed to Ensure Validity and Equity of Fitness Standards*. Washington, DC: U.S. Government Printing Office.

Gibson SA. 2000. Associations between energy density and macronutrient composition in the diets of pre-school children: Sugars vs. starch. *Int J Obes Relat Metab Disord* 24:633–638.

Gilliat-Wimberly M, Manore MM, Woolf K, Swan P, Carrol S. 2001. Effects of habitual physical activity on the resting metabolic rates and body compositions of women aged 35 to 50 years. *J Am Diet Assoc* 101:1181–1188.

Glass JN, Miller WC, Szymanski M, Fernhall B, Durstine JL. 2002. Physiological responses to weight-loss intervention in inactive obese African-American and Caucasian women. *J Sports Med Phys Fitness* 42:56–64.

Goldstein DJ, Rampey AH Jr, Dornseif BE, Levine LR, Potvin JH, Fludzinski LA. 1993. Fluoxetine: A randomized clinical trial in the maintenance of weight loss. *Obes Res* 1:92–98.

Goldstein DJ, Rampey AH Jr, Roback PJ, Wilson MG, Hamilton SH, Sayler ME, Tollefson GD. 1995. Efficacy and safety of long-term fluoxetine treatment of obesity—maximizing success. *Obes Res* 3:481S–490S.

Goodman MT, Nomura AM, Wilkins LR, Hankin J. 1992. The association of diet, obesity, and breast cancer in Hawaii. *Cancer Epidemiol Biomarkers Prev* 1:269–275.

Goran MI. 2001. Metabolic precursors and effects of obesity in children: A decade of progress, 1990–1999. *Am J Clin Nutr* 73:158–171.

Goris AHC, Westerterp-Plantenga MS, Westerterp KK. 2000. Undereating and underrecording of habitual food intake in obese men: Selective underreporting of fat intake. *Am J Clin Nutr* 71:130–134.

Gortmaker SL, Must A, Perrin JM, Sobol AM, Dietz WH. 1993. Social and economic consequences of overweight in adolescence and young adulthood. *N Engl J Med* 329:1008–1012.

Gosztonyi G, Ludwig H. 1995. Borna disease: Neuropathology and pathogenesis. *Curr Top Microbiol Immunol* 190:39–73.

Gould BS. 1979. *Investigations into the Military and Anthropological Statistics of American Soldiers.* New York: Arno Press. P. 418.

Graham DJ, Green L. 1997. Further cases of valvular heart disease associated with fenfluramine-phentermine. *N Engl J Med* 337:635.

Grant KE, Chandler RM, Castle AL, Ivy JL. 1997. Chromium and exercise training: Effect on obese women. *Med Sci Sports Exerc* 29:992–998.

Gray AS, Raab CA. 1999. 'On-line to healthy weighs': Employed women's responses to electronic messages on weight management. *J Nutr Educ* 31:56–59.

Greenway FL. 2001. The safety and efficacy of pharmaceutical and herbal caffeine and ephedrine use as a weight loss agent. *Obes Rev* 2:199–211.

Griffen L, Anchors M. 1998. The "phen-pro" diet drug combination is not associated with valvular heart disease. *Arch Intern Med* 158:1278–1279.

Griffiths RR, Brady JV, Bradford LD. 1979. Predicting the abuse liability of drugs with animal drug self-administration procedures: Psychomotor stimulants and hallucinogens. *Adv Behav Pharm* 2:163–208.

Gunay-Aygun M, Cassidy SB, Nicholls RD. 1997. Prader-Willi and other syndromes associated with obesity and mental retardation. *Behav Genet* 27:307–324.

Guo SS, Zeller C, Chumlea WC, Siervogel RM. 1999. Aging, body composition, and lifestyle: The Fels Longitudinal Study. *Am J Clin Nutr* 70:405–411.

Guo SS, Huang C, Maynard LM, Demerath E, Towne B, Chumlea WC, Siervogel RM. 2000. Body mass index during childhood, adolescence and young adulthood in relation to adult overweight and adiposity: The Fels Longitudinal Study. *Int J Obes* 24:1628–1635.

Gurrici S, Hartriyanti Y, Hautvast JG, Deurenberg P. 1998. Relationship between body fat and body mass index: Differences between Indonesians and Dutch Caucasians. *Eur J Clin Nutr* 52:779–783.

Gütersohn A, Naber C, Müller N, Erbel R, Siffert W. 2000. G protein β-3 subunit 825 TT genotype and post-pregnancy weight retention. *Lancet* 355:1240–1241.

Gutin B, Islam S, Manos T, Cucuzzo N, Smith C, Stachura ME. 1994. Relation of percentage of body fat and maximal aerobic capacity to risk factors for atherosclerosis and diabetes in black and white seven- to eleven-year-old children. *J Pediatr* 125:847–852.

Halaas JL, Gajiwala KS, Maffei M, Cohen SL, Chair BT, Rabinowitz D, Lallone RL, Burley SK, Friedman JM. 1995. Weight-reducing effects of the plasma protein encoded by the obese gene. *Science* 269:543–546.

Hallberg D, Backman L, Espmark S. 1975. Surgical treatment of obesity. *Prog Surg* 14:46–83.

Haller CA, Benowitz NL. 2000. Adverse cardiovascular and central nervous system events associated with dietary supplements containing ephedra alkaloids. *N Engl J Med* 343:1833–1838.

Hallmark MA, Reynolds TH, de Souza CA, Dotson CO, Anderson RA, Rogers MA. 1996. Effects of chromium and resistive training on muscle strength and body composition. *Med Sci Sports Exerc* 28:139–144.

Han TS, Bijnen FCH, Lean MEJ, Seidell JC. 1998. Separate associations of waist and hip circumference with lifestyle factors. *Int J Epidemiol* 27:422–430.

Hanotin C, Thomas F, Jones SP, Leutenegger E, Drouin P. 1998a. A comparison of sibutramine and dexfenfluramine in the treatment of obesity. *Obes Res* 6:285–291.

Hanotin C, Thomas F, Jones SP, Leutenegger E, Drouin P. 1998b. Efficacy and tolerability of sibutramine in obese patients: A dose-ranging study. *Int J Obes* 22:32–38.

Hara H, Egusa G, Yamakido M. 1996. Incidence of non-insulin-dependent diabetes mellitus and its risk factors in Japanese-Americans living in Hawaii and Los Angeles. *Diabet Med* 13:S133–S142.

Haraldsdottir J, Andersen LB. 1994. Dietary factors related to fitness in young men and women. *Prev Med* 23:490–497.

Hart J, Einav C, Weingarten MA, Stein M. 1990. The importance of family support in a behavior modification weight loss program. *J Am Diet Assoc* 90:1270–1271.

He Q, Karlberg J. 2002. Probability of adult overweight and risk change during the BMI rebound period. *Obes Res* 10:135–140.

Heal DJ, Ashley S, Prow MR, Jackson HC, Martin KF, Cheetham SC. 1998. Sibutramine: A novel anti-obesity drug. A review of the pharmacological evidence to differentiate it from d-amphetamine and d-fenfluramine. *Int J Obes Relat Metab Disord* 22:S18–S28.

Heber D, Ashley JM, Wang HJ, Elashoff RM. 1994. Clinical evaluation of a minimal intervention meal replacement regimen for weight reduction. *J Am Coll Nutr* 13:608–614.

Hennrikus DJ, Jeffery RW. 1996. Worksite intervention for weight control: A review of the literature. *Am J Health Promot* 10:471–498.

Hertzler AA, Schulman RS. 1983. Employed women, dieting, and support groups. *J Am Diet Assoc* 82:153–158.

Heshka S, Greenway F, Anderson JW, Atkinson RL, Hill JO, Phinney SD, Miller-Kovach K, Pi-Sunyer FX. 2000. Self-help weight loss versus a structured commercial program after 26 weeks: A randomized controlled study. *Am J Med* 109:282–287.

Heymsfield SB, Allison DB, Vasselli JR, Pietrobelli A, Greenfield D, Nunez C. 1998. Garcinia cambogia (hydroxycitric acid) as a potential antiobesity agent: A randomized controlled trial. *J Am Med Assoc* 280:1596–1600.

Heymsfield SB, Greenberg AS, Fujioka K, Dixon RM, Kushner R, Hunt T, Lubina JA, Patane J, Self B, Hunt P, McCamish M. 1999. Preliminary communication. Recombinant leptin for weight loss in obese and lean adults: A randomized, controlled, dose-escalation trial. *J Am Med Assoc* 282:1568–1575.

HHS (U.S. Department of Health and Human Services). 1996. *Physical Activity and Health. A Report of the Surgeon General*. Washington, DC: U.S. Government Printing Office.

HHS. 2001. *The Surgeon General's Call to Action to Prevent and Decrease Overweight and Obesity.* Washington, DC: U.S. Government Printing Office.

HHS/FDA. 1997. Dietary supplements containing ephedrine alkaloids; Proposed rule. *Fed Reg* 62:30677–30724.

Hill JO. 2000. Long-term weight control with meal replacements. *Nutrition* 16:385.

Hill JO, Peters JC. 1998. Environmental contributions to the obesity epidemic. *Science* 280:1371–1374.

Hill JO, Saris WHM. 1998. Energy expenditure in physical activity. In: Bray GA, Bouchard C, James WPT, eds. *Handbook of Obesity*. New York: Marcel Dekker. Pp. 457–474.

Hjermann I. 1992. The metabolic cardiovascular syndrome: Syndrome X, Reaven's syndrome, insulin resistance syndrome, atherothrombogenic syndrome. *J Cardiovasc Pharmacol* 20:S5–S10.

Hodgdon JA. 1992. Body composition in the military services: Standards and methods. In: Marriott BM, Grumstrup-Scott J, eds. *Body Composition and Physical Performance.* Washington, DC: National Academy Press. Pp. 57–70.

Hodgdon JA. 1999. *A History of the U.S. Navy Physical Readiness Program from 1976 to 1999.* NHRC Publication 99-6F. San Diego, CA: Naval Health Research Center.

Hodgdon JA, Fitzgerald PI, Vogel JA. 1990. *Relationships Between Fat and Appearance Ratings of U.S. Soldiers*. NHRC Publication 90-1. San Diego, CA: Naval Health Research Center.

Hoerr SM, Louden VA. 1993. Can nutrition information increase sales of healthful vended snacks? *J Sch Health* 63:386–390.

Hoiberg A, McNally MS. 1991. Profiling overweight patients in the U.S. Navy: Health conditions and costs. *Mil Med* 156:76–82.

Hollander PA, Elbein SC, Hirsch IB, Kelley D, McGill J, Taylor T, Weiss SR, Crockett SE, Kaplan RA, Comstock J, Lucas CP, Lodewick PA, Canovatchel W, Chung J, Hauptman J. 1998. Role of orlistat in the treatment of obese patients with type 2 diabetes. A 1-year randomized double-blind study. *Diabetes Care* 21:1288–1294.

Holle F, Bauer H. 1978. The definitive technique of selective proximal vagotomy with pyloroplasty appropriate to form and function in surgery of peptic ulcer disease. *Surg Ann* 10:387–416.

Hu FB, Stampfer MJ, Manson JE, Rimm E, Colditz GA, Speizer FE, Hennekens CH, Willett WC. 1999. Dietary protein and risk of ischemic heart disease in women. *Am J Clin Nutr* 70:221–227.

Hubbard VS, Hall WH. 1991. Gastrointestinal surgery for severe obesity. *Obes Surg* 1:257–265.

Hughes J, Todorovic V, Kemp H. 1999. 'The Sugar Buddies': An intervention programme for 'obese' patients with poorly controlled diabetes. *J Hum Nutr Diet* 12:71–78.

IOM (Institute of Medicine). 1990. *Nutrition During Pregnancy. Part I–Weight Gain. Part II–Nutrient Supplements.* Washington, DC: National Academy Press.

IOM. 1992a. *Body Composition and Physical Performance*. Washington, DC: National Academy Press.

IOM. 1992b. *Nutrition During Pregnancy and Lactation. An Implementation Guide*: Washington, DC: National Academy Press.

IOM. 1995. *Weighing the Options: Criteria for Evaluating Weight-Management Programs*. Washington, DC: National Academy Press.

IOM. 1998. *Assessing Readiness in Military Women. The Relationship of Body Composition, Nutrition, and Health*. Washington, DC: National Academy Press.

IOM. 2002. *Dietary Reference Intakes for Energy, Carbohydrate, Fiber, Fat, Fatty Acids, Cholesterol, Protein, and Amino Acids.* Washington, DC: National Academy Press.

Jackson AA, Langley-Evans SC, McCarthy HD. 1996. Nutritional influences in early life upon obesity and body proportions. *Ciba Found Symp* 201:118–129.

Jakicic JM, Wing RR, Butler BA, Robertson RJ. 1995. Prescribing exercise in multiple short bouts versus one continuous bout: Effects on adherence, cardiorespiratory fitness, and weight loss in overweight women. *Int J Obes Relat Metab Disord* 19:893–901.

Jakicic JM, Winters C, Lang W, Wing RR. 1999. Effects of intermittent exercise and use of home exercise equipment on adherence, weight loss, and fitness in overweight women: A randomized trial. *J Am Med Assoc* 282:1554–1560.

Jakicic JM, Clark K, Coleman E, Donnelly JE, Foreyt J, Melanson E, Volek J, Volpe SL. 2001. American College of Sports Medicine position stand. Appropriate intervention strategies for weight loss and prevention of weight regain for adults. *Med Sci Sports Exerc* 33:2145–2156.

James LC, Folen RA, Garland FN, Edwards C, Noce M, Gohdes D, Williams D, Bowles S, Kellar MA, Supplee E. 1997. The Tripler Army Medical Center LEAN program: A healthy lifestyle model for the treatment of obesity. *Mil Med* 162:328–332.

James LC, Earles J, Folen RA. 1999a. *The Tripler L^2E^3AN Program: A Current Update*. Presented at the Institute of Medicine Workshop on Military Weight-Management Programs: State of the Art and Future Initiatives, Washington, DC, October 25–26. Subcommittee on Military Weight Management.

James LC, Folen RA, Page H, Noce M, Brown J, Britton C. 1999b. The tripler LE^3AN program: A two-year follow-up report. *Mil Med* 164:389–395.

James WP, Avenell A, Broom J, Whitehead J. 1997. A one year trial to assess the value of orlistat in the management of obesity. *Int J Obes* 21:S24–S30.

Jeffery RW. 1996. Bias in reported body weight as a function of education, occupation, health and weight concern. *Addict Behav* 21:217–222.

Jeffery RW, French SA. 1999. Preventing weight gain in adults: The Pound of Prevention Study. *Am J Public Health* 89:747–751.

Jeffery RW, Bjornson-Benson WM, Rosenthal BS, Lindquist RA, Kurht CL, Johnson SL. 1984. Correlates of weight loss and its maintenance over two years of follow-up among middle-aged men. *Prev Med* 13:155–168.

Jenkins DJ, Kendall CW, Axelsen M, Augustin LS, Vuksan V. 2000. Viscous and nonviscous fibres, nonabsorbable and low glycaemic index carbohydrates, blood lipids and coronary heart disease. *Curr Opin Lipidol* 11:49–56.

Jensen EX, Fusch C, Jaeger P, Peheim E, Horber FF. 1995. Impact of chronic cigarette smoking on body composition and fuel metabolism. *J Clin Endocrinol Metab* 80:2181–2185.

Jequier E, Schutz Y. 1983. Long-term measurements of energy expenditure in humans using a respiration chamber. *Am J Clin Nutr* 38:989–998.

Jick H, Vasilakis C, Weinrauch LA, Meier CR, Jick SS, Derby LE. 1998. A population-based study of appetite-suppressant drugs and the risk of cardiac-valve regurgitation. *N Engl J Med* 339:719–724.

Johnson NA. 1997. The history of the army weight standards. *Mil Med* 162:564–570.

Johnston EM. 1991. Weight changes during pregnancy and the postpartum period. *Prog Food Nutr Sci* 15:117–157.

Jonderko K, Kucio C. 1989. Extra-anorectic actions of mazindol. *Israel J Med Sci* 25:20–24.

Jones BH, Bovee MW, Knapik JJ. 1992. Associations among body composition, physical fitness, and injury in men and women Army trainees. In: Mariott BM, Grumstrup-Scott J, eds. *Body Composition and Physical Performance*. Washington, DC: National Academy Press. Pp. 141–173.

Kalman D, Incledon T, Gaunaurd I, Schwartz H, Krieger D. 2002. An acute clinical trial evaluating the cardiovascular effects of an herbal ephedra-caffeine weight loss product in healthy overweight adults. *Int J Obes Relat Metab Disord* 26:1363–1366.

Kanders BS, Blackburn GL. 1994. Very-low-calorie diets for the treatment of obesity. In: Blackburn GL, Kanders BS, eds. *Obesity: Pathophysiology, Psychology and Treatment*. New York: Chapman Hall. Pp. 197–216.

Katzmarzyk PT, Malina RM, Song TM, Bouchard C. 1998. Television viewing, physical activity, and health-related fitness of youth in the Quebec Family Study. *J Adolesc Health* 23:318–325.

Katzmarzyk PT, Pérusse L, Rao DC, Bouchard C. 2000. Familial risk of overweight and obesity in the Canadian population using the WHO/NIH criteria. *Obes Res* 8:194–197.

Kayman S, Bruvold W, Stern JS. 1990. Maintenance and relapse after weight loss in women: Behavioral aspects. *Am J Clin Nutr* 52:800–807.

Kendall A, Levitsky DA, Strupp BJ, Lissner L. 1991. Weight loss on a low-fat diet: Consequences of the imprecision of the control of food intake in humans. *Am J Clin Nutr* 53:1124–1129.

Kesaniemi YA, Danforth E Jr, Jensen MD, Kopelman PG, Lefebvre P, Reeder BA. 2001. Dose-response issues concerning physical activity and health: An evidence-based symposium. *Med Sci Sports Exerc* 33:S351–S358.

Khan MA, Herzog CA, St. Peter JV, Hartley GG, Madlon-Kay R, Dick CD, Asinger RW, Vessey JT. 1998. The prevalence of cardiac valvular insufficiency assessed by transthoracic echocardiography in obese patients treated with appetite-suppressant drugs. *N Engl J Med* 339:713–718.

Kimmel SE, Keane MG, Crary JL, Jones J, Kinman JL, Beare J, Sammel M, Sutton MS, Strom BL. 1999. Detailed examination of fenfluramine-phentermine users with valve abnormalities identified in Fargo, North Dakota. *Am J Cardiol* 84:304–308.

Klem ML, Wing RR, McGuire MT, Seagle HM, Hill JO. 1997. A descriptive study of individuals successful at long-term maintenance of substantial weight loss. *Am J Clin Nutr* 66:239–246.

Kneip JK, Fox HM, Fruehling JK. 1985. A weight-control program for bank employees. *J Am Diet Assoc* 85:1489–1491.

Knuiman JT, West CE. 1982. The concentration of cholesterol in serum and in various serum lipoproteins in macrobiotic, vegetarian, and non-vegetarian men and boys. *Atherosclerosis* 43:71–82.

Kogon MM, Krauchi K, van der Velde P, van der Werf H, Keller U. 1994. Psychological and metabolic effects of dietary carbohydrates and dexfenfluramine during a low-energy diet in obese women. *Am J Clin Nutr* 60:488–493.

Koplan JP, Dietz WH. 1999. Caloric imbalance and public health policy. *J Am Med Assoc* 282:1579–1581.

Kral JG. 1989. Surgical treatment of obesity. *Med Clin North Am* 73:251–264.

Kral JG. 1998. Surgical treatment of obesity. In: Bray GA, Bouchard C, James WPT, eds. *Handbook of Obesity*. New York: Marcel Dekker. Pp. 977–993.

Kramer MS, Lane DA. 1998. Aminorex, dexfenfluramine, and primary pulmonary hypertension. *J Clin Epidemiol* 51:361–364.

Kris-Etherton PM, Binkoski AE, Zhao G, Coval SM, Clemmer KF, Hecker KD, Jacques H, Etherton TD. 2002. Dietary fat: Assessing the evidence in support of a moderate-fat diet; the benchmark based on lipoprotein metabolism. *Proc Nutr Soc* 61:287–298.

Kuczmarski RJ, Flegal KM, Campbell SM, Johnson CL. 1994. Increasing prevalence of overweight among U.S. adults. *J Am Med Assoc* 272:205–211.

Kuczmarski RJ, Carroll MD, Flegal KM, Troiano RP. 1997. Varying body mass index cutoff points to describe overweight prevalence among U.S. adults: NHANES III (1988 to 1994). *Obes Res* 5:542–548.

Kumanyika S, Wilson JF, Guilford-Davenport M. 1993. Weight-related attitudes and behaviors of black women. *J Am Diet Assoc* 93:416–422.

Kurz X, van Ermen A. 1997. Valvular heart disease associated with fenfluramine-phentermine. *N Engl J Med* 337:1772–1773.

Kushi LH, Lew RA, Stare FJ, Ellison CR, Lozy M, Bourke E, Daly L, Graham I, Hickey N, Mulcohy R, Kevaney J. 1985. Diet and 20-year mortality from coronary heart disease: Irish-Boston Diet-Heart Study. *N Engl J Med* 312:811–818.

Larsen J. 2000. Point Paper: Accession Weight Standards (AR 40-501). May 24. Photocopy.

Latner JD, Stunkard AJ, Wilson GT, Jackson ML, Zelitch DS, Labouvie E. 2000. Effective long-term treatment of obesity: A continuing care model. *Int J Obes Relat Metab Disord* 24:893–898.

Lawson KD, Middleton SJ, Hassal CD. 1997. Olestra, a nonabsorbed, noncaloric replacement for dietary fat: A review. *Drug Metab Rev* 29:651–703.

Layman DK, Boileau RA, Erickson DJ, Painter JE, Shiue H, Sather C, Christou DD. 2003a. A reduced ratio of dietary carbohydrate to protein improves body composition and blood lipid profiles during weight loss in adult women. *J Nutr* 133:411–417.

Layman DK, Shiue H, Sather C, Erickson DJ, Baum J. 2003b. Increased dietary protein modifies glucose and insulin homeostasis in adult women during weight loss. *J Nutr* 133:405–410.

Lee A, Morley JE. 1998. Metformin decreases food consumption and induces weight loss in subjects with obesity with type II non-insulin-dependent diabetes. *Obesity Res* 6:47–53.

Lee CD, Blair SN, Jackson AS. 1999. Cardiorespiratory fitness, body composition, and all cause and cardiovascular disease mortality in men. *Am J Clin Nutr* 69:373–380.

Lee L, Kumar S, Leong LC. 1994. The impact of five-month basic military training on the body weight and body fat of 197 moderately to severely obese Singaporean males aged 17 to 19 years. *Int J Obes Relat Metab Disord* 18:105–109.

Leeds AR. 1987. Dietary fibre: Mechanisms of action. *Int J Obes* 11:3–7.

Leibel RL, Hirsch J, Appel BE, Checani GC. 1992. Energy intake required to maintain body weight is not affected by wide variation in diet composition. *Am J Clin Nutr* 55:350–355.

Leibel RL, Rosenbaum M, Hirsch J. 1995. Changes in energy expenditure resulting from altered body weight. *N Engl J Med* 332:621–628.

Leibowitz SF. 1995. Brain peptides and obesity: Pharmacologic treatment. *Obes Res* 3:573S–589S.

Levine JA, Eberhardt NL, Jensen MD. 1999. Role of nonexercise activity thermogenesis in resistance to fat gain in humans. *Science* 283:212–214.

Lin P-Y, Romsos DR, van der Tuig JG, Leveille GA. 1979. Maintenance energy requirements, energy retention and heat production of young obese (ob/ob) and lean mice fed a high-fat or a high-carbohydrate diet. *J Nutr* 109:1143–1153.

Lindquist CH, Bray RM. 2001. Trends in overweight and physical activity among U.S. military personnel, 1995–1998. *Prev Med* 32:57–65.

Linner JH. 1982. Comparative effectiveness of gastric bypass and gastroplasty. A clinical study. *Arch Surg* 117:695–700.

Liu YL, Toubro S, Astrup A, Stock MJ. 1995. Contribution of β_3-adrenoceptor activation to ephedrine-induced thermogenesis in humans. *Int J Obes* 19:678–685.

Loper JF, Barrows KK. 1985. A nutrition and weight-control program in industry. *J Am Diet Assoc* 85:1487–1488.

Love AG, Hamilton EL, Hellman IL. 1958. *Tabulating Equipment and Army Medical Statistics.* Washington, DC: U.S. Department of the Army, Office of the Surgeon General. Pp. 78–79.

LSRO (Life Sciences Research Office). 1987. *Physiological Effects and Health Consequences of Dietary Fiber.* Bethesda, MD: LSRO Federation of American Societies for Experimental Biology. Pp. 74–79.

Luepker RV. 1999. How physically active are American children and what can we do about it? *Int J Obes Relat Metab Disord* 23:S12–S17.

Lukaski HC, Bolonchuk WW, Siders WA, Milne DB. 1996. Chromium supplementation and resistance training: Effects on body composition, strength, and trace element status of men. *Am J Clin Nutr* 63:954–965.

Lyons MJ, Faust IM, Hemes RB, Buskirk DR, Hirsch J, Zabriskie JB. 1982. A virally induced obesity syndrome in mice. *Science* 216:82–85.

MacCluer JW, Stern MP, Almasy L, Atwood LA, Blangero J, Comuzzie AG, Bennett D, Haffner SM, Henkel RD, Hixson JE, Kammerer CM, Mahaney MC, Mitchell BD, Rainwater DL, Samollow PB, Sharp RM, VandeBerg JL, Williams JT. 1999. Genetics of atherosclerosis risk factors in Mexican Americans. *Nutr Rev* 575:S59–S65.

Macdiarmid JI, Cade J, Burley VJ, Blundell JE. 1994. Leeds high fat study: First analysis of the characteristics of high fat consumers. *Int J Obes* 18:135.

Macdiarmid JI, Vail A, Cade JE, Blundell JE. 1998. The sugar-fat relationship revisited: Differences in consumption between men and women of varying BMI. *Int J Obes Rel Metab Disord* 22:1053–1061.

MacDonald KG, Long SD, Swanson MS, Brown BM, Morris P, Dohm GL, Pories WJ. 1997. The gastric bypass operation reduces the progression and mortality of non-insulin-dependent diabetes mellitus. *J Gastrointest Surg* 1:213–220.

MacLean LD, Rhode BM, Sampalis J, Forse RA. 1993. Results of the surgical treatment of obesity. *Am J Surg* 165:155–162.

Maffeis C, Schutz Y, Grezzani A, Provera S, Piacentini G, Tato L. 2001. Meal-induced thermogenesis and obesity: Is a fat meal a risk factor for fat gain in children? *J Clin Endocrinol Metab* 86:214–219.

Manson JE, Faich GA. 1996. Pharmacotherapy for obesity—Do the benefits outweigh the risks? *N Engl J Med* 335:659–660.

Mason EE. 1982. Vertical banded gastroplasty for obesity. *Arch Surg* 117:701–706.

McCann U, Hatzidimitriou G, Ridenour A, Fischer C, Yuan J, Katz J, Ricaurte G. 1994. Dexfenfluramine and serotonin neurotoxicity: Further preclinical evidence that clinical caution is indicated. *J Pharm Exp Ther* 269:792–798.

McGinnis JM, Foege WH. 1993. Actual causes of death in the United States. *J Am Med Assoc* 270:2207–2212.

McGuire MT, Wing RR, Klem ML, Seagle HM, Hill JO. 1998. Long-term maintenance of weight loss: Do people who lose weight through various weight loss methods use different behaviors to maintain weight? *Int J Obes Relat Metab Disord* 22:572–577.

McGuire MT, Wing RR, Klem ML, Hill JO. 1999. Behavioral strategies of individuals who have maintained long-term weight losses. *Obes Res* 7:334–341.

McIntyre A, Vincent RM, Perkins AC, Spiller RC. 1997. Effect of bran, ispaghula, and inert plastic particles on gastric emptying and small bowel transit in humans: The role of physical factors. *Gut* 40:223–227.

McKeigue PM, Pierpoint T, Ferrie JE, Marmot MG. 1992. Relationship of glucose intolerance and hyperinsulinaemia to body fat pattern in south Asians and Europeans. *Diabetologia* 35:785–791.

McNeely W, Benfield P. 1998. Orlistat. *Drugs* 56:241–249.

McNulty PA. 1997a. Prevalence and contributing factors of eating disorder behaviors in a population of female Navy nurses. *Mil Med* 162:703–706.

McNulty PA. 1997b. Prevalence and contributing factors of eating disorder behaviors in active duty navy men. *Mil Med* 162:753–758.

McNulty PA. 2001. Prevalence and contributing factors of eating disorder behaviors in active duty service women in the Army, Navy, Air Force, and Marines. *Mil Med* 166:53–58.

Melby CL, Ho RC, Jeckel K, Beal L, Goran M, Donahoo WT. 2000. Comparison of risk factors for obesity in young, nonobese African-American and Caucasian women. *Int J Obes* 24:1514–1522.

Miles J, Petrie C, Steel M. 2000. Slimming on the Internet. *J Royal Society Med* 93:254–257.

Miller AB. 1988. Cancer and obesity. In: Frankle RT, Yang M-U, eds. *Obesity and Weight Control: The Health Professional's Guide to Understanding and Treatment.* Rockville, MD: Aspen Publishers. Pp. 445–456.

Miller WC, Lindeman AK. 1997. The role of diet and exercise in weight management. In: Dalton S, ed. *Overweight and Weight Management: The Health Professional's Guide To Understanding and Practice*. Gaithersburg, MD: Aspen Publishers. Pp. 405–438.

Mokdad AH, Serdula MK, Dietz WH, Bowman BA, Marks JS, Koplan JP. 1999. The spread of the obesity epidemic in the United States, 1991–1998. *J Am Med Assoc* 282:1519–1522.

Molarius A, Seidell JC, Sans S, Tuomilehto J, Kuulasmaa K. 2000. Educational level, relative body weight, and changes in their association over 10 years: An international perspective from the WHO MONICA Project. *Am J Public Health* 90:1260–1268.

Morgan KJ, Goungetas B. 1986. Snacking and eating away from home. In: *What is America Eating?* Washington, DC: National Academy Press. Pp. 91–125.

Murata M. 2000. Secular trends in growth and changes in eating patterns of Japanese children. *Am J Clin Nutr* 72:1379S–1383S.

Must A, Jacques PF, Dallal GE, Bajema CJ, Dietz WH. 1992. Long-term morbidity and mortality of overweight adolescents: A follow-up of the Harvard Growth Study of 1922–1935. *New Engl J Med* 327:1350–1355.

Must A, Spandano J, Coakley EH, Field AE, Colditz G, Dietz WH. 1999. The disease burden associated with overweight and obesity. *J Am Med Assoc* 282:1523–1529.

Nagashima K, Zabriskie JB, Lyons MJ. 1992. Virus-induced obesity in mice: Association with a hypothalamic lesion. *J Neuropath Exp Neuro* 51:101–109.

NCHS (National Center for Health Statistics). 1998. *Health, United States 1998 with Socioeconomic Status and Health Chart Book*. PHS 98-1232. Hyattsville, MD: HHS. P. 283.

NHLBI (National Heart, Lung and Blood Institute). 1998. Clinical guidelines on the identification, evaluation, and treatment of overweight and obesity in adults—The evidence report. *Obes Res* 6:51S–209S.

Nides M, Rand C, Dolce J, Murray R, O'Hara P, Voelker H, Connett J. 1994. Weight gain as a function of smoking cessation and 2-mg nicotine gum use among middle-aged smokers with mild lung impairment in the first 2 years of the Lung Health Study. *Health Psychol* 13:354–361.

Nielsen SJ, Popkin BM. 2003. Patterns and trends in food portion sizes, 1977–1998. *J Am Med Assoc* 289:450–453.

NIH (National Institutes of Health). 1992. Consensus development conference statement on gastrointestinal surgery for severe obesity. *Am J Clin Nutr* 55:615S–619S.

Nolte R, Franckowiak SC, Crespo CJ, Andersen RE. 2002. U.S. military weight standards: What percentage of U.S. young adults meet the current standards. *Am J Med* 113:486–490.

Noppa H, Andersson M, Bengtsson C, Bruce A, Isaksson B. 1980. Longitudinal studies of anthropometric data and body composition. The population study of women in Goteborg, Sweden. *Am J Clin Nutr* 33:155–162.

Novak LP. 1972. Aging, total body potassium, fat-free mass, and cell mass in males and females between ages 18 and 85 years. *J Gerontol* 27:438–443.

O'Brien TP, Walley PB, Anderson-Smith S, Drabman RS. 1982. Naturalistic observation of the snack-selecting behavior of obese and nonobese children. *Addict Behav* 7:75–77.

Ogden CL, Flegal KM, Carroll MD, Johnson CL. 2002. Prevalence and trends in overweight among U.S. children and adolescents, 1999–2000. *J Am Med Assoc* 288:1728–1732.

Okada S, York DA, Bray GA, Erlanson-Albertsson C. 1991. Enterostatin (Val-Pro-Asp-Pro-Arg), the activation peptide of procolipase selectively reduces fat intake. *Physiol Behav* 49:1185–1189.

Oken E, Gillman MW. 2003. Fetal origins of obesity. *Obes Res* 11:496–506.

Ornish D. 1993. *Eat More, Weigh Less*. New York: Harper Collins.

Ortiz O, Russell M, Daley TL, Baumgartner RN, Waki M, Lichtman S, Want J, Pierson RN, Heymsfield SB. 1992. Differences in skeletal muscle and bone mineral mass between black and white females and their relevance to estimates of body composition. *Am J Clin Nutr* 55:8–13.

Owens JF, Matthews KA, Wing RR, Kuller LH. 1992. Can physical activity mitigate the effects of aging in middle-aged women? *Circulation* 85:1265–1270.

Parker JD, Abrams B. 1993. Differences in postpartum weight retention between black and white mothers. *Obstet Gynecol* 81:768–774.

Pasman WJ, Saris WH, Wauters MA, Westerterp-Plantenga MS. 1997a. Effect of one week of fibre supplementation on hunger and satiety ratings and energy intake. *Appetite* 29:77–87.

Pasman WJ, Westerterp-Plantenga MS, Muls E, Vansant G, van Ree J, Saris WH. 1997b. The effectiveness of long-term fibre supplementation on weight maintenance in weight-reduced women. *Int J Obes Relat Metab Disord* 21:548–555.

Pasman WJ, Westerterp-Plantenga MS, Saris WH. 1997c. The effectiveness of long-term supplementation of carbohydrate, chromium, fibre and caffeine on weight maintenance. *Int J Obes* 21:1143–1151.

Pate RR, Pratt M, Blair SN, Haskell WL, Macera CA, Bouchard C, Buchner D, Ettinger W, Heath GW, King AC, Kriska A, Leon AS, Marcus BH, Morris J, Pafenbarger RS, Patrick K, Pollock ML, Rippe JM, Sallis J, Wilmore JH. 1995. Physical activity and public health. A recommendation from the Centers for Disease Control and Prevention and the American College of Sports Medicine. *J Am Med Assoc* 273:402–407.

Pavlou KN, Drey S, Steffee WP. 1989a. Exercise as an adjunct to weight loss and maintenance in moderately obese subjects. *Am J Clin Nutr* 49:1115–1123.

Pavlou KN, Whatley JE, Jannace PW, DiBartolomeo JJ, Burrows BA, Duthie EA, Lerman RH. 1989b. Physical activity as a supplement to a weight-loss dietary regimen. *Am J Clin Nutr* 49:1110–1114.

Payne JH, DeWind LT. 1969. Surgical treatment of obesity. *Am J Surg* 118:141–147.

Pelleymounter MA, Cullen MJ, Baker MB, Hecht R, Winters D, Boone T, Collins F. 1995. Effects of the obese gene product on body weight regulation in ob/ob mice. *Science* 269:540–543.

Perkins KA. 1993. Weight gain following smoking cessation. *J Consult Clin Psychol* 61:768–777.

Perri MG, Sears SF, Clark JE. 1993. Strategies for improving maintenance of weight loss. Toward a continuous care model of obesity management. *Diabetes Care* 16:200–209.

Perri MG, Nezu AM, McKlvey WF, Shermer RL, Renjilian DA, Viegener BJ. 2001. Relapse prevention training and problem-solving therapy in the long-term management of obesity. *J Consult Clin Psychol* 69:722–726.

Pérusse L, Bouchard C. 1999. Genotype-environment interaction in human obesity. *Nutr Rev* 57:S31–S37.

Pérusse L, Chagnon YC, Weisnagel J, Bouchard C. 1999. The human obesity gene map: The 1998 update. *Obes Res* 7:111–129.

Peterson AL, Talcott GW, Kelleher WJ, Smith SD. 1995. Bulimic weight-loss behaviors in military versus civilian weight-management programs. *Mil Med* 160:616–620.

Phillips DF. 1998. Leptin passes safety tests, but effectiveness varies. *J Am Med Assoc* 280:869–870.

Phinney S. 1992. Exercise in the treatment of obesity. *J Fla Med Assoc* 79:400–402.

Phinney SD, Horton ES, Sims EA, Hanson JS, Danforth E Jr, LaGrange BM. 1980. Capacity for moderate exercise in obese subjects after adaptation to a hypocaloric, ketogenic diet. *J Clin Invest* 66:1152–1161.

Pi-Sunyer FX. 1988. Obesity. In: Shils ME, Young VR, eds. *Modern Nutrition in Health and Disease.* 7th ed. Philadelphia: Lea & Febiger. Pp. 795–816.

Pi-Sunyer FX. 1993. Medical hazards of obesity. *Ann Intern Med* 119:655–660.

Piatti PM, Monti LD, Magni F, Fermo I, Baruffaldi L, Nasser R, Santambrogio G, Librenti MC, Galli-Kienle M, Pontiroli AE, Pozza G. 1994. Hypocaloric high-protein diet improves glucose oxidation and spares lean body mass: Comparison to hypocaloric high-carbohydrate diet. *Metabolism* 43:1481–1487.

Pittler MH, Abbot NC, Harkness EF, Ernst E. 1999. Randomized, double-blind trial of chitosan for body weight reduction. *Eur J Clin Nutr* 53:379–381.

Poehlman ET, Tchernof A. 1998. Traversing the menopause: Changes in energy expenditure and body composition. *Coron Art Dis* 9:799–803.

Poirier P, Despres JP. 2001. Exercise in weight management of obesity. *Cardiol Clin* 19:459–470.

Pories WJ, MacDonald KG, Morgan EJ, Sinha MK, Dohm GL, Swanson MS, Barakat HA, Khazanie PG, Leggett-Frazier N, Long SD, O'Brien KF, Caro JF. 1992. Surgical treatment of obesity and its effect on diabetes: 10 Year followup. *Am J Clin Nutr* 55:582S–585S.

Pories WJ, Swanson MS, MacDonald KG, Long SB, Morris PG, Brown BM, Barakat HA, de Ramon RA, Israel G, Dolezal JM, Dohm L. 1995. Who would have thought it? An operation proves to be the most effective therapy for adult-onset diabetes mellitus. *Ann Surg* 222:339–352.

Prewitt TE, Schmeisser D, Brown PE, Aye P, Dolecek TA, Langenberg P, Cole T, Brace L. 1991. Changes in body weight, body composition, and energy intake in women fed high- and low-fat diets. *Am J Clin Nutr* 54:304–310.

Pritikin N. 1982. *The Pritikin Permanent Weight Loss Manual*. New York: Bantam Books.

Putnam JJ, Allshouse JE. 1999. *Food Consumption, Prices, and Expenditures, 1970–97.* Statistical Bulletin No. 965. Food and Rural Economics Division, Economic Research Service. Washington, DC: U.S. Department of Agriculture.

Quesenberry CP Jr, Caan B, Jacobson A. 1998. Obesity, health services use, and health care costs among members of a health maintenance organization. *Arch Intern Med* 158:466–472.

Raben A, Christensen NJ, Madsen J, Holst JJ, Astrup A. 1994. Decreased postprandial thermogenesis and fat oxidation but increased fullness after a high-fiber meal compared with a low-fiber meal. *Am J Clin Nutr* 59:1386–1394.

Rankinen T, Pérusse L, Weisnagel SJ, Snyder EE, Chagnon YC, Bouchard C. 2002. The human obesity gene map: The 2001 update. *Obes Res* 10:196–243.

Rasmussen MH, Andersen T, Breum L, Gotzsche PC, Hilsted J. 1993. Cimetidine suspension as adjuvant to energy restricted diet in treating obesity. *Br Med J* 306:1093–1096.

Ravelli GP, Stein, ZA, Susser MW. 1976. Obesity in young men after famine exposure in utero and early infancy. *N Engl J Med* 295:349–353.

Ravussin E, Burnand B, Schutz Y, Jequier E. 1982. Twenty-four-hour energy expenditure and resting metabolic rate in obese, moderately obese, and control subjects. *Am J Clin Nutr* 35:566–573.

Ravussin E, Lillioja S, Knowler WC, Christin L, Freymond D, Abott WG, Boyce V, Howard BV, Bogardus C. 1988. Reduced rate of energy expenditure as a risk factor for body-weight gain. *N Engl J Med* 318:467–472.

Reed DR, Ding Y, Xu W, Cather C, Price RA. 1995. Human obesity does not segregate with the chromosomal regions of Prader-Willi, Bardet-Biedl, Cohen, Borjeson or Wilson-Turner syndromes. *Int J Obes Relat Metab Disord* 19:599–603.

Ricaurte GA, Molliver ME, Martello MB, Katz JL, Wilson MA, Martello AL. 1991. Dexfenfluramine neurotoxicity in brains of non-human primates. *Lancet* 338:1487–1488.

Ricca V, Mannucci E, Di Bernardo M, Rizzello SM, Cabras PL, Rotella CM. 1997. Sertraline enhances the effects of cognitive-behavioral treatment on weight reduction of obese patients. *J Endocrinol Invest* 19:727–733.

Rice T, Sjostrom CD, Pérusse L, Rao DC, Sjostrom L, Bouchard C. 1999. Segregation analysis of body mass index in large sample selected for obesity: The Swedish Obese Subjects Study. *Obes Res* 7:246–255.

Rigaud D, Paycha F, Meulemans A, Merrouche M, Mignon M. 1998. Effect of psyllium on gastric emptying, hunger feeling and food intake in normal volunteers: A double blind study. *Eur J Clin Nutr* 52:239–245.

Riva A, Smigelski C, Friedman R. 2000. *WebDietAID: An Interactive Web-Based Nutritional Counselor*. In: *Converging Information, Technology, and Health Care: Proceedings of the 2000 AMIA Annual Symposium*. Bethesda, MD: American Medical Informatics Association. Pp. 709–713.

Robbins AS, Chao SY, Fonseca VP, Snedecor MR, Knapik JJ. 2001. Predictors of low physical fitness in a cohort of active-duty U.S. Air Force members. *Am J Prev Med* 20:90–96.

Robbins AS, Chao SY, Russ CR, Fonseca VP. 2002. Costs of excess body weight among active duty personnel, U.S. Air Force, 1997. *Mil Med* 167:393–397.

Rogers I. 2003. The influence of birthweight and intrauterine environment on adiposity and fat distribution in later life. *Int J Obes Relat Metab Disord* 27:755–777.

Rolland-Cachera MF, Deheeger M, Akrout M, Bellisle F. 1995. Influence of macronutrients on adiposity development: A follow up study of nutrition and growth from 10 months to 8 years of age. *Int J Obes Relat Metab Disord* 19:573–578.

Rolls BJ. 2000. The role of energy density in the overconsumption of fat. *J Nutr* 130:268S–271S.

Rolls BJ, Hammer VA. 1995. Fat, carbohydrate, and the regulation of energy intake. *Am J Clin Nutr* 62:1086S–1095S.

Rolls BJ, Shide DJ, Thorwart ML, Ulbrecht JS. 1998. Sibutramine reduces food intake in non-dieting women with obesity. *Obes Res* 6:1–11.

Rolls BJ, Bell A, Castellanos VH, Chow M, Pelkman CL, Thorwart ML. 1999. Energy density but not fat content of foods affected energy intake in lean and obese women. *Am J Clin Nutr* 69:863–871.

Romieu I, Willett WC, Stampfer MJ, Colditz GA, Sampson L, Rosner B, Hennekens CH, Speizer FE. 1988. Energy intake and other determinants of relative weight. *Am J Clin Nutr* 47:406–412.

Root MP. 1990. Disordered eating in women of color. *Sex Roles* 22:525–546.

Rosenfeld WE, Kanner A, Jacobson N, Kretschmar P. 1997. Topiramate and concomitant weight loss. PADS Investigator Group. *Epilepsia* 38:98.

Rothacker DQ. 2000. Five-year self-management of weight using meal replacements: Comparison with matched controls in rural Wisconsin. *Nutrition* 16:344–348.

Rudman D, Feller AG, Nagraj HS, Gergans GA, Lalitha PY, Goldbery AF, Schlenker RA, Cohn L, Rudman IW, Amattson DE. 1990. Effects of human growth hormone in men over 60 years old. *N Engl J Med* 323:1–6.

Russ CR, Fonseca VP, Peterson AL, Blackman LR, Robbins AS. 2001. Weight gain as a barrier to smoking cessation among military personnel. *Am J Health Promot* 16:79–84.

Sacks FM, Castelli WP, Donner A, Kass EH. 1975. Plasma lipids and lipoproteins in vegetarians and controls. *N Engl J Med* 292:1148–1151.

Samaras K, Kelly PJ, Chiano MN, Spector TD, Campbell LV. 1999. Genetic and environmental influences on total-body and central abdominal fat: The effect of physical activity in female twins. *Ann Intern Med* 130:873–888.

Scalfi L, D'Arrigo E, Carandente V, Coltorti A, Contaldo F. 1993. The acute effect of dexfenfluramine on resting metabolic rate and postprandial thermogenesis in obese subjects: A double-blind placebo-controlled study. *Int J Obes Relat Metab Disord* 17:91–96.

Schoeller DA, Shay K, Kushner RF. 1997. How much physical activity is needed to minimize weight gain in previously obese women? *Am J Clin Nutr* 66:551–556.

Schonfeld J, Evans DF, Wingate DL. 1997. Effect of viscous fiber (guar) on postprandial motor activity in human small bowel. *Dig Dis Sci* 42:1613–1617.

Schutz Y, Munger R, Deriaz O, Jequier E. 1992. Effect of dexfenfluramine on energy expenditure in man. *Int J Obes Relat Metab Disord* 16:S61–S66.

Schwartz RS, Shuman WP, Larson V, Cain KC, Fellingham GW, Beard JC, Kahn SE, Stratton JR, Cerqueira MD, Abrass IB. 1991. The effect of intensive endurance exercise training on body fat distribution in young and older men. *Metabolism* 40:545–551.

Scopinaro N, Gianetta E, Civalleri D, Bonalumi U, Bachi V. 1979. Biliopancreatic bypass for obesity: II. Initial experience in man. *Br J Surg* 66:618–620.

Scopinaro N, Adami GF, Marinari GM, Gianetta E, Traverso E, Friedmen D, Camerini G, Baschieri G, Simonelli A. 1998. Biliopancreatic diversion. *World J Surg* 22:936–946.

Seagle HM, Bessesen DH, Hill JO. 1998. Effects of sibutramine on resting metabolic rate and weight loss in overweight women. *Obes Res* 6:115–121.

Sears B, Lawren B. 1998. *The Zone.* New York: Harper Collins.

Senauer B. 1986. Economics and nutrition. In: *What is America Eating?* Washington, DC: National Academy Press. Pp. 46–57.

Serdula MK, Williamson DF, Anda RF, Levy A, Heaton A, Byers T. 1994. Weight control practices in adults: Results of a multistate telephone survey. *Am J Pub Health* 84:1821–1824.

Shah M, Garg A. 1996. High-fat and high-carbohydrate diets and energy balance. *Diabetes Care* 19:1142–1152.

Sharp MA, Nindl BC, Westphal KA, Friedl KE.1994. The physical performance of female army basic trainees who pass and fail the army body weight and percent body fat standards. In: Aghazadeh F, ed. *Advances in Industrial Ergonomics and Safety VI.* Washington, D.C.: Taylor & Francis. Pp. 743–750.

Shekelle PG, Herdy ML, Morton SC, Maglione M, Mojica WA, Surttorp MJ, Rhodes SL, Jungvig L, Gagne J. 2003. Efficacy and safety of ephedra and ephedrine for weight loss and athletic performance. A meta-analysis. *J Am Med Assoc* 289:1537–1545.

Sheppard L, Kristal AR, Kushi LH. 1991. Weight loss in women participating in a randomized trial of low-fat diets. *Am J Clin Nutr* 54:821–828.

Silverstone T. 1992. Appetite suppressants: A review. *Drugs* 43:820–836.

Sims EAH, Danforth E Jr, Horton ES, Bray GA, Glennon JA, Salans LB. 1973. Endocrine and metabolic effects of experimental obesity in man. *Rec Prog Horm Res* 29:457–464.

Singer B, Palmer B, Rogers B, Smith J. 2002. *Military Services Physical Fitness and Weight Management Database: A Review and Analysis.* HSIAC-RA-2002-001. Wright-Patterson Air Force Base, OH: Human Systems IAC.

Sjostrom L, Rissanen A, Anderson T, Boldrin M, Golay A, Koppeschaar HP, Krempf M. 1998. Randomised placebo-controlled trial of orlistat for weight loss and prevention of weight regain in obese patients. European Multicentre Orlistat Study Group. *Lancet* 352:167–172.

Skender ML, Goodrick GK, Del Junco DJ, Reeves RS, Darnell L, Gotto AM, Foreyt JP. 1996. Comparison of 2-year weight loss trends in behavioral treatments of obesity: Diet, exercise, and combination interventions. *J Am Diet Assoc* 96:342–346.

Skov AR, Toubro S, Bulow J, Krabbe K, Parving HH, Astrup A. 1999a. Changes in renal function during weight loss induced by high vs low-protein low-fat diets in overweight subjects. *Int J Obes Relat Metab Disord* 23:1170–1177.

Skov AR, Toubro S, Ronn B, Holm L, Astrup A. 1999b. Randomized trial on protein vs carbohydrate in ad libitum fat reduced diet for the treatment of obesity. *Int J Obes Relat Metab Disord* 23:528–536.

Smith GP, Gibbs J. 1984. Gut peptides and postprandial satiety. *Federation Proc* 43:2889–2892.

Sorensen TI, Holst C, Stunkard AJ. 1998. Adoption study of environmental modifications of the genetic influences on obesity. *Int J Obes Relat Metab Disord* 22:73–81.

Sothern MS, Loftin JM, Udall JN, Suskind RM, Ewing TL, Tang SC, Blecker U. 1999. Inclusion of resistance exercise in a multidisciplinary outpatient treatment program for preadolescent obese children. *South Med J* 92:585–592.

Spahn JM. 1999. *The Sensible Weigh Lifestyle Change Program: an Air Force Weight-Management Program.* Presented at the Institute of Medicine Workshop on Military Weight-Management Programs: State of the Art and Future Initiatives, Washington, DC, October 25–26. Subcommittee on Military Weight Management.

Sperry L. 1985. Family processes in health promotion: Applications to weight management. Individual psychology. *J Adlerian Theory Res Practice* 41:544–551.

Stalonas PM, Perri MG, Kerzner AB. 1984. Do behavioral treatments of obesity last? A five-year follow-up investigation. *Addict Behav* 9:175–183.

Stanner SA, Bulmer K, Andres C, Lantseva OE, Borodina V, Poteen VV, Yudkin JS. 1997. Does malnutrition in utero determine diabetes and coronary heart disease in adulthood? Results from the Leningrad Siege Study, a cross sectional study. *Br Med J* 315:1342–1348.

Steen B, Isaksson B, Svanborg A. 1979. Body composition at 70 and 75 years of age: A longitudinal study. *J Clin Exp Gerontol* 1:185–200.

Stein TP, Scholl TO, Schluterm MD, Schroeder CM. 1998. Plasma leptin influences gestational weight gain and postpartum weight retention. *Am J Clin Nutr* 68:1236–1240.

Stevens J, Kumanyika SK, Keil JE. 1994. Attitudes toward body size and dieting: Differences between elderly black and white women. *Am J Public Health* 84:1322–1325

Stillman IM, Baker SS. 1978. *The Doctor's Quick Weight Loss Diet*. New York: Dell Publishing.

Stoa-Birketvedt G. 1993. Effect of cimetidine suspension on appetite and weight in overweight subjects. *Br Med J* 306:1091–1093.

Stock MJ. 1996. Potential for β_3–adrenoceptor agonists in the treatment of obesity. *Int J Obes* 20:4–5.

Strain GW, Zumoff B. 1992. The relationship of weight-height indices of obesity to body fat content. *J Am Coll Nutr* 11:715–718.

Strauss RS. 1999. Comparison of measured and self-reported weight and height in a cross-sectional sample of young adolescents. *Int J Obes Relat Metab Disord* 23:904–908.

Stunkard A, Sorensen TI, Hanis C, Teasdale TW, Chakraborty R, Schull WK, Schulsinger F. 1986. An adoption study of human obesity. *N Engl J Med* 314:193–198.

Stunkard AJ, Harris JR, Pedersen NL, McLearn GE. 1990. The body-mass index of twins who have been reared apart. *N Engl J Med* 322:1483–1487.

Sugerman HJ. 1987. Pulmonary function in morbid obesity. *Gastroenterol Clin North Am* 16:225–237.

Sugerman HJ, Fairman RP, Baron PL, Qwentus JA. 1986. Gastric surgery for respiratory insufficiency of obesity. *Chest* 90:81–86.

Sugerman HJ, Baron PL, Fairman RP, Evans CR, Betrovec GW. 1988. Hemodynamic dysfunction in obesity hypoventilation syndrome and the effects of treatment with surgically induced weight loss. *Ann Surg* 207:604–613.

Sugerman HJ, Londrey GL, Kellum JM, Wolf L, Liszka T, Engle KM, Birkenhauer R, Starkey JV. 1989. Weight loss with vertical banded gastroplasty and roux-y gastric bypass for morbid obesity with selective versus random assignment. *Am J Surg* 157:93–102.

Sugerman HJ, Felton WL 3rd, Salvant JB Jr, Sismanis A, Kellum JM. 1995. Effects of surgically induced weight loss on idiopathic intracranial hypertension in morbid obesity. *Neurology* 45:1655–1659.

Sugerman HJ, Felton WL 3rd, Sismanis A, Kellum JM, deMaria EJ, Sugerman EL. 1999. Gastric surgery for pseudotomor cerebri associated with severe obesity. *Ann Surg* 229:634–640.

Susser M, Stein Z. 1994. Timing in prenatal nutrition: A reprise of the Dutch Famine Study. *Nutr Rev* 52:84–94.

Takada H, Harrell J, Deng S, Bandgiwala S, Washino K, Iwata H. 1998. Eating habits, activity, lipids and body mass index in Japanese children: The Shiratori Children Study. *Int J Obes Relat Metab Disord* 22:470–476.

Tanasescu M, Ferris AM, Himmelgreen DA, Rodriguez N, Perez-Escamilla R. 2000. Biobehavioral factors are associated with obesity in Puerto Rican children. *J Nutr* 130:1734–1742.

Tanner CJ, Barakat HA, Dohm GL, Pories WJ, MacDonald KG, Cunningham PRG, Swanson MS, Houmard JA. 2002. Muscle fiber type is associated with obesity and weight loss. *Am J Physiol Endocrinol Metab* 282:E1191–E1196.

Tataranni PA, Larson DE, Snitkre S, Ravussin E. 1995. Thermic effect of food in humans: Methods and results from use of a respiratory chamber. *Am J Clin Nutr* 61:1013–1019.

Taylor CB, Fortmann SP, Flora J, Kayman S, Barrett DC, Jatulis D, Farquhar JW. 1991. Effect of long-term community health education on body mass index. The Stanford five-city project. *Am J Epidemiol* 134:235–249.

Thomas KT, Keller CS, Holbert KE. 1997. Ethnic and age trends for body composition in women residing in the U.S. southwest: II. total fat. *Med Sci Sports Exerc* 29:90–98.

Tonstad S, Pometta D, Erkelens DW, Ose L, Moccetti T, Schouten JA, Golay A, Reitsma J, Del Bufalo A, Pasotti E, van der Wal P. 1994. The effect of the gastrointestinal lipase inhibitor, orlistat, on serum lipids and lipoproteins in patients with primary hyperlipidaemia. *Eur J Clin Pharmacol* 46:405–410.

Toubro S, Astrup AV, Breum L, Quaade F. 1993. Safety and efficacy of long-term treatment with ephedrine, caffeine, and an ephedrine/caffeine mixture. *Int J Obes* 17:S69–S72.

Tremblay A, St. Pierre S. 1996. The hyperphagic effect of a high-fat diet and alcohol intake persists after control for energy density. *Am J Clin Nutr* 63:479–482.

Tremblay A, Wouters E, Wenker M, St. Pierre S, Bouchard C, Despres JP. 1995. Alcohol and a high-fat diet: A combination favoring overfeeding. *Am J Clin Nutr* 62:639–644.

Trent LK, Stevens LT. 1993. Survey of the Navy's three-tiered obesity treatment program. *Mil Med* 158:614–618.

Trent LK, Stevens LT. 1995. Evaluation of the Navy's obesity treatment program. *Mil Med* 160:326–330.

Trent LK, Thieding-Cencel D. 1995. Effects of chromium picolinate on body composition. *J Sports Med Phys Fitness* 35:273–280.

Troiano RP, Levitsky DA, Kalkwarf HJ. 1990. Effect of d,l-fenfluramine on thermic effect of food in humans. *Int J Obes* 14:647–655.

Troiano RP, Briefel RR, Carroll MD, Bialostosky K. 2000. Energy and fat intakes of children and adolescents in the United States: Data from the National Health and Nutrition Examination Surveys. *Am J Clin Nutr* 72:1343S–1353S.

Tzankoff SP, Norris AH. 1977. Effect of muscle mass decrease on age-related BMR changes. *J Appl Physiol* 43:1001–1006.

Tzankoff SP, Norris AH. 1978. Longitudinal changes in basal metabolism in man. *J Appl Physiol* 45:536–539.

USAF (U.S. Air Force). 1975. *Analysis of Human Body Composition Data as Related to Height and Age.* Report SAM-TR-75-38. October. USAF School of Aerospace Medicine, Brooks Air Force Base, Texas. San Antonio: USAF.

USAF. 2002. *The Weight and Body Fat Management Program.* Air Force Instruction 40-502. April 3. Washington, DC: U.S. Government Printing Office.

U.S. Army. 1987. *The Army Weight Control Program.* Army Regulation 600-9. June 10. Washington, DC: U.S. Government Printing Office.

U.S. Army. 1998. *Standards of Medical Fitness.* Army Regulation 40-501. February 27. Washington, DC: U.S. Government Printing Office

U.S. Census Bureau. 2003. *National Population Estimates-Characteristics.* Online. Available at http://eire.census.gov/popest/data/national/asro.php. Accessed July 11, 2003.

USMC (U.S. Marine Corps). 1995. *Marine Corps Uniform Regulations.* Marine Corps Order P1020.34F. January 27. Washington, DC: U.S. Government Printing Office. Chapter 8.

USMC. 2002. *Marine Corps Physical Fitness Test and Body Composition Program Manual.* Marine Corps Order 6100.12. May 10. Washington, DC: U.S. Government Printing Office.

U.S. Navy. 2002. *Physical Readiness Program.* Office of Personnel Navy Instruction 6110.1G. October 10. Washington, DC: U.S. Government Printing Office.

van Gaal LF, Broom JI, Enzi G, Toplak H. 1998. Efficacy and tolerability of orlistat in the treatment of obesity: A 6-month dose-ranging study. Orlistat Dose-Ranging Study Group. *Eur J Clin Pharmacol* 54:125–132.

van Puijenbroek EP, Meyboom RH. 1998. Semen-like urethral discharge during the use of mazindol. *Int J Eating Disorders* 24:111–113.

Vincent R, Roberts A, Frier M, Perkins AC, MacDonald IA, Spiller RC. 1995. Effect of bran particle size on gastric emptying and small bowel transit in humans: A scintigraphic study. *Gut* 37:216–219.

Vogel JA, Friedl KE. 1992. Body fat assessment in women. Special considerations. *Sports Med* 13:245–269.

Vorachek T. 1999. October 25. *The Air Force LEAN Program.* Presented at the Institute of Medicine Workshop on Military Weight-Management Programs: State of the Art and Future Initiatives, Washington, DC, October 25–26. Subcommittee on Military Weight Management.

Wadden TA. 1993. Treatment of obesity by moderate and severe caloric restriction. *Ann Intern Med* 119:688–693.

Wadden TA. 1995. Very-low-calorie diets: Appraisal and recommendations. In: Brownell KD, Fairburn CG, eds. *Eating Disorders and Obesity: A Comprehensive Handbook.* New York: Guilford Press. Pp. 484–490.

Wadden TA, Sarwer DB. 1999. Behavioral treatment of obesity: New approaches to an old disorder. In: Goldstein DJ, ed. *The Management of Eating Disorders and Obesity.* Totowa, NJ: Humana Press.

Wadden TA, Sternberg JA, Letizia KA, Stunkard AJ, Foster GD. 1989. Treatment of obesity by very low calorie diet, behavior therapy, and their combination: A five year perspective. *Int J Obes* 13:39–46.

Wadden TA, Bartlett SJ, Foster GD, Greenstein RA, Wingate BJ, Stunkard AJ, Letizia KA. 1995. Sertraline and relapse prevention training following treatment by very–low-calorie diet: A controlled clinical trial. *Obesity Res* 3:549–557.

Wang J, Thornton JC, Burastero S, Shen J, Tanenbaum S, Heymsfield SB, Pierson RN Jr. 1996. Comparisons for body mass index and body fat percent among Puerto Ricans, blacks, whites and Asians living in the New York City area. *Obes Res* 4:377–384.

Wannamethee SG, Shaper AG. 2003. Alcohol, body weight, and weight gain in middle-aged men. *Am J Clin Nutr* 77:1312–1317.

Wee CC, Phillips RS, Aurigemma G, Erban S, Kriegel G, Riley M, Douglas PS. 1998. Risk for valvular heart disease among users of fenfluramine and dexfenfluramine who underwent echocardiography before use of medication. *Ann Intern Med* 129:870–874.

Wei M, Macera CA, Hornung CA, Blair SN. 1997. Changes in lipids associated with changes in regular exercise in free-living men. *J Clin Epidemiol* 50:1137–1142.

Wei M, Kampert JB, Barlow CE, Nichaman MZ, Gibbons LW, Paffenbarger RS Jr, Blair SN. 1999. Relationship between low cardiorespiratory fitness and mortality in normal-weight, overweight, and obese men. *J Am Med Assoc* 282:1547–1553.

Weinsier RL, Nagy TR, Hunter GR, Darnell BE, Hensrud DD, Weiss HL. 2000. Do adaptive changes in metabolic rate favor weight regain in weight-reduced individuals? An examination of the set-point theory. *Am J Clin Nutr* 72:1088–1094.

Weintraub M. 1992. Long-term weight control study III (weeks 104 to 156): An open-label study of dose adjustment of fenfluramine and phentermine. *Clin Pharmacol Ther* 51:602–607.

Weintraub M, Hasday JD, Mushlin AI, Lockwood DH. 1984. A double blind clinical trial in weight control: Use of fenfluramine and phentermine alone and in combination. *Arch Intern Med* 144:1143–1148.

Weissman NJ, Tighe JF Jr, Gottdiener JS, Gwynne JT. 1998. An assessment of heart-valve abnormalities in obese patients taking dexfenfluramine, sustained-release dexfenfluramine, or placebo. *N Engl J Med* 339:725–732.

Wheeler DC. 1965. Physical standards in allied and enemy armies in WW II. *Mil Med* 130:899.

Whitaker RC, Wright JA, Pepe MS, Seidel KD, Dietz WH. 1997. Predicting obesity in young adulthood from childhood and parental obesity. *N Engl J Med* 337:869–873.

Wilbur J, Naftzger-Kang L, Miller AM, Chandler P, Montgomery A. 1999. Women's occupations, energy expenditure, and cardiovascular risk factors. *J Womens Health* 8:377–387.

Willett WC. 1998a. Dietary fat and obesity: An unconvincing relation. *Am J Clin Nutr* 68:1149–1150.

Willett WC. 1998b. Is dietary fat a major determinant of body fat? *Am J Clin Nutr* 67:556S–562S.

Williams PT. 1997. Evidence for the incompatibility of age-neutral overweight and age-neutral physical activity standards from runners. *Am J Clin Nutr* 65:1391–1396.

Williamson DF, Madans J, Pamuk E, Flegal KM, Kendrick JS, Serdula MK. 1994. A prospective study of childbearing and 10-year weight gain in U.S. white women 25 to 45 years of age. *Int J Obes* 18:561–569.

Wilson GT. 1995. Behavioral approaches to the treatment of obesity. In: Brownell DK, Fairburn CG, eds. *Eating Disorders and Obesity: A Comprehensive Handbook*. New York: Guilford Press. Pp. 479–483.

Wing RR. 1992. Behavioral treatment of severe obesity. *Am J Clin Nutr* 55:545S–551S.

Wing RR. 1998. Behavioral approaches to the treatment of obesity. In: Bray GA, Bouchard C, James WPT, eds. *Handbook of Obesity*. New York: Marcel Dekker. Pp. 855–873.

Wing RR, Greeno CG. 1994. Behavioural and psychosocial aspects of obesity and its treatment. *Baillieres Clin Endocrinol Metab* 8:689–703.

Winick C, Rothacker DQ, Norman RL. 2002. Four worksite weight loss programs with high-stress occupations using a meal replacement product. *Occup Med* 52:25–30.

Wolever TM, Chiasson JL, Josse RG, Hunt JA, Palmason C, Rodger NW, Ross SA, Ryan EA, Tan MH. 1997. Small weight loss on long-term acarbose therapy with no change in dietary pattern or nutrient intake of individuals with non-insulin-dependent diabetes. *Int J Obes* 21:756–763.

Wolfe BM, Giovannetti PM. 1991. Short-term effects of substituting protein for carbohydrate in diets of moderately hypercholesterolemic human subjects. *Metabolism* 40:338–343.

Wolfe RR. 1998. Fat metabolism in exercise. In: Richter EA, Kiens B, Galbo H, Saltin B, eds. *Skeletal Muscle Metabolism in Exercise and Diabetes.* New York: Plenum Press. Pp. 147–156.

Wuolijoki E, Hirvela T, Ylitallo P. 1999. Decrease in serum LDL cholesterol with microcrystalline chitosan. *Methods Find Exp Clin Pharmacol* 21:357–361.

Wurtman JJ, Wurtman RJ, Reynolds S, Tsay R, Chew B. 1987. Fenfluramine suppresses snack intake among carbohydrate cravers but not among non-carbohydrate cravers. *Int J Eating Disorders* 6:687–699.

Wylie-Rosett J. 1988. Obesity and type II diabetes. In: Frankle RT, Yang M-U, eds. *Obesity and Weight Control: The Health Professional's Guide to Understanding and Treatment.* Rockville, MD: Aspen Publishing. Pp. 425–440.

Wylie-Rosett J, Swencionis C, Ginsberg M, Cimino C, Wassertheil-Smoller S, Caban A, Segal-Isaacson CJ, Martin T, Lewis J. 2001. Computerized weight loss intervention optimizes staff time: The clinical and cost results of a controlled clinical trial conducted in a managed care setting. *J Am Diet Assoc* 101:1155–1162.

Yale CE. 1989. Gastric surgery for morbid obesity. *Arch Surg* 124:941–946.

Yen TT. 1995. ß-Agonists as antiobesity, antidiabetic and nutrient partitioning agents. *Obes Res* 3:531S–536S.

Young LR, Nestle M. 2002. The contribution of expanding portion sizes to the U.S. obesity epidemic. *Am J Public Health* 92:246–249.

Young LR, Nestle M. 2003. Expanding portion sizes in the U.S. marketplace: Implications for nutrition counseling. *J Am Diet Assoc* 103:231–234.

Zed C, James WP. 1986. Dietary thermogenesis in obesity: Fat feeding at different energy intakes. *Int J Obes* 10:375–390.

Zhi J, Melia AT, Guerciolini R, Chung J, Kinberg J, Hauptman JB, Patel IH. 1994. Retrospective population-based analysis of the dose-response (fecal fat excretion) relationship of orlistat in normal and obese volunteers. *Clin Pharmacol Ther* 56:82–85.

Ziegler RG, Hoover RN, Nomura AM, West DW, Wu AH, Pike MC, Lake AJ, Horn-Ross PL, Kolonel LN, Siiteri PK, Fraumeni JF Jr. 1996. Relative weight, weight change, height, and breast cancer risk in Asian-American women. *J Natl Cancer Inst* 88:650–660.

Zurlo F, Ferraro RT, Fontvielle AM, Rising R, Bogardus C, Ravussin E. 1992. Spontaneous physical activity and obesity: Cross-sectional and longitudinal studies in Pima Indians. *Am J Physiol* 263:E296–E300.

A

Workshop Agenda and Abstracts

Military Weight-Management Program Workshop
State of the Art and Future Initiatives

Subcommittee on Military Weight Management
Committee on Military Nutrition Research
Food and Nutrition Board
Institute of Medicine
The National Academies

October 25–26, 1999

Monday October 25, 1999

9:00 Welcome on Behalf of the Food and Nutrition Board
Dr. Allison A. Yates, Director, Food and Nutrition Board

9:05 Welcome on Behalf of the Subcommittee on Military Weight Management
Dr. Richard Atkinson, Chair, Subcommittee

9:15 Opening Comments on Behalf of the Military
LTC Karl E. Friedl, U.S. Army Medical Research and Materiel Command, Fort Detrick, Frederick, MD

9:30 Important Historical Military Data: Obesity and Mortality
Dr. William Page, Medical Follow-Up Agency, The National Academies

Part I: Weight Management in the Military Today (Moderator: Richard Atkinson)

9:45 Panel: Current Military Policies and Approaches to Body-Weight Management
LCDR Sue Hite, Health and Physical Fitness Branch, USN
LTC Francine LeDoux, Health Promotion Policy Officer, USA
LTC Leon Pappa, Training Program Branch, USMC
COL Esther Myers/LTC Regina Watson, Health Promotion, USAF
Discussion

11:00 Break

11:15 Challenges to Military Weight Standards and Maladaptive Practices of Service Members to Meet These Weight Standards
MAJ Stephen Bowles, M.D., U.S. Army Soldier Support Institute, Ft. Jackson, SC

12:30 Lunch

Part II: Current Military Weight-Loss/Management Programs (Moderator: John Vanderveen)

1:30 Panel: Effective Military Programs
Air Force Weight-Management Program – LTC Joanne Spahn, Elmendorf AFB, Alaska
The Air Force LEAN Program – CAPT Trisha Vorachek, McConnell AFB
Impact of a Shipboard Weight-Control Program - Dr. Karen E. Dennis, Veterans Affairs Medical Center, University of MD School of Medicine
Nutrition and Diet Aboard Submarines – LT Deborah White, Naval Submarine Medical Research Lab, Groton, CT
The Army's LEAN Program: Current Update – LTC Larry James, Walter Reed Army Medical Center
Army Weight-Management Instruction to Master Fitness Trainers – Dr. Lou Tomasi, LT Kerryn Davidson, Army Physical Fitness School, Ft. Benning, GA
Discussion

3:45 Break

Part III. Factors Affecting Weight Management (Moderator: John Fernstrom)

4:00 Behavior
Dr. Patrick O'Neil, Medical University of South Carolina
Dr. Gary Foster, University of Pennsylvania
Discussion

5:30 Adjourn

Tuesday, October 26, 1999

Part III. Factors Affecting Weight Management (cont.) (Moderator: William Dietz)

9:00 Genetic Influences on Obesity
Dr. Anthony Comuzzi, Southwestern Foundation for Biomedical Research
Effects of Age, Gender, and Ethnicity on Ideal Weight
Dr. June Stevens, University of North Carolina – Chapel Hill
Discussion

10:30 Break

Pharmacological Aids (Moderator: Steven Heymsfield)

11:00 The Pharmacology of Weight Loss and Its Potential Application in the Military Setting
MAJ H. Glenn Ramos, M.D., Fort Gordon, GA
Use of Pharmacologic Aids in Weight Management
Dr. Frank Greenway, Pennington Biomedical Research Center
Discussion

12:00 Lunch

Physiology – Physical Activity (Moderator: Barbara Hansen)

1:00 Effects of Exercise, Diet, and Weight Loss on Lipid Metabolism
Dr. Marcia Stefanick, Stanford University
Reproductive Health Issues in Fitness and Weight-Control Programs
Dr. Anne Loucks, Ohio University

2:00 **Obesity: An Infectious Disease?**
Dr. Nikhil Dhurandhar, Wayne State University
Discussion

Part IV: Factors Affecting Long-Term Maintenance of Weight Loss (Moderator: Arthur Frank)

2:45 *Dr. George Blackburn, Harvard Medical School*
Dr. John Jakicic, Miriam Hospital and Brown University
Discussion

3:45 Break

Part V: Effective Strategies for the Military Setting (Moderator: Gail Butterfield)

4:00 Panel Discussion
Military Speakers:
CAPT Trisha Vorachek (USAF)
LT Deborah White (USN)
Dr. H. Glenn Ramos (USA)
LT Kerryn Davidson (USA)
Civilian Speakers:
Dr. Frank Greenway
Dr. John Jakicic
Dr. Patrick O'Neil

5:00 Summary of the Workshop
Dr. Richard Atkinson, Subcommittee Chair
Dr. John Vanderveen, Vice-Chair

5:30 Adjourn

WORKSHOP ABSTRACTS

THE ARMY WEIGHT CONTROL PROGRAM (AR 600-9)

LTC Francince M. LeDoux, Health Promotion Policy Officer

The primary objective of the Army Weight Control Program (AWCP) is to ensure that all personnel are able to meet the physical demands of their duties under combat conditions and to present a trim military appearance at all times. Proper weight control assists Army personnel in establishing and maintaining discipline, operational readiness, optimal physical readiness, and effectiveness. The regulation establishes appropriate body-fat standards and provides procedures by which personnel are counseled to assist them in meeting the prescribed standards.

Historical Perspective

Prior to 1981, height/weight tables and a physician's assessment were used to determine body-fat standards. In 1981 DOD implemented the Physical Fitness and Weight Control Program (DOD Directive 1308.1). This program stated that various tests were acceptable for use in determining body fat. Between 1983 and 1986, the Army used the "pinch test" to determine body fat. Beginning in 1987, the DOD revised Directive 1308.1 stating that the skinfold measurement test would no longer be used, and that only the "Tape" measurement method should be used to measure body fat. The Army Weight Control Program (U.S. Army, 1986) was published in 1986. In 1994, Interim Change 101 specified that all soldiers were to be issued Handbook/Issue 15. In 1995, DOD Directive 1308.1 was revised, changing the body-fat standards and establishing fat standards for pregnant soldiers (DOD, 1995).

Rationale

The AWCP is based on body composition (body fat vs. total body mass). Physical fitness is key to body composition. Fit soldiers are better able to carry their load. They have less body fat and more muscle mass. In contrast, overfat soldiers are: less able to perform physical tasks, are at greater risk of developing injury, and have lower Army Physical Fitness Test scores. Excessive body fat also detracts from soldierly appearance.

Key Requirements

Soldiers are weighed every 6 months. If a soldier is overweight (exceeds the weight-for-height standard) he or she will be measured for percent body fat using the "tape test" circumference method. The measurement sites for males are: abdomen, neck with a range of 20–26 percent body fat (maximum); and for females: neck, forearm, wrist, and hip with a range of 20–36 percent body fat (maximum). If a soldier is overfat he or she is enrolled in the AWCP.

AWCP Enrollment

Soldiers enrolled in the AWCP will have a permanent record on file. Each soldier enrolled is required to attend nutritional counseling and is weighed on a monthly basis. A soldier may only be removed from the program when body-fat standards have been achieved. The height/weight table standards will not be used. The standard requires a loss of 3–8 lb per month. If a soldier fails to make satisfactory progress in two consecutive months, he or she can be discharged per AR 635-200, Chapter 18, Personnel Separations (U.S. Army, 2000).

Medical Limitations and Pregnant Soldiers

Medical limitations include pregnancy, hospitalization, prolonged medical treatment, and positive profiles according to Mandatory Medical Review Boards.

Once a female soldier is diagnosed as pregnant, she is exempt from the standards of AR 600-9 during pregnancy and for 6 months postpartum. The soldier will remain in the program if she was enrolled previously. After 6 months postpartum, she will continue on the AWCP with physician clearance. Postpartum soldiers may request to be weighed anytime before 6 months. This standard implements DOD Directive 1308.1, July 20, 1995.

References

DOD (U.S. Department of Defense). 1995. *DOD Physical Fitness and Body Fat Program Procedures*. Department of Defense Directive 1308.1. July 20. Washington, DC: U.S. Government Printing Office.

U.S. Army. 1986. *The Army Weight Control Program*. Army Regulation 600-9. September 1. Washington, DC: U.S. Government Printing Office.

U.S. Army (U.S. Department of the Army). 2000. *Enlisted Personnel*. Army Regulation 635-200. November 1. Washington, DC: U.S. Government Printing Office.

CHALLENGES TO MILITARY WEIGHT STANDARDS AND MALADAPTIVE PRACTICES OF SERVICE MEMBERS TO MEET THESE WEIGHT STANDARDS

MAJ Stephen V. Bowles, PhD, United States Army Soldier Support Institute, Director, USAREC Command Psychological Operations, Fort Jackson, South Carolina

At the time this abstract was written, no information on service members who exceed weight standards or have been discharged from the service in 1999 could be obtained from DOD or individual services. It has been reported that as many as 40 percent of the soldiers discharged from the Army was due to service members being overweight (James et al., 1997). The military faces several challenges to include: overweight accessions into the military, lifestyle practices of overweight service members, and command awareness of lifestyle change programs.

Challenges to Military Weight Standards

With current recruitment shortfalls, the number of overweight recruits (meeting accession standards but not the services retention standard for weight) may be increasing due to a smaller applicant pool. This can translate into a considerable number of overweight personnel entering yearly that meet accession standards but do not meet military retention standards at that time. This may place extra strain on the system to get personnel physically fit, while preparing new service members for the complexities of the military. In addition, this also places increased stress on young service members who are in many cases away from home for the first time in their first job.

With this in mind, educating recruiters on healthy lifestyle changes for new recruits may be beneficial. This may help reduce the time spent on new overweight service members and retain more personnel. Recruiters can be provided with lifestyle change training in recruiting school and provide recruits with approaches to healthy lifestyle change. Similarly, military academies and ROTC programs can provide training to new officers throughout their school years. Students must be trained in maintaining healthy lifestyles in accordance with military weight guidelines. These are important preventative measures in stressful academic environments, which may preclude students from engaging in maladaptive eating behaviors.

Eating on the run is sometimes dictated by our mission. When training new service members today we have attempted to offer adequate time to eat in dinning facilities. This is different from the past where older, overweight service members have identified early dining experiences as eating as much as they can in as little time as possible. This set the pattern of their eating over the course of their military careers. When providing new personnel training and education on healthy lifestyle behaviors, we must incorporate these changes into our training structures as best we can. As a tradition, service members have complained about the food provided to them in the mess hall or galley. However, great improvements have been made in the quality of foods. More effort needs to be initiated in educating cooks (James et al., 1999) to provide more variety in the low-fat main dishes served for lunch and dinner. Furthermore, there should be uniformity across dining facilities in the education of customers on calorie and fat gram amounts per food served.

Maladaptive Practices of Service Members

While there are differences in each of the services' military weight/body-fat standards, the goal of each service member twice a year is to meet the weight standard and pass the physical fitness test. The family is well aware of the borderline or overweight service member's plight at these times of the year. There is often tension in the home emanating from the service member's desire and actions to stay off the weight program. This may involve physical fitness training five times or more a week. Additionally, a service member will attempt to lose weight by using over-the-counter medication. They may go to the local health food store and purchase different herbal supplements or attend a local weight-reduction clinic and get on prescription medication. They will sit in the sauna, or they may obtain laxatives through the local drug store or their medical facility if they are on the hospital staff. If they are looking for the more popular diets, they can choose from protein, blood, cabbage, grapefruit or what ever the most recent diet is. Of the 108 applicant records examined for the Eisenhower LIFE Program, 34 percent reported starving or fasting, 33 percent reported using laxatives or over-the-counter medication, and 4 percent reported purging at some time in their career.

Meeting Military Weight Standards: Lifestyle Change Programs

Across the services there is a need to become more familiar with various programs available in local areas and encourage the use of these programs. Units that have used local lifestyle change (weight) programs are able to save financial resources for their organizations and save units time if their armed service program is several hours or states away from where they are located.

As a group, the medical field must educate the commanders in their area on services available to assist service members in weight reduction. Commanders, after seeing the results of their service members in lifestyle change programs, will be a steady referral source to programs. The Eisenhower LIFE Program (a week-long day-treatment program and 1 year follow-up) disseminated an 11 question survey asking commanders and supervisors for their feedback on the program. The results of 9 of the questions from the survey are found in Figure 1. Ninety percent of the respondents were from the Army, while the remainder of the respondents were from the Air Force, Navy, and Marines.

The results of the survey indicate that 22 out of 24 commanders/ supervisors responding, were satisfied with the program. Most respondents agreed that the program saved their unit time (81 percent), prevented the service member from separation from the military (91 percent), taught the service member new information for weight management (96 percent), and provided a comprehensive multidisciplinary program for weight reduction (91 percent). In addition, 96 percent believed a specialized physical training program is helpful for weight reduction, while 86 percent supported a specialized LIFE physical training program. While 95 percent believed weekly support groups are helpful, only 73 percent supported service members attending weekly support groups. Though some commanders/supervisors prefer to operate their own physical training and follow-up support (perhaps due to unit esprit de corps or due to shortage of work personnel), these results suggest that overall, commanders support this lifestyle change program.

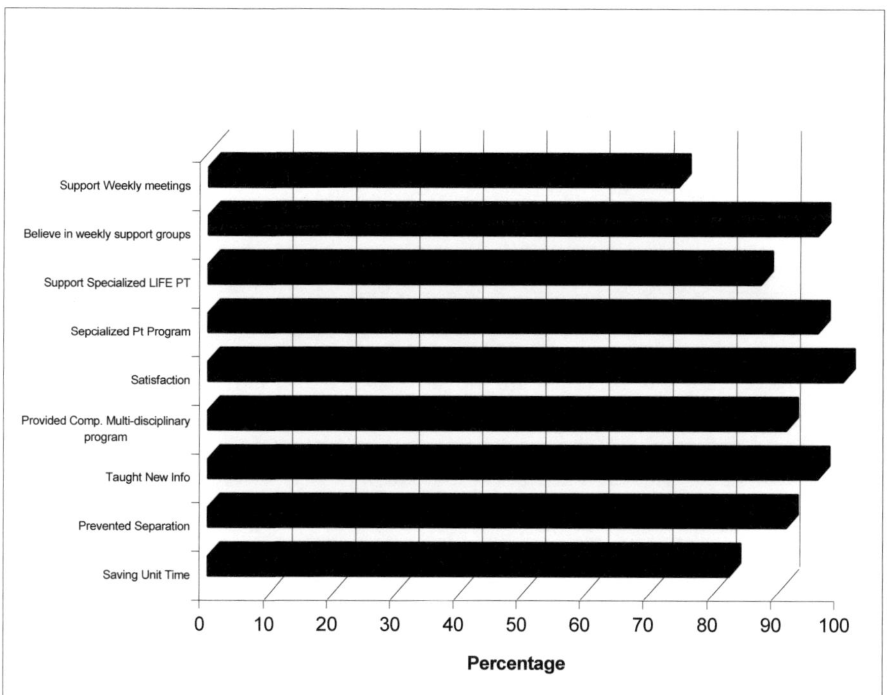

FIGURE 1 Command Satisfaction Survey.

These findings suggest that commands are open to assistance from weight-reduction programs to maintain readiness levels in their organizations. Similar education and training can be provided across the services to assist service members in meeting their organizations' weight standards. The training provided to service members and in support of service members can be provided through healthy lifestyle change programs.

References

James LC, Folen RA, Garland FN, Edwards C, Noce M, Gohdes D, Williams D, Bowles S, Kellar MA, Supplee E. 1997. The Tripler Army Medical Center LEAN program: A healthy lifestyle model for the treatment of obesity. *Mil Med* 162:328–332.

James LC, Folen RA, Page H, Noce M, Brown J, Britton C. 1999. The Tripler LEAN program: A two-year follow-up report. *Mil Med* 164:389–395.

THE SENSIBLE WEIGH LIFESTYLE CHANGE PROGRAM: AN AIR FORCE WEIGHT-MANAGEMENT PROGRAM

Joanne M. Spahn, Lt Col, USAF, BSC, MS, RD

The health risks associated with overweight and obesity are well established (NHLBI, 1998; Van Itallie, 1985) and the incidence of overweight continues to rise (Kuczmarski et al., 1994). In the military, sustained overweight can end an otherwise successful career. An increased operations tempo, decreased physical activity, and easy availability of calorie-dense foods may frustrate earnest weight-management efforts. Until the 1990s, the typical Air Force treatment program for overweight entailed a single group class where military members were given instruction on a low calorie diet, typically 1,200–1,800 calories, information on behavior modification, and counseled to exercise three to five times a week for 30 minutes. In the late 1980s and early 1990s, numerous published or home-grown multisession programs were established at a variety of sites. These programs for the most part emphasized increased physical activity, modest calorie restriction, skill development in selecting and preparing healthy foods, and behavior modification techniques. At most sites, these programs could accommodate few participants. There was fear among active duty personnel that weight loss would be too slow to meet weight-loss requirements.

In the early 1990s, the National Institutes of Health held a Technology Assessment Conference on Methods for Voluntary Weight Loss and Control. In 1995, *Weighing the Options: Criteria for Evaluating Weight-Management Programs* was published (IOM, 1995). These materials were utilized to guide development of The Sensible Weigh Program initiated in 1997. Practical managerial constraints and Weight Management Program (WMP) guidelines factored into program development. Specifically, this included the need for military members to loss 3 to 5 lb the first month identified as overweight to avoid disciplinary action and the need for Wing and Army Commander support of treatment incorporating increased use of duty time. Deployment of The Sensible Weigh to a large number of bases with varying levels of manpower support has also shaped program implementation across the Air Force.

The Sensible Weigh is a lifestyle change program aimed at optimizing weight and fitness of military members and their families. It is a science-based protocol designed to prevent weight gain, facilitate weight loss, and the maintenance of weight loss. It was developed to support the Air Force WMP and as an avenue for commanders and health care providers to intervene with concerned individuals early, before negative consequences occur. This multi-disciplinary program offers participants a variety of strategies from which to choose to improve their nutrition, fitness, and health. Program materials are available on the web at the following site: http://afmam.satx.disa.mil.

Clients enrolling in The Sensible Weigh can either self-refer, be sent by their squadron, or be referred by a medical provider. The protocol begins with a thorough assessment of anthropometric, biochemical parameters, comorbidities, medications, family history, weight and dieting history, exercise habits, diet readiness, and evaluation of the Physical Activity Readiness Questionnaire. Nursing personnel review the assessment form with clients and use standardized guidelines to refer clients to medical providers when the need arises. Assessment data is used to tailor the program to meet client needs, discuss the benefits of weight management in terms other than pounds lost, and to facilitate measurement of program efficacy.

Program length varies from 4 to 12 weeks. The first four core classes are taken by all participants in The Sensible Weigh and provide a foundation of information and skills. The first class orients clients to the concept of lifestyle change, the diverse benefits of weight management, addresses relapse prevention and diet readiness, and encourages increased physical activity. Clients are instructed on how to complete a food and exercise diary and are required to monitor their eating habits for the coming week. This is an important class for establishing rapport, venting anger, and building a trusting relationship. This was a difficult class to implement because of the immediate penalties incurred if members did not lose the prescribed weight in the first 30 days. Members and supervisors were concerned that the member did not "get the diet."

During the second class, each client receives a calorie and fat budget following Step I diet recommendations. Clients are offered a variety of strategies from which to choose to modify their diet. Strategies include calorie counting, fat gram counting, following food guide pyramid guidelines, and following a calorie controlled meal plan. Pros and cons of each method are discussed and clients select the strategy they feel best meets their needs. The food and exercise diary is used to track progress. Instructors, called coaches, review food diaries at each visit and provide individualized coaching on strategies to improve the healthfulness of the client's diet and fitness regimen and provide encouragement. It takes a few weeks for many clients to become proficient in maintaining a food diary.

Class three is taught by an exercise physiologist who covers the basic components of a personal fitness program targeted at reducing body fat. American Academy of Sports Medicine fitness guidelines are used. A strong emphasis on fitness is crucial in this young, moderately overweight and healthy population (IOM, 1995). Members are encouraged to have a personalized fitness prescription designed for them by the exercise physiologist. The forth class covers the basics of behavior modification and the concept of behavior chains. During the final core class, clients sign-up for their next four electives. Client goals and Diet Readiness Test results are utilized in deciding which electives might be most beneficial.

Electives are taught by a variety of people from diverse disciplines and may include skill development classes on dining out, supermarket tours and cooking demonstrations, stress management and classes covering relapse prevention, cognitive-behavioral therapy, and a variety of fitness topics. Support groups are offered weekly and participants are encouraged to attend one elective or one support group per week. This modular approach facilitates tailoring the program to the diverse needs of a population and allows for more flexible use of limited manpower resources. Electives are typically scheduled two times per month.

Outcome statistics have been maintained on The Sensible Weigh. Between February 1997 and June 1998, 656 clients enrolled in The Sensible Weigh. Of this group, 24 percent were active duty, 38 percent were family members of active duty personnel, 8.9 percent were retirees, and 28 percent were spouses of retired personnel. Thirty-three percent were self-referrals and 49 percent were referred by the Family Practice Clinic. At the 3-month follow-up, 163 (25 percent) returned and the average weight loss was 11.2 pounds. At the 6-month follow-up, 50 (10 percent) of clients returned for follow-up with an average weight loss of 15.7 pounds. Between October 1998 and February 1999, 94 active duty personnel were enrolled in The Sensible Weigh. Fifty-two (55 percent) returned for 3-month follow-up (21 Air Force, 21 Army personnel), and an average of 11.5 pounds was lost.

The Sensible Weigh represents incremental improvement in weight-management treatment in the Air Force. The program has been exported to many Air Force bases worldwide and a 1-week training program has been developed to train The Sensible Weigh coaches. Recent changes in Air Force WMP guidance have made implementation of The Sensible Weigh easier, particularly the requirement for a 90-day fitness and dietary program and the official implementation of a warning or cautionary zone prior to enrollment into the program. The withholding of promotions during this cautionary phase however, is still considered a significant program penalty. The new 90-day period, provided for a fitness and exercise program, allows members more time to address readiness to change issues. Few members referred due to the Weight and Body Fat Management Program come voluntarily and many would fall into Prochaska's precontemplation and contemplation stages of change (DiPietro, 1995). Most programs currently offered are tailored for clients in the preparation and action stage.

Posting The Sensible Weigh materials on the Air Force Medical Applications Model web site has facilitated implementation of the program at multiple sites and allows for a certain degree of standardization of weight-management treatment at numerous sites. Standardized treatment programs have many benefits, including the potential to improve staff training, improve continuity of care in a highly mobile population, facilitate increased collaboration, testing of hypotheses which could lead to program improvement, and allows for efficient program updates. Use of one standardized program however, is not sufficient to meet the needs of the entire population.

Availability of a variety of standardized programs using a variety of educational modalities would provide increased flexibility for service members, particularly those frequently deployed or on field duty. Research should describe characteristics of personnel on the weight-management program, barriers, enabling factors, stage of change information, current diet and fitness habits, typical lapse situations, strategies currently used for weight loss, sources of weight-management information, and preferred modes of education. This would be helpful in the development of programs tailored to the unique needs of military personnel and their families. Community programs, which address both prevention and treatment of overweight in military communities, are essential. The Sensible Weigh provides treatment on the individual level, but community programs that address environmental support for health and fitness are crucial.

References

DiPietro L. 1995. Physical activity, body weight, and adiposity: An epidemiological perspective. *Exerc Sport Sci Rev* 23:275–303.

IOM (Institute of Medicine). *Weighing the Options: Criteria for Evaluating Weight-Management Programs.* Washington, DC: National Academy Press.

Kuczmarski RJ, Flegal KM, Campbell SM, Johnson CL. 1994. Increasing prevalence of overweight among U.S. adults: The National Health and Nutrition Examination Surveys, 1960 to 1991. *J Am Med Assoc* 272:205–211.

NHLBI (National Heart, Lung and Blood Institute). 1998. Clinical guidelines on the identification, evaluation, and treatment of overweight and obesity in adults—The evidence report. In: Pi-Sunyer XP, Rosenhouse-Romeo H, eds. *Obes Res* 6:51S–209S.

Van Itallie TB. 1985. Health implications of overweight and obesity in the United States. *Ann Internal Med* 103:983– 988.

THE AIR FORCE LEAN PROGRAM

CAPT Trisha Vorachek, McConnell AFB

Prior to the July 1999 policy changes in the Air Force (AF) weight management program (WMP), most AF members identified as overfat received only a 2-hour nutrition class, taught by a registered dietitian or nutrition certified dietitian or medical technician, before officially entering the WMP. The overfat AF members were also monitored for successful weight loss progress. Once placed in the WMP, members were required monthly to lose either 3 pounds if female or 5 pounds if male or percent body fat until the body-fat standard was reached. If members did not make satisfactory progress, punitive action was taken, and after four failures, members were discharged from the AF. With only an insufficient 2-hour nutrition class to assist members in successfully attempting to reach their body-fat percentage goal, WMP discharges and frustrations of members and commanders were high. Therefore, in response to commanders' requests to develop a more positively focused WMP, the Lifestyle, Exercise, Attitude and Nutrition (LEAN) weight-loss program was developed and implemented at McConnell Air Force Base (AFB) in October 1995.

After reviewing the current research on weight-loss programs, the LEAN program was developed by a multidisciplinary team that included a physician, registered dietitian, psychologist, mental health technician, fitness specialist and the base health promotion manager. The newly created LEAN program was a mandatory, multidisciplinary 4-week program for all active duty (AD) members identified for the WMP after 15 Oct 1995. The LEAN program met weekly for 2 ½ to 3 ½ hours and, during each session, nutrition, behavior change and exercise were taught by a registered dietitian, psychologist, and exercise physiologist, respectively. Each member was required to attend all four sessions prior to officially being placed in the WMP. While in the LEAN program, members were not allowed to go on temporary duty or leave, except for emergency situations. Squadron commanders or first sergeants were notified of all missed appointments, and the member was automatically scheduled for the missed class in the next month's LEAN program. A new LEAN program started each month, and 1 week prior to the start of a new program, any remaining open slots were opened to AD volunteers, dependents, and retirees. After completing the LEAN program, members were required to attend a monthly group follow-up session until they met their body-fat standard.

The nutrition component of the LEAN program included guidelines on healthy weight loss, principles of the Food Guide Pyramid, food label reading, calorie and fat gram counting, self monitoring, dangers of fad dieting, low-fat cooking techniques, and healthy dining out. The behavior change portion of the LEAN program consisted of assessing stage of readiness, stimulus control, breaking associations, generating social support, realistic goal setting, stress management, and relapse prevention. Finally, the exercise component included recommendations and hands-on training regarding proper exercise warm-up and cool-down, stretching, aerobic conditioning, and strength training. The monthly group follow-up sessions expanded on the already discussed LEAN program topics, and monthly rotated between each discipline.

Only 9 months after the initial implementation of LEAN program, the program experienced great success. There was a 50 percent decrease in the percent of AD population on the WMP and over a 60 percent decrease in the monthly failure rate in the WMP. The LEAN program was also cited as one of the top three best things about McConnell AFB at the Senior Enlisted Advisor's Enlisted Call. Without a doubt, the greatest strengths of the LEAN program were the multidisciplinary approach and the length of the program. It was the first AF program to provide members with increased education, skills and support in all the disciplines necessary for successful weight loss *prior* to official placement in the WMP. The success of the LEAN program was a key factor in the current AF policy of members receiving 3 months of weight-loss counseling prior to starting the WMP.

Although I strongly agree that the military individual WMP needs improvement, I would also highly encourage the committee to consider making recommendations for environmental approaches to improving the military's WMP. Broad policy changes in regards to nutrition and exercise can have a much greater impact on the military's population as a whole then even the best individual focused weight-loss programs. For example, we know from current research that availability, taste, and price are three of the greatest factors affecting food selection today (Colby et al., 1987; French et al., 1999; Glanz et al., 1998; National Restaurant Association, 1984; National Restaurant Association and Gallop Organization, 1986). Therefore, example policies could be: all base eating establishments must have at least 30 percent of their menu as low-fat selections; or all low-fat foods in vending machines and cafeterias must cost 30 percent less than the high-fat food choices; or all food service personnel receive at least 1 week of low-fat cooking training during their technical school; or for at least 1 week every quarter, the food service workers on base receive additional training on low-fat cooking from a certified executive chef and culinary trainer. I commend the committee for addressing the need for changes to the counseling portion of the WMP, and I challenge the committee to take the next step and recommend policy changes that modify the military's environment to decrease barriers and enable the population as a whole to become more fit and healthy.

References

Colby JJ, Elder JP, Peterson Q, Knisley PK, Carleton RA. 1987. Promoting the selection of health food through menu item description in a family-style restaurants. *Am J Prev Med* 3:171–177.

French SA, Story K, Hannan P, Breitlow KK, Jeffery RW, Baxter JS, Snyder W. 1999. Cognitive and demographic correlates of low-fat vending snack choices among adolescents and adults. *J Am Diet Assoc* 99:471–475.

Glanz K, Basil K, Malibach E, Goldberg J, Snyder D. 1998. Why Americans eat what they do: Taste, nutrition, cost, convenience, and weight control concerns as influences on food consumption. J *Am Diet Assoc* 98:1118–1126.

National Restaurant Association. 1984. *Consumer Restaurant Behavior: A View based on Occasion Segmentation.* Washington, DC: NRA.

National Restaurant Association and Gallup Organization. 1986. *Changes in Consumer Eating Habits*. Washington, DC: NRA.

Additional Recommended Resources

Battle EK, Brownell KD. 1996. Confronting a rising tide of eating disorders and obesity: Treatment vs prevention and policy. *Addict Behav* 21:755–765.

French SA, Jeffrey RW, Story K Hannan P, Snyder MP. 1997. A pricing strategy to promote low-fat snack choices through vending machines. *Am J Public Health* 97:849–851.

French SA, Story K Jeffery RW, Snyder P, Eisenberg K, Sidebottom A, Murray D. 1997. Pricing strategy to promote fruit and vegetable purchase in high school cafeterias. *J Am Diet Assoc* 97:1008–1010.

Jeffrey RW. 1998. Prevention of obesity. In: Bray GA, Bouchard C, James WPT, eds. *Handbook of Obesity*. New York: Marcel Dekker. Pp. 819–829.

Jeffery RW, French SA, Raether C, Baxter JE. 1994. An environmental intervention to increase fruit and salad purchases in a cafeteria. *Prev Med* 23:788–792.

THE IMPACT OF A SHIPBOARD WEIGHT-CONTROL PROGRAM

Karen E. Dennis, PhD, RN, FAAN, and CAPT, NC, USNR[1,2,3], Karen W. Pane, MPA, RN, and LT, NC, USNR[3], Douglas D. Bradham, DrPH[1,2], Brett R. South, BS[1,2], Heather J. Saunders, MBA[1,2], Mark D. Heuser, MD, MS[1,2], Bing Bing Qi, MS[2]

[1]*University of Maryland, Baltimore, School of Medicine;*
[2]*Geriatric Research Education and Clinical Center at the Maryland VA Health Care System, Baltimore;*
[3]*US Navy-Reserve*

Background

Superimposed on obesity's risk factors for cardiovascular disease (CVD), Navy personnel who fail to meet Physical Readiness Test (PRT) and body-weight standards are subject to potentially serious administrative sanctions such as ineligibility for promotion or potential termination of their military careers. With impact beyond the well being of the individual service member, these administrative actions may signify the Navy's forfeiture of its investment in the development of personnel's unique knowledge, skills, and services. Although obesity has been projected to cost the Navy considerable dollars in inpatient bed days (Hoiberg and McNally, 1991), to our knowledge, health care expenses due to this particular condition and its associated sequelae among Navy personnel have never been quantified. Yet this is only a portion of the total economic impact of obesity (Colditz, 1992).

To assist its obese service members in attaining weight and fitness standards, the Navy implemented a multiple-tiered obesity treatment program. However, this remedial approach is not standardized and it typically fails to bring the majority of participants within weight standards (Trent and Stevens, 1993). In addition, over 80 percent of program time is devoted to physical activity even though 63 percent of enrollees are obese (Trent and Stevens, 1993) who need state-of-the-art, multi-faceted weight-loss programs (Goodrick and Foreyt, 1991; Wadden and Bell, 1990).

Aims

This study assessed whether a multi-faceted approach to weight loss and physical readiness could be implemented onboard ship, evaluated factors at sea that could affect the program's implementation, and determined its relative effectiveness in helping obese service members meet weight and physical fitness standards. Uniquely, this study also documented the economic impact (cost-effectiveness and cost-savings) of the shipboard weight-control program relative to the current Command Level program.

Methods, Intervention Component

Thirty-nine men (31 ± 6 years old, mean ± sd) assigned to the USS ENTERPRISE (CVN 65) during a 6-month Mediterranean deployment who had failed their previous PRT due to excessive body weight (108 ± 11 kg overweight) were randomly assigned to: (1) an experimental treatment of weekly sessions on diet, behavior modification, psychosocial issues, plus the current Command Level program of exercise, or (2) a usual care control treatment comprised of the existing Command Level program of exercise alone.

The goal of the experimental treatment was to educate participants in effective, realistic, and acceptable ways to adopt lifestyle, lifetime behaviors conducive to healthy nutrition, long-term weight control, and physical activity. The format was small group lecture/discussion conducted by a Navy dietitian. Groups of 10–12 individuals met in hour-long, weekly sessions for 16 weeks of the 6-month deployment to fit within the constraints of deployment time, departure from and return-to-port activities, as well as data collection onboard. The diet followed NCEP Step I (Heart Healthy) guidelines for dietary composition, with portions controlled to decrease energy intake by 500 calories per day to promote weight loss of 0.5–1 kg per week. The dietitian used a standardized instructor manual, and each participant received a notebook of course material generated and used in numerous studies in the Geriatric Research Education and Clinical Center at the VA Maryland Health Care System, Baltimore (Dengel et al., 1995; Dennis and Goldberg, 1996; Dennis et al., 2001; Landkammer et al., 1992; Nicklas et al., 1997a, 1997b). Behavior modification consisted of teaching participants well-documented behavioral modification techniques, such as dealing with external stimuli associated with eating occasions, and managing holidays and special events, including shore liberty. Combining a greater knowledge of food choices with an understanding of behavioral techniques enabled participants to select foods from a wider variety of alternatives, fully consider the consequences of each one, and structure the environment for success. Self-monitoring was introduced as a new lifestyle behavior that is central to achieving the desired weight-loss outcomes. Interpersonal processes were designed to build camaraderie and group support as participants were guided to creatively problem solve and adopt a series of small, achievable steps that had a cumulative impact on body weight.

The exercise program for the experimental group was the mandated program already being conducted for Command Level remediation (i.e., "Navy usual care"), which consisted of 1 hour of exercise 4 days per week. Established exercises included curl-ups, push-ups, walking, jogging, and other aerobic exercises conducive to successful completion of the PRT. PRT in the Navy involves sit-reach, curl-ups, push-ups, and a 1.5 mile run. Although standards are age- and gender-based, the "average" 31-year-old male participating in this study would need to touch his toes with legs out-stretched, perform 32 curl-ups and 23 push-ups, and run 1.5 miles in 15 minutes/30 seconds to pass the PRT. Exercise was not experimentally controlled because the intent of the study was to evaluate the addition of a standardized dietary behavioral modification component to the Navy's existing program.

Like the experimental group, men in the "usual care" control group (i.e., existing Command Level remediation program) knew that weight loss was requisite to continue their Navy careers beyond an 18-month grace period. While these men were provided nutrition fact sheets and brochures if requested, they did not receive group or individual counseling. The control group received "usual care" by participating, as required, in the current Command Level I program of exercise described above for the treatment group.

Methods and Results

Intervention Component

Prior to treatment there were no significant differences in body composition parameters (weight, BMI, percent body fat, waist and hip girths, waist/hip ratio) between men in the treatment and control groups. However, outcomes for the treatment group were significantly better than the controls, with 8.6 ± 5.0 vs 5.0 ± 4.1 kg weight loss, 8 percent versus 5 percent reduction in original body weight, and body-fat loss of 7 percent versus 5 percent. Moreover, 10 men in the treatment group vs only 2 in the control group lost at least 10 kg of their initial body weight. Prior to treatment, most CVD risk factors reflected values that were within NCEP guidelines. The exception was high-density lipoprotein cholesterol, which averaged 35 ± 8 mg/dl for the total group, and was low enough to place these men at increased CVD risk. With weight loss and exercise, triglycerides declined significantly greater in the treatment group than the controls (145 to 109 mg/dl vs 146 to 145 mg/dl, $p < .05$)

At baseline, despite random assignment, men in the treatment group reported significantly greater binge eating symptoms, less use of eating behaviors conducive to weight loss, and more difficulty controlling overeating at times of negative affect than men in the control group. At the end of the program, however, treated men had significant improvements in all of these elements, as well as a significant improvement in the difficulty they experienced controlling overeating in certain social circumstances. Beginning worse than the control group, men in the treatment group finished the study with similar or better eating behaviors than their counterparts. These outcomes hold even when controlling for significant differences pretreatment.

Problematic environmental factors were the limited variety of heart healthy foods in the galley, short meal breaks and long mess hall lines that led to eating snacks from vending machines, and frequent port calls. Although greater weight loss than would be expected of a Command Level remedial group diluted the treatment effect, the treated men still fared significantly better (Dennis et al., 1999).

Intervention Cost-Effectiveness

To examine the cost-effectiveness of the standardized shipboard weight-control program (SBWC) vs the Navy's current exercise-only Physical Readiness Test (PRT) remediation, costs were examined from the Navy (long-term) and Command (short-term) perspectives. The Navy's costs, both direct (i.e., intervention and personnel replacement) and indirect (i.e., participant's obesity-related health care savings), formulated the cost-effectiveness analysis. The frequency and probability of medical events in the Navy active duty population, valued at Medicare cost rates, generated total inpatient and outpatient obesity-related expected per person health care costs to calculate cost-saving from the effects of the innovative shipboard weight control and the current Command-Level interventions.

The SBWC was more expensive to deliver than the PRT-exercise only remediation. The per-person expense for the SBWC was $1,269, which consisted of $509 for the conduct of the intervention plus $722 in the participants' indirect costs. The Command-Level, PRT exercise-only cost per-person was $760, with $38 for the intervention and the same $722 of indirect costs. Additionally, $65,561 is required to replace the average service member when dismissed for PRT non-compliance. However, these PRT-intervention and replacement costs apply only to personnel in PRT remediation or those who are discharged, so the probability of these events is accounted for in the final calculation of expected per person costs of: $143 for the PRT exercise-only and $195 for the SBWC remediations, at the Command Level. The "effect" measure is the percent of weight loss, which is the most meaningful clinical outcome achieved by the two interventions under scrutiny. The SBWC and PRT groups on average achieved weight reductions of 7.8 percent and 4.6 percent, respectively, indicating that the SBWC is more effective.

The simple or "average" cost-effectiveness ratios indicate that the SBWC is cheaper to deliver, considering the gains achieved, under either the Command or Navy perspective. Exercise-alone remediation annually costs the Command (per person) $31 per percent weight loss achieved, while the SBWC costs $25. In the Navy's perspective, PRT-exercise-only obtains a ratio of $19 per percent weight-loss achieved while SBWC obtains a value of $13. These ratios indicate the SBWC is "dominant" across perspectives with consistently lower average annual per person costs per effect unit achieved.

Because the SBWC is an enhancement of the PRT-exercise remediation, the cost effectiveness analysis (CEA) also can examine the preferred cost-effectiveness of program efficiency, the incremental cost-effectiveness. That incremental CEA comparison examines whether the additional costs achieve an additional effect, which makes the SBWC incrementally more cost-effective. The SBWC program is estimated to annually save approximately $1 per percentage weight loss per person over the PRT-exercise-only remediation from both the Command and Navy perspectives. Thus, the estimated annual impact would be a savings of $675,198 with an investment of $24,363 twice annually, assuming the probabilities of PRT failures and discharges are maintained. These findings were sustained under sensitivity analysis that tests the influence of the assumptions and inclusiveness of the CEAs.

This study documents the average cost-effectiveness of the Navy's current Command Level PRT exercise-only program and the improved cost-effectiveness when that intervention is standardized and augmented with nutrition and behavioral modification interventions (SBWC), even while onboard the Navy's sea-going vessels. These findings are based on conservative assumptions and valuation techniques at each stage of the analysis underlying the comparisons. The consistent dominance of the SBWC over the PRT-exercise-only remediation across both Command and Navy perspectives further confirms the findings that SBWC should be implemented Navy-wide (Bradham et al., in press).

Obesity-Related Hospitalization Costs

The objective to estimate the cost to the U.S. Navy for obesity-related hospital admissions was examined by: (1) the inpatient utilization associated with obesity; (2) the rank order, probability, and total facility costs of obesity-related Diagnosis Related Groups (DRG); and (3) the expected inpatient expenses. The analysis was structured by age groups (18–24, 25–34, 35–44, and 45–64 years old) that are commonly used in the Navy's central health care data system. Stratification by age also permitted documentation of increased cardiovascular disease incidence over life span. Detailed hospital event data were extracted from the Retrospective Case Mix Analysis System (RCMAS). The RCMAS database provides several descriptors of the admission and associated treatment including up to 20 diagnostic classifications (ICD9 codes), the DRG for the admission, the length of the hospital stay, and procedures (ICD9 codes) delivered during the admission. Having a CVD diagnosis ICD9 code in the primary or lower-order diagnosis fields for a 1995 or 1996 admission identified patients who were entered into this analysis. The candidate CVD diagnoses were determined from both empirical evidence and expert judgment.

Among patents admitted with an ICD9 of CVD as one of the diagnoses, advancing age was associated with more admissions for chest pain and circulatory disorders. Coronary bypass began to appear in the top five obesity-related DRGs in the 45–64 year old age group. The number of CVD admissions in that oldest age group drops markedly, which is consistent with military retirement and the number of personnel of that age who remain on active duty. Expected facility costs per obesity-related admission for active duty Navy personnel increased by age group from $3,328 for 18–24 year olds to $5,746 for 45–64 year olds. Annual avoidable inpatient for the Navy was estimated to be $5,842,627 for the top ten obesity-related DRGs (Bradham et al., 2001).

Clinical Significance

Results of the standardized shipboard weight-control program support the ability to conduct multifaceted weight-control programs on deployed naval vessels and are important to the Navy because of their potential to positively impact Navy policy on obesity treatment. Through extension and replication, the effect of this program conducted on other types of operational platforms and at shore-based facilities may result in a feasible and effective approach to improving the health and well-being of the Navy's service members. Pilot data from a refinement of this shipboard weight-control program that uses indigenous shipboard personnel rather than a Navy dietitian to conduct the intervention are very promising.

Obesity extracts a large economic cost from the Navy in terms of health care services (inpatient and outpatient) and premature discharges for failure to maintain body composition and physical readiness standards. These costs are high in aggregate, and no less significant at the individual level. Importantly, these costs are avoidable if innovative and cost-effective remedial treatments are implemented. Improvements to the Navy's physical readiness remedial program and other health promotion interventions that might reduce weight, cardiovascular risks, obesity-related health care, and personnel discharges should be examined rigorously before adoption. Those that are efficacious and cost-effective should be implemented to reduce the public's economic burden.

References

Bradham DD, South BR, Saunders HJ, Heuser MD, Pane KW, Dennis KE. In press. The cost effectiveness of a shipboard weight control program.

Bradham DD, South BR, Saunders HJ, Heuser MD, Pane KW, Dennis KE. 2001. Obesity-related hospitalization costs to the U.S. Navy, 1993 to 1998. *Mil Med* 166:1–10.

Colditz GA. 1992. Economic costs of severe obesity. *Am J Clin Nutr* 55:503S–507S.

Dengel JL, Katzel LI, Goldberg AP. 1995. Effect of an American Heart Association diet, with or without weight loss, on lipids in obese middle-aged and older men. *Am J Clin Nutr* 62:715–721.

Dennis KE, Goldberg AP. 1996. Weight control self-efficacy types and positive transitions affect weight loss in obese women. *Addict Behav* 21:103–116.

Dennis KE, Pane KW, Adams BK, Qi BB. 1999. The impact of a shipboard weight control program. *Obes Res* 7:60–67.

Dennis KE, Tomoyasu N, Goldberg AP, McCrone SH, Bunyard L, Qi BB. 2001. Self-efficacy targeted treatments for weight loss in postmenopausal women. *Sch Inq Nurs Pract* 15:259–276.

Goodrick GK, Foreyt JP. 1991. Why treatments for obesity don't last. *J Am Diet Assoc* 91:1243–1247.

Hoiberg A, McNally MS. 1991. Profiling overweight patients in the U.S. Navy: Health conditions and costs. *Mil Med* 156:76–82.

Landkammer J, Katzel L, Engelhardt S, Simpson K, Goldberg A. 1992. Cardiovascular risk factors modification after dietary therapy of obese older men. 32:71A.
Nicklas BJ, Katzel LI, Bunyard LB, Dennis KE, Goldberg AP. 1997a. Effects of an American Heart Association diet and weight loss on lipoprotein lipids in obese, postmenopausal women. *Am J Clin Nutr* 66:853–859.
Nicklas BJ, Katzel LI, Ryan AS, Dennis KE, Goldberg AP. 1997b. Gender differences in the response of plasma leptin concentrations to weight loss in obese older individuals. *Obes Res* 5:62–68.
Trent LK, Stevens LT. 1993. Survey of the Navy's three-tiered obesity treatment program. *NEI Med* 158:614–618.
Trent LK, Stevens LT. 1995. Evaluation of the Navy's obesity treatment program. *Mil Med* 160:326–330.
Wadden TA, Bell ST. 1990. Obesity. In: Bellack AS, Hersen M, Kazdin AE, eds. *International Handbook of Behavior Modification and Therapy*. New York: Plenum. Pp. 449–473.

THE TRIPLER L^2E^3AN PROGRAM: A CURRENT UPDATE

Larry C. James, PhD, ABPP, Jay Earles, PsyD LTC MS USA CPT(P) MS USA, Raymond A. Folen, PhD, ABPP

As obesity has effected the civilian population over the last two decades, so have the rates of obesity increased in the U.S. military. In 1994, many service members were administratively discharged for their inability to maintain weight standards. Moreover, as the armed services downsizes, loss of trained and skilled personnel due to weight problems has taken on increased importance. As a result of the problems associated with obesity and other behavioral disorders and lifestyle diseases (such as obesity, essential hypertension, type II diabetes, and hyperlipidemia), Tripler Army Medical Center developed a healthy lifestyle program to treat any of these diseases. Coined the **L^2E^3AN PROGRAM** (emphasizing healthy **L**ifestyles, health for **L**ife, **E**xercise, **E**motions, **E**xpectations that are reasonable, **A**ttitudes and **N**utrition), its major emphasis is on short bout, low intensity exercise consuming three well-balanced meals each day rather than fad diets or painful exercise. Additionally, the programs six psychologists teach patients how to cope with the wide array of emotions associated with food and eating. The presentation will discuss the conceptualization behind the program's development as well as major components and ideas for program implementation, and highlight practical problems. An emphasis will be placed on key aspects of the program curriculum that are most efficacious and helpful in assisting military patients in managing their weight. Demographics of weight loss by age, gender, race, military ranks, and occupation will be provided. The results suggest that at 18 months post-treatment, patients maintained 8 to 10 percent weight loss. Of particular interest was the fact that minority men did equally well as nonminority men in the program. Although these programs are very promising, the researchers had difficulty testing out quantifiable reasons for the success of the minority men, a pattern inconsistent with studies on minorities (U.S. African-American women on the other hand, had great difficulty achieving even modest weight loss). This finding has been demonstrated in some previous studies. A practical problem for potential program participants is that this program requires 12 months of follow-up. It involves 3 weeks of day treatment and 12 months of weekly follow-up. Thus, patients unable to follow the year-long follow-up regimen are not admitted to the program. The exclusion criteria eliminates many active duty navy patients from participation. To offset this problem, the researchers developed and pioneered behavioral health telemedicine treatment. An inter-active webpage was developed and coupled with the use of low-cost video teleconferencing. Currently, all service members who can attend the day treatment phase of the program can participate in the program. The researchers have compared the finding between patients ($n = 30$) who participate in follow-up via the interactive web page and those who attend weekly follow-up sessions. The weight-loss slopes are nearly identical for both groups. To date, the L^2E^3AN Program and its innovative telemedicine web page offers promise for the treatment of obesity and it related diseases. The authors of this study will continue to develop similar programs at other military medical facilities and hope to find innovative ways to treat obesity.

ARMY WEIGHT-MANAGEMENT INSTRUCTION TO MASTER FITNESS TRAINERS (MFTS),

Lou Tomasi, EdD and 1LT Kerryn Davidson, RD, US Army Physical Fitness School, Ft. Benning, GA

Introduction

The United States Army Physical Fitness School (APFS) is located in Ft. Benning, GA, Home of the US Army Infantry Training Center. The APFS is responsible for writing operational physical fitness doctrine, conducting physical fitness research, and providing physical training support to the Army. Writing the fitness doctrine includes composing, staffing, reviewing and publishing Field Manual 21-20, *Physical Fitness Training* (U.S. Army, 1992) and the on-going responsibility of updating changes and authoring articles for Army publications.

The APFS also conducts operational research. For example, APFS personnel designed the protocol and administered the research procedures to set the 1995 Army Physical Fitness Test (APFT) Standards Update Study, 1997

APFT Validation Study, 1998 Entrance and Exit Requirements for the Army Basic Combat Training (BCT) Fitness Training Units, 1999 Impact of the New APFT Standards on Attrited Soldiers from BCT, and 1999 Upper Body Strength Needed to Complete Army Airborne Training.

Providing training support to the Army includes conducting many mid-length and short physical training courses. The most visible course is the Master Fitness Trainer (MFT) course, a 101-hour course that begins with some basic anatomy, muscle and exercise physiology, strength, flexibility, and cardio-respiratory training techniques. Additionally, other topics include nutrition, unit and individual exercise prescriptions, and teaching the MFTs the Army Weight Control Program.

MFT Instruction

The agenda of this presentation is to provide the audience with an overview of the Army Weight Control Program instruction provided to the MFTs, and the role of the MFT in the Army Weight Control Program. This instruction is segmented in two parts: Army Regulation (AR) 600-9 (4 hours) (U.S. Army, 1986), and nutrition (4 hours). The purpose of the regulation is to establish policy and procedure for the implementation of the Army Weight Control Program. The objectives include: meeting the physical demands of their duties under combat conditions and presenting a trim military appearance at all times. The commanders' responsibilities include the following: program implementation, personnel monitoring, exercise programs, and providing education programs to the soldiers enrolled in the Army Weight Control Program.

The MFTs have an integral role in the Army Weight Control Program. They conduct weight-ins when the APFT is administered (i.e., biannually). Soldiers are placed in the Army Weight Control Program when they exceed the set weight for their height as determined by the AR 600-9 Screening Table Weight (U.S. Army, 1986). The MFT's role is to assess the identified soldiers, write an exercise prescription, assist with the maintenance of personal weight and body composition goals, assist the commander in the development of proactive fitness programs, and provide dietary and nutritional guidance. Soldiers are monitored monthly, weigh-ins are conducted by the commander or designee, body fat is evaluated regularly. Satisfactory progress is 3–8 lb per month weight loss.

Identified soldiers are removed from the program by the commanders and supervisors when body-fat standards are met, and the AR 600-9 Screening Table Weight is not used for removal. When there is unsatisfactory progress, the soldiers are screened for a medical condition. When there is a medical condition, hospital personnel provide medical treatment. When there is no medical condition, Army administrative personnel bar the soldier from reenlistment, other favorable actions, and administrative separation procedures begin.

Soldiers are monitored for 36 months upon removal from the program. If a soldier again exceeds body fat within 12 months of removal date, the soldier is separated. If soldier again exceeds the body-fat standards after the twelfth month, but within 36 months, the soldier is allowed 90 days to meet the standard.

The Army Weight Control Program uses separate circumference measurement sites for females and males. The males' measurement sites are at the abdomen at the level of the navel and around the neck, just below the larynx. The females' measurement sites are: at the hip where the point of the gluts protrude the most, forearm at the largest point, neck just below the larynx, and the wrist between the bones of the wrist and the forearm.

During MFT instruction, APFS instructors teach the MFT students Lean Body Mass and Target Weight Formulae, that is, Lean Body Mass = Present Body Weight X (1 – % present body fat) and Target Weight = Lean Body Mass ÷ (1 – % target body fat). The concept of energy balance is presented. For example these formulae are taught to the MFT students:

Energy Input = Energy Output = Stable Body Weight;
Energy Input > Energy Output = Increase Body Weight;
Energy Input < Energy Output = Decrease Body Weight.

During MFT instruction, APFS instructors teach the MFT students energy balance manipulation for effective weight loss. These include:

- Reduce caloric intake below daily energy requirements;
- Maintain caloric intake and increase caloric output through exercise;
- *Ideally*, reduce caloric intake below daily energy requirements and increase caloric output through exercise.

To determine weight-maintenance formula, the activity factors of sedentary: 12–14 calories per lb (desk job, little/no exercise), active: 15 calories per lb (regular exercise program) and highly active: 16–18 calories per lb (physically demanding work and/or high level of physical training) are used. MFT instruction presents safe minimum calorie intakes of no less than 1,500 kcal for males and no less than 1,200 kcal for females. Nutrition in the MFT course is directly linked to weight management through the dietary guidelines; nutrients, class, characteristics, function; interpreting food labels, conducting a dietary recall; and calculating of per cent calories from carbohydrate, protein, and fat.

Mandatory requirements for nutrition education prior to or shortly after enrollment in Army Weight Control Program includes instruction by a registered dietitian in which soldiers learn proper diet for weight control. Follow-up with the RD is encouraged; however, it is not required under the provisions of AR 600-9 (U.S. Army, 1986).

Summary

In summary, the overview of Army weight-management instruction to Master Fitness Trainers includes: program implementation, personnel monitoring, exercise programs, and education programs.

References

U.S. Army. 1986. *The Army Weight Control Program*. Army Regulation 600-9. September 1. Washington, DC: U.S. Government Printing Office.

U.S. Army. 1992. *Physical Fitness Training.* Field Manual 21-20. September 30. Washington, DC: U.S. Government Printing Office.

THE GENETICS OF OBESITY

Anthony G. Comuzzie

The understanding of the genetic influences on obesity in humans has recently increased at a tremendous rate. It is now well established that obesity has a significant genetic component. In humans approximately 50 to 70 percent of the within-population variation in a variety of obesity-related phenotypes appears to be due to within-population genetic variation. Several single gene defects leading to massive obesity have been found in animal models, but very few humans appear to be obese due to mutations in single obesity genes. As a result, investigators are actively searching for oligogenic influences on human adiposity.

One of the greatest challenges in biomedical research today is the elucidation of the underlying genetic architecture of complex phenotypes such as obesity. In contrast to simple Mendelian disorders, in which there is generally a one-to-one relationship between genotype at a single locus and the presence or absence of the disorder, obesity rises as a result of numerous behavioral, environmental, and genetic factors (i.e., obesity is multifactoral in origin).

Twin, adoption, and family status have long established that an individual's risk of obesity is increases when he/she has relatives who are obese. In fact, it has been shown repeatedly that a substantial portion (≈ 40 to 70 percent) of the variation in obesity related phenotypes, such as body mass index (BMI), sum of skinfolds thickness, fat mass, and leptin levels, is heritable (Comuzzie et al., 1993, 1994, 1996). Finally, numerous segregation analyses (studies evaluating the evidence and mode or transmission for a major gene based on observed patterns of phenotypic inheritance among related individuals) have provided evidence that among the genes influencing the expression of these obesity-related phenotypes, there are at least a few with relatively large measurable contributions. For example ≈ 40 percent of the variation in fat mass has been attributed to the effects of such a major gene (Comuzzie et al., 1995; Rice et al., 1993). These segregation analyses reveal that there are genes with major effects on the amount and distribution of body fat, and that these genes appear to exert their affects across various ethnic populations. In addition, segregation analysis of longitudinal changes in percent body fat over a 5-year period has yielded evidence for a major gene effect (Comuzzie et al., 1999).

Most recently the emphasis has shifted from the question of whether human obesity has a genetic component to the question of which specific genes are responsible. Currently the major effect in the search for specific genes contributing to human obesity is based on the use of genome scanning. In a genome scan, linkage analysis is conducted using a series of anonymous polymorphisms, spaced at a relatively constant interval over the entire genome (for example ≅ 350–370 markers with an average spacing of 10cM), to identify quantitative trait loci (QTLs) affecting the phenotype under study. In contrast to the typical candidate gene approach, with genome scanning there are no a priori assumptions about the potential importance of specific genes or chromosomal regions. Instead, the results of the scan are used to identify candidate chromosomal regions, or in some cases, positional candidate genes, which then become the focus of more intensive follow-up analyses. A positional candidate gene differs from a traditional candidate gene in that it is only considered as a candidate after the establishment of its proximity to a QTL identified via linkage in a genome scan. Thus, the genomic scan approach offers the potential of identifying previously unknown, or unsuspected, genes influencing the phenotype of interest.

In the case of our work in the San Antonio Family Heart Study, ten extended families of Mexican Americans (representing 459 individuals comprising 5,667 relative pairs ranging from parent-offspring to double second cousins) were evaluated for several obesity related phenotypes in a 20 cM genomic span (Comuzzie et al., 1997). Significant linkages were detected for QTLs on chromosome 2 (≈ 74 cM from the tip of the short arm) and chromosome 8 (≈ 65 cM from the tip of the short arm) and leptin levels (LOD scores = 4.3 and 2.2, respectively). A significant linkage was also detected between fat mass (FM) and the chromosome 2 QTL (LOD score = 1.9). Multipoint analysis of the leptin linkages increased the LOD score to 4.95 for the QTL on chromosome 2 and 2.2 for the chromosome 8 QTL (Comuzzie et al., 1997). In the case of the chromosome 2 linkages, this QTL is estimated to account for 47 percent of the variation in serum leptin levels and 32 percent of the variation in fat mass. Recent follow-up work in this region of chromosome 2 has now boosted the LOD score for the leptin linkage to 7.5 (Hixon et al., 1999).

The areas of linkage on chromosome 2 and chromosome 8 contain strong positional candidate genes for obesity. For example, the region on chromosome 2 encompasses *POMC*, which codes for the prohormone pro-opiomelanocortin, which is post-transcriptionally processed to produce a number of hormones in the hypothalamic-pituitary axis such as melanocyte-stimulating hormones and adrenocorticotrophic hormone, which have long been suspected of being involved in obesity. POMC was originally identified as a candidate gene based on its location, and its gene product has now been implicated in appetite regulation (Boston et al., 1997; Schwartz et al., 1997; Seeley et al., 1996, 1997). We have now identified two polymorphisms in *POMC* that are associated with variation in leptin levels in this population of Mexican Americans (Hixon et al., 1999). The region of linkage on chromosome 8 encompasses ADRB3, for the β-3Adrenergic receptor, which represents a previously identified candidate based on its physiological activity with respect to the regulation of energy expenditure. Although the cumulative evidence of linkage between the well-known tryptophan to arginine mutation (trp64Arg) in ADRB3 and BMI is weak, the argument that *ADRB3* is a human obesity gene has been strengthened by the follow-up analyses in this same sample of Mexican Americans (Mitchell et al., 1998). These analyses have revealed an association between *ADRB3* variants and BMI, FM, and waist circumference after first continuing on the stronger QTL signal on chromosome 2.

In addition to our work in humans, our preliminary genome scanning efforts in primates (i.e., baboons) have also begun to reveal additional QTLs with significant effects on obesity-related phenotypes. At present, we have detected suggestive evidence of linkage for QTLs influencing body weight (LOD = 2.12) and fat cell number (LOD = 2.15). In both cases, the confidence intervals surrounding these two QTLs contain two strong positional candidates. The QTL for body weight is located near *NPY* and QTL for fat cell number is near IGF-1.

While there are undoubtedly single genes that produce massive phenotypic effects on obesity-related phenotypes in isolated individuals or families, the identification of at least a few loci with common alleles with measurable effects on the general population has significant implications for public health. Work to date suggests the existence of roughly a dozen genes with measurable effects of the expression of obesity-related phenotypes at the population level. As a result, there is now not only strong evidence for a genetic component in the variation of body weight across individuals, but we are beginning to identify specific genes with measurable effects.

References

Boston BA, Blaydon KM, Varnerin J, Cone RD. 1997. Independent and additive effects of central POMC and leptin pathways on murine obesity. *Science* 278:1641–1644.

Comuzzie AG, Blangero J, Mahaney MC, Mitchell BD, Stern MP, MAcCluer JW. 1993. The quantitative genetics of sexual dimorphism in body fat measurements. *Am J Hum Biol* 5:725–734.

Comuzzie AG, Blangero J, Mahaney MC, Mitchell BD, Stern MP, MacCluer JW. 1994. Genetic and environmental correlations among skinfold measures. *Int J Obes Relat Metab Disord* 18:413–418.

Comuzzie AG, Blangero J, Mahaney MC, Mitchell BD, Hixson JE, Samollow PB, Stern MP, MacCluer JW. 1995. Major gene with sex-specific effects influences fat mass in Mexican Americans. *Genet Epidemiol* 12:475–488.

Comuzzie AG, Blangero J, Mahaney MC, Haffner SM, Mitchell BD, Stern MP, MacCluer JW. 1996. Genetic and environmental correlations among hormone levels and measures of body fat accumulation and topography. *J Clin Endocrinol Metabol* 81:597–600.

Comuzzie AG, Hixson JE, Almasy L, Mitchell BD, Mahaney MC, Dyer TD, Stern MP, MacCluer JW, Blangero J. 1997. A major quantitative trait locus determining serum leptin levels and fat mass is located on human chromosome 2. *Nat Genet* 15:273–276.

Comuzzie AG, Mitchell BD, Blangero J, MacCluer JW, Stern MP. 1999. Evidence for genetic influences on the change in percent body fat over time in Mexican Americans. *Genet Epidemiol* 17:221–222.

Hixon JE, Almasy L, Cole S, Birnbaum S, Mitchell BD, Mahaney MC, Stern MP, MacCluer JW, Blangero J, Comuzzie AG. 1999. Normal variation in leptin levels in associated with polymorphisms in the proopiomelanocortin gene, POMC. *J Clin Endocrinol Metab* 84:3187–3191.

Mitchell BD, Blangero J, Comuzzie AG, Almasy LA, Shuldiner AR, Silver K, Stern MP, MacCluer JW, Hixson JE. 1998. A paired sibling analysis of the beta-3 adrenergic receptor and obesity in Mexican Americans. *J Clin Invest* 101:584–587.

Rice T, Borecki IB, Bouchard C, Rao DC. 1993. Segregation analysis of fat mass and other body composition measures derived from underwater weighing. *Am J Human Genet* 52:967–973.

Schwartz MW, Seeley RJ, Woods SC, Weigle DS, Campfield LA, Burn P, Baskin DG. 1997. Leptin increases hypothalamic pro-opiomelanocortin mRNA expression in the rostral arcuate nucleus. *Diabetes* 46:2119–2123.

Seeley RJ, van Dijk G, Campfield LA, Smith FJ, Burn P, Nelligan JA, Bell SM, Baskin DG, Woods SC, Schwartz MW. 1996. Intraentricular leptin reduces food intake and body weight of lean rats but not obese Zucker rats. *Horm Metab Res* 28:664–668.

Seeley RJ, Yagaloff KA, Fisher SL, Burn P, Thiele TE, van Dijk G, Baskin DG, Schwartz MW. 1997. Melanocortin receptors in leptin effects. *Nature* 390:349.

THE PHARMACOTHERAPY OF WEIGHT LOSS AND ITS POTENTIAL APPLICATION IN THE MILITARY SETTING

MAJ H. Glenn Ramos, Fort Gordon, GA

General Information

Only a small percentage of obese patients are able to achieve their weight goals and an even smaller percentage are able to maintain such weights over time. The majority of those who lose weight return to their initial obese state or gain more (Turner et al., 1995).

This is particularly well illustrated by Kramer (Kramer et al., 1999) who, in a 5-year study, demonstrated that only 5.3 percent of women and 0.9 percent of men were able to maintain all the weight that they had lost. Forty percent in general gained weight at least to baseline levels or above at some point during the follow-up.

The "bright" side of Kramer's study was that there were measurable residual benefits from behavioral weight-management programs 4–5 years beyond termination of initial treatment—18.5 percent maintained at least half of their losses throughout follow-up, and 34 percent kept off at least 25 percent.

The view that short-term interventions will cure a chronic condition has hampered the development of methods for controlling weight. The major challenge facing obese patients and health care providers is to improve the ability to sustain, rather than to achieve, weight loss.

The definition of success that is applied in evaluating weight-loss programs should be broadened and made more realistic based on the research to date that small weight losses can reduce the risks of developing chronic diseases. Specifically, the goal of obesity treatment should be refocused from weight loss alone to weight management, achieving the best weight possible in the context of overall health. In contrast to weight loss, the primary purpose of weight management is to achieve and maintain good health. This concept includes weight loss but is not limited to it (IOM, 1995).

In this light, pharmacotherapy for obesity must be seriously considered in the acute, and chronic, management of this disease.

Anorectics and Weight Loss/Weight Maintenance

The following are the three currently available classes of anorectics:

1. Catecholamine-like agents
2. Serotonin re-uptake inhibitors
3. Lipase inhibitors

The following two additional classes are undergoing research:

1. Leptin
2. Metabolic enhancers

The catecholarnine-like agents include phentermine (Fastin/Adipex), diethylproprion (Tenuate), and the phenopropanalamines (Accutrim and Dexatrim). These are the oldest agents available and are very effective.

Sympathomimetic amines have actions that include symptoms similar to the fight or flight syndrome, to include central nervous system stimulation and anorexia. This is also the source of most of the medication's side-effects that include insomnia, palpitations, tachycardia, dry mouth, dizziness, euphoria and headache, elevation of blood pressure, and tachycardia,.

The average weight loss is around 10 kg at 6 months. Studies of greater than 6 months are lacking with the exception of the combination Phen-Fen, which was studied out to 3.5 years, and will be discussed later.

The rate of weight loss associated with the use of phentermine tends to be greatest in the first weeks of therapy, and decrease with succeeding weeks, to an eventual plateau around the sixth month of treatment.

Use of these agents is contraindicated in advanced atherosclerotic coronary artery disease, moderate to severe hypertension, hyperthyroidism, glaucoma, agitated states, pregnancy, and in eating disorders.

- Fecal urgency 10.0–29.0 percent
- Fecal incontinence 5.0–11.8 percent

Both high fiber meals and low-fat diets have reduced the frequency of intestinal complaints by producing fewer liquid or oily stools.

In some the fat-soluble vitamins (A, D, E, K, and beta-carotene) are reduced and need to be supplemented (2 hours before or after use of Xenical).

Since orlistat undergoes minimal systemic absorption, the primary drug interaction concern has been its influence on the absorption of coadministered drugs. Orlistat has been found to increase the half-life of farosernide and the time to peak concentration of sustained-release nifedipine (adalat/procardia XL), although these increases were not considered to be clinically significant. The concomitant administration of pravastatin and orlistat increased pravastatin's bioavailability and lipid-lowering effect modestly. The combination has also been shown to increase the risk of rhabdomyolosis. Because of the decreased absorption of vitamin K, Coumadin use must be monitored closely during coadministration with Xenical.

Orlistat is contraindicated in patients with chronic malabsorption syndrome, or cholestasis, and in patients with known hypersensitivity to Xenical.

Leptin is a natural human protein produced by fat that has few or no apparent significant adverse side effects. Currently this medication is experimental, and given subcutaneously, with its most common adverse effect being moderate skin reaction (redness, itching, swelling) at the injection site.

It appears to act as a chemical messenger from fat cells to the brain to indicate the level of fat in the body. By complex endocrine controls that may include decreasing levels of a hormone called neuropeptide Y, the Leptin tells the brain to decrease fat intake and increase energy use. Theoretically, the lateral hypothalmus of an individual taking Leptin would not realize that the body is losing weight, and compensatory mechanisms would not be put into effect.

In animals it not only reduces food intake, but also increases basal metabolic rate with selective promotion of fat metabolism.

In contrast to the Leptin-deficient lab mice upon which this was initially tested, most obese mammals have elevated plasma concentrations of Leptin and insulin, and appear to be resistant to leptin-induced anorexia. This resistance is similar to a type II diabetic resistance to insulin. Thus, Leptin's effect in humans has not been as dramatic as in animals. It is modestly effective, causing an average weight loss of 16 lb over 6 months.

Thyroid hormone is one prototype of a thermogenic drug. It produces a log-dose increase in metabolic expenditure. Pharmacologic doses of thyroid hormone, however, are associated with increased breakdown of protein, increased calcium loss from bone, and an increased risk of cardiovascular dysfunction.

Interest in triiodothyronine (T_3) as a treatment for obesity has been revived by the observation that T_3 falls in very low-calorie diets (as well as in anorexics and bulemics), and the administration of T_3 can prevent the decline in metabolic rate that occurs. However, the reduction in T_3 when dieting may be a compensatory effort by the body to conserve visceral proteins since it has been found that up to 75 percent of the extra weight lost on T_3 replacement can be accounted for by the loss of fat-free mass.

Brown fat stimulants show much promise in the future, but are only in the beginning phases of animal research. Currently there are no agents on the market that have been proven to increase the metabolism of dieting patients (despite all the "health food" claims to the opposite).

Barriers to Drug Treatment

The view that obese people need "only to close their mouths" has caused us to demand a higher standard for medications used in treating obesity than we do for treatments of any other chronic condition. In many conditions we accept that the condition will relapse following the cessation of therapy. Even in the absence of cure, patients and physicians still view ocular hypotensive agents, anti-hypertensive agents, cholesterol-lowering medications, antidepressants, and H2-blockers as valuable. However, the failure of a medication to "cure" obesity is found to be unacceptable. The anorexiants are labeled as failures when the patient regains weight after treatment has ended.

References

IOM (Institute of Medicine). 1995. *Weighing the Options; Criteria for Evaluating Weight Management Programs*. Washington, DC: National Academy Press. Pp. 122.

Kramer FM, Jeffery RW, Forster JL, Snell MK. 1989. Long-term follow-up of behavioral treatment for obesity: Patterns of weight regain among men and women. *Int J Obes* 13:123–136.

Turner LW, Wang MQ, Wasterfield RC. 1995. Preventing relapse in weight control: A discussion of cognitive and behavioral strategies. *Psychol Rep* 77:651–656.

Additional References

Griffiths RR, Brady JV, Bradford LD. 1979. Predicting the abuse liability of drugs with animal drug self-administration procedures: Psychomotor stimulants and hallucinogens. *Adv Behav Pharmacol* 2:163–208.

James WP, Avenell A, Broom J, Whitehead J. 1997. A one-year trial to assess the value of orlistat in the management of obesity. *Int J Obes* 21:S24–S30.

Lean ME. 1997. Sibutramine—A review of clinical efficacy. *Int J Obes Relat Metab Disord* 21:S30–S36.

Marston AR, Criss J. 1984. Maintenance of successful weight loss: Incidence and prediction. *Int J Obes* 8:435–439.

Perri MG, McAllister DA, Gange JJ, Jordan RC, McAdoo G, Nezu AM. 1988. Effects of four maintenance programs on the long-term management of obesity. *J Consult Clin Psychol* 56:529–534.

Perri MG, Nezu AM, Patti ET, McCann KL. 1989. Effect of length of treatment on weight loss. *J Consult Clin Psychol* 57:450–452.

Perri MG, McAdoo WG, Spevak PA, Newlin DB. 1984. Effect of a multicomponent maintenance program on long-term weight loss. *J Consult Clin Psychol* 52:480–481.

Reddy P, Chow SS. 1998. Focus on orlistat: A nonsystemic inhibitor of gastrointestinal lipase for weight reduction in the management of obesity. *Formulary* 33:943–959.

Safer DJ. 1991. Diet, behavior modification, and exercise: A review of obesity treatments from a long-term perspective. *South Med J* 84:1470–1474.

Van Gaal LF, Broom JI, Enzi G, Toplak H. 1998. Efficacy and tolerability of orlistat in the treatment of obesity: A 6-month dose ranging study. *Eur J Clin Pharmacol* 54:125–132.

Weintraub M, Sundaresan RP, Madan M, Schuster B, Balder A, Lasagna L, Cox C. 1992. Long-term weight control study I (weeks 0 to 34). The enhancement of behavior modification, caloric restriction, and exercise by fenfluramine plus phentermine versus placebo. *Clin Pharmaco Ther* 51:586–594.

Weintraub M, Sundaresan RP, Schuster B, Ginsberg G, Madan M, Balder A, Stein EC, Byrne L. 1992. Long-term weight control study II (weeks 34 to 104). An open-labeled study of continuous fenfluramine plus phentermine versus targeted intermittent medication as adjuncts to behavior modification, caloric restriction, and exercise. *Clin Pharmaco Ther* 51:595–601.

Weintraub M, Sundaresan RP, Schuster B, Moscucci M, Stein EC. 1992. Long-term weight control study III (weeks 104 to 156). An open-labeled study of dose adjustment of fenfluramine and phentermine. *Clin Pharmaco Ther* 51:602–607.

Weintraub M, Sundaresan RP, Schuster B, Averbuch M, Stein EC, Cox C, Byrne L. 1992. Long-term weight control study IV (weeks 156 to 190). The second double-blind phase. *Clin Pharmaco Ther* 51:608–614.

Weintraub M, Sundaresan RP, Schuster B, Stein EC, Byrne L. 1992. Long-term weight control study V (weeks 190 to 210). Follow-up of participants after cessation of medication. *Clin Pharmaco Ther* 51:615–618.

Weintraub M, Sundaresan RP, Cox C. 1992. Long-term weight control study VI. Individual participant response patterns. *Clin Pharmaco Ther* 51:619–633.

Weintraub M, Sundaresan RP, Schuster B. 1992. Long-term weight control study VII (weeks 0 to 210). Serum lipid changes. *Clin Pharmaco Ther* 51:634–641.

USE OF PHARMACOLOGICAL AIDS IN WEIGHT MANAGEMENT

Frank Greenway, MD

Obesity is now recognized as a chronic disease. Although the NIH Consensus Conference declared such as early as 1985 (Anonymous, 1985), it was not until the identification of the leptin gene (Halaas et al., 1995) and the other single-gene mutations causing rodent obesity that the chronic disease model of obesity gained wider acceptance. Like hypertension and other chronic medical conditions, obesity will, in all likelihood, require chronic pharmacological treatment in a stepped-care approached when diet and lifestyle modification alone are inadequate.

Treatment of any medical condition involves weighing risks of the disease against the risks and benefits of treatment. Evidence-based national guidelines have evaluated these risks and benefits. They suggest that medications be a consideration in obesity treatment programs for individuals with a BMI greater than 30 kg/m^2 or greater than 27 kg/m^2 when complicated by diabetes or other medical conditions likely to improve with weight loss (NHLBI, 1998). Although individuals less than 30 years of age have a lower mortality risk from obesity than individuals over 50, this difference is not clinically significant until the BMI exceeds kg/m^2 (Calle et al., 1999).

Although obesity is now recognized in the medical community as a chronic disease, the public is much more concerned about the cosmetic aspects of being obese. The average American woman has a BMI of 24 kg/m^2, while the average fashion model, the ideal to which many women aspire, has a BMI of 16 kg/m^2. The upper limits of military standards for weight correspond to a BMI of 22–25 kg/m^2 for women and 23–28 kg/m^2 for men. The stated reasons for these standards are to maintain a trim military appearance.

It could be argued that, like national guidelines for obesity treatment, military weight standards should be based upon medical risks rather than cosmetic considerations. Since one-third of the American population has a BMI greater than 27 kg/m^2, the military may be losing the services of many healthy and talented people who would like to serve in their nation's military service. The military service draws its ranks disproportionately from minority groups. Minority groups bear a disproportionate obesity burden making the potential loss of talent to the military even greater (NHLBI, 1998).

The basis of any weight-loss program is diet and lifestyle change. When these modalities by themselves are not sufficient, and the BMI is 27–30 kg/m^2 depending on the presence or absence of comorbid diseases, medications for obesity can be justified. Therefore, except in the case of unequal application of military standards, individuals with this degree of obesity will be discharged from the military service. Thus, the indications for obesity medications in the military are vanishingly small.

There are two medications approved for the long-term treatment of obesity. Sibutramine is a norepinephrine and serotonin reuptake inhibitor that inhibits food intake centrally, and orlistat is an inhibitor of pancreatic lipase that functions within the intestinal lumen. Both drugs give a 7–10 percent weight loss over 6 months that is maintained at 1 year (Bray et al., 1999; Sjostrom et al., 1998). Orlistat gives a drop of cholesterol in excess of that predicted from the weight loss it induces, but sibutramine does not give the blood pressure drop expected from weight loss. In other respects, cardiovascular risk factors are reduced in proportion to weight loss.

If serotonin reuptake inhibitors are excluded from the military formulary, sibutramine may not qualify for use in the military. Although generally well tolerated, orlistat can give gastrointestinal symptoms such as abdominal cramps, soft stools, and fecal urgency. If these symptoms were to occur in a military field exercise, training disruptions could result. Due to the loss of fat-soluble vitamins in the stool, a vitamin supplement is recommended with orlistat. The only other prescription medications indicated for weight loss are scheduled by the DEA, since all of them have at least some potential for abuse. In addition, they have only been approved and tested for use over periods up to 12 weeks. Therefore, the approved prescription medications for weight loss have little utility in the military service.

The criteria for using nonprescription drugs in the treatment of obesity have received much less attention from groups forming guidelines for obesity treatment. Phenylpropanolamine is sold without a prescription for the treatment of obesity. Ephedrine with a methylxanthine is sold without a prescription for the treatment of asthma, but is approved and sold for the treatment of obesity in Denmark. At least in the 1970s, phenylpropanolamine was on the military formulary as a decongestant and ephedrine with theophylline was on the military formulary for asthma. These two pharmacological approaches deserve further comment.

Phenylpropanolamine is approved for the short-term treatment of obesity (less than 12 weeks). Phenylpropolamine is a central alpha-1 adrenergic stimulator that has no addictive potential and gives weight loss equivalent to prescription anorectic drugs during the first 4 weeks of treatment. The longest study with this medication lasted 20 weeks and was small, but the phenylpropanolamine group lost 6.5 percent of their body weight (Schteingart, 1992). Phenylpropanolamine has a remarkable record of safety. It gives a small increase in blood pressure that is statistically, but not clinically, significant. The dose approved to treat obesity is 75 mg/d. Phenylpropanolamine is approved for use without a prescription in cough and cold preparations in twice that dose. Short-term treatment of a long-term disease is not logical, but it is unlikely that approval of phenylpropanolamine for the long-term treatment of obesity will be pursued unless financed by the government, since the drug is no longer covered by patent. The wholesale price of 1 month of treatment with phenylpropanolamine is less than $0.50 per month.

Caffeine and theophylline are both methylxanthines. Two mg of caffeine has the potency of 1 mg of theophylline, but they are otherwise equivalent. Ephedrine 24 mg combined with 125 mg of theophylline is sold without a prescription for the treatment of asthma in the dose of one or two tablets three times a day. This combination was the first-line treatment for asthma in both adults and children in the 1970s. Caffeine 200 mg with ephedrine 20 mg given three times a day is an approved obesity medication in Denmark. In a trial conducted in Denmark, the combination gave a 16 percent weight loss over 6 months that was maintained with continued treatment at 1 year (Toubro et al., 1993). Caffeine and ephedrine is also inexpensive. A month of treatment at wholesale prices runs less than $2.50, but not being covered by patent, is unlikely to be approved for the long-term treatment of obesity without government subsidy.

Not only are the risks and benefits of using even nonprescription medications to treat obesity in a population of healthy individuals with a BMI less than 28 kg/m^2 unclear, but dietary treatments may have greater long-term efficacy than the available obesity medications. A recent study lasting 3 months demonstrated that a 1,200-calorie balanced diet was many times more effective in causing weight loss when it included calorie-controlled portions substituted for two meals and two snacks per day compared to the standard 1,200-calorie diet utilizing an exchange system (Ditschuneit et al., 1999). Individuals replacing one meal and one snack with calorie controlled portions following this 3-month weight-loss program lost 9 percent of their body weight at 1 year and 11 percent at 2 years.

Studies with sibutramie, orlistat, and phenylpropanolarnine give a 6–10 percent weight loss at 1 year. The military appears to be in an ideal position to exploit this new information. Meals Ready to Eat (MREs), the military field rations perfected through military nutrition research, could easily be modified for a weight-loss program using a 1,200-calorie diet and calorie controlled portions.

Epidemiological studies such as the Framingham study show a higher mortality in those individuals losing weight. Since the risk factors for cardiovascular disease improve with weight loss, this finding has remained a paradox. Recently, Allison et al. reanalyzed the Framingham and Tecumseh studies and demonstrated that mortality increases by 29 percent for every standard deviation (4.6–6.7 kg) of weight loss but decreases 15 percent for every standard deviation of fat loss (4.8–10 mm of skin-fold thickness) (Allison et al., 1999). This suggests that losing lean tissue during weight loss carries a mortality risk. Therefore, the ideal weight-loss medication should cause fat loss and spare lean tissue.

When people gain weight, 75 percent of the weight gain is fat and 25 percent is lean tissue. Weight is lost with diet or appetite suppressing medications in these same proportions of fat and lean tissue. Exercise and caffeine with ephedrine, both of which increase catacholamine turnover, induce a selective loss of body fat. Not only does a selective fat loss have the potential to impact in a positive way upon mortality risk, but preservation of lean tissue is likely to reduce injury and contribute positively to the fighting strength in a military setting.

In conclusion:

- The military may be paying a price in lost talent for its stringent weight requirements aimed at maintaining a trim military appearance.
- Given that military personnel have a BMI less than 28 kg/M2, there is little place for the pharmacological treatment of obesity in the military.
- Caffeine and ephedrine give preferential fat loss and might deserve further consideration as a military obesity treatment if military weight standards are liberalized.
- Calorie-controlled portions combined into a 1,200-calorie balanced diet may give better sustained weight loss than presently available obesity medi-

cations, and these calorie-controlled portions could be created for the military through modification of existing field rations (MREs).

References

Allison DB, Zannolli R, Faith MS, Heo M, Pietrobelli A, Vanltallie TB, Pi-Sunyer FX, Heymsfield SB. 1999. Weight loss increases and fat loss decreases all-cause mortality rate: Results from two independent cohort studies. *Int J Obes* 23:603–611.

Anonymous. 1985. Health implications of obesity. National Institutes of Health Consensus Developed Conference Statement. *Ann Int Med* 103:1073–1077.

Bray GA, Blackburn GL, Ferguson JM, Greenway FL, Jain AK, Mendel CM, Mendels J, Ryan DH, Schwartz SL, Scheinbaum ML, Seaton TB. 1999. Sibutramine produces dose-related weight loss. *Obes Res* 7:189–198.

Calle EE, Thim MJ, Petrelli JM, Rodriguez C, Heath CW. 1999. Body-mass index and mortality in a prospective cohort of U.S. adults. *N Engl J Med* 241:1097–1105.

Ditschuneit HH, Flechtner-Mors M, Johnson TD, Adler G. 1999. Metabolic and weight loss effects of a long-term dietary intervention in obese patients. *Am J Clin Nutr* 69:198–204.

Halaas JL, Gajiwala KS, Maffei M, Cohen SL, Chait BT, Rabinowitz D, Lallone RL, Burley SK, Friedman JM. 1995. Weight-reducing effects of the plasma protein encoded by the obese gene. *Science* 269:543–546.

NHLBI (National Heart, Lung and Blood Institute). 1998. *Clinical Guidelines of the Identification, Evaluation, and Treatment of Overweight and Obesity in Adults - The Evidence Report. Obes Res* 6:51S–209S.

Sjostrom L, Rissanan A, Andersen T, Boldrin M, Golay A, Koppeschaar HP, Krempf M. 1998. Randomised placebo-controlled trial of orlistat for weight loss and prevention of weight regain in obese patients. *Lancet* 352:167–172.

Schteingart DE. 1992. Effectiveness of phenylpropanolamine in the management of moderate obesity. *Int J Obes Relat Metab Disord* 16:487–493.

Toubro S, Astrup AV, Breum L, Quaade F. 1993. Safety and efficacy of long-term treatment with ephedrine, caffeine, and an ephedrine/caffeine mixture. *Int J Obes Relat Metab Disord* 17:S69–S72.

EFFECTS OF EXERCISE, DIET, AND WEIGHT LOSS ON LIPID METABOLISM IN WOMEN

Marcia L. Stefanick, PhD, Associate Professor of Medicine, and of Obstetrics and Gynecology, Stanford University

Consensus has been reached within the past 5 years that sedentary status and overweight are each independent risk factors for coronary heart disease

(CHD) in adults, despite their strong associations with other established CHD risk factors, including low levels of high-density lipoprotein (HDL) cholesterol, elevated triglycerides, hypertension, and diabetes (HHS, 1996; NHLBI, 1998). Many observational and prospective cohort studies have shown that physical inactivity (Blair et al., 1989; HHS, 1996; Kushi et al., 1997; Manson et al., 1999) and excess body weight (Manson et al., 1990; NHLBI, 1998) are each associated with a two- to threefold increased risk of CHD in women compared with active and/or normal-weight women. In addition to low HDL cholesterol, it is generally accepted that elevated low-density lipoprotein (LDL) cholesterol is a major CHD risk factor in women, and that a diet high in fat, especially saturated fat, raises LDL-cholesterol levels; furthermore, adoption of a low-fat diet is recommended as the initial step in managing an adverse lipoprotein profile before resorting to a pharmacological approach (NHLBI, 1993). The role of exercise, diet, and weight loss on lipid metabolism is, therefore, of major interest for women.

Recent national surveys report that over a third of U.S. women aged ≥ 45 years participate in no leisure-time physical activity and less than 20 percent participate in regular, sustained physical activity at the recommended level (≥ 5 days per week for ≥ 30 minutes) (HHS, 1996); while nearly two-thirds of women aged ≥ 50 years are overweight (BMI ≥ 25.0 kg/m^2), half of whom are obese (BMI ≥ 30.0 kg/m^2) (NHLBI, 1998). It has been suggested that adoption of the recommended level of physical activity could reduce the risk of coronary events by 30–40 percent in women (Manson et al., 1999) and that as much as 70 percent of the coronary disease observed in obese women and 40 percent of that among women overall is attributable to overweight and is therefore preventable (Manson et al., 1990). A combined intervention of caloric reduction (emphasizing reduction of dietary fat, especially saturated fat, simple carbohydrates, and alcohol), physical activity, and behavior therapy, provide the most successful therapy for weight loss, (with a goal of losing 10 percent of body weight over a period of about 6 months), and weight maintenance (NHLBI, 1998).

Although trials of exercise, diet, or weight loss for prevention of CHD morbidity or mortality have not been completed, to date, the effects of diet and exercise by initially sedentary or overweight women on specific CHD risk factors, such as HDL and LDL cholesterol, have been reported in several randomized, controlled clinical trials (Duncan et al., 1991; King et al., 1991, 1995; McCarron et al., 1997; Stefanick, 1999; Stefanick et al., 1998; Svendsen et al., 1993; Wood et al., 1991). While several such studies have reported an HDL-lowering effect of a low-fat diet in women, when LDL cholesterol is lowered, or no significant lipoprotein improvements of diet alone, for women with initially unfavorable lipoproteins, the addition of exercise to the low-fat diet has been shown to result in significantly greater lipoprotein improvements in both pre- and postmenopausal women, even in the absence of greater weight loss with the addition of exercise to the diet (Stefanick, 1999; Stefanick et al.,

1998; Wood et al., 1991). There is little evidence, however, that aerobic or resistance exercise alone can improve obesity-related lipoprotein problems; therefore, diet, and if appropriate, weight loss, should be a focus of intervention as well (Stefanick, 1999). In general, these trials suggest that a lifestyle approach (diet, exercise, and weight loss) can substantially reduce CHD risk in women by reducing body weight and improving HDL and LDL cholesterol, triglycerides, blood pressure, and blood glucose.

Physical activity need not be of high intensity to reduce CHD risk substantially (HHS, 1996; Manson et al., 1999) and lower-intensity activity may result in better adherence over the long term (King et al., 1995). For weight loss, women randomized to three 10 minute bouts appeared to do better than those randomized to one 30 minute bout (Stefanick, 1999). Finally, for both improvement in cardiovascular fitness (King et al., 1991) and in weight loss (Perri et al., 1997), home-based programs seem to be more effective than group-based programs for women, although this will certainly depend on the individual. Whether lifestyle in combination with hormone replacement therapy (HRT) is superior in improving lipoproteins in postmenopausal women compared with HRT alone is unknown, but is being explored in the Women's Healthy Lifestyle Project (Simkin-Silverman et al., 1998).

References

Blair SN, Kohl HW III, Paffenbarger RS Jr, Clark DG, Cooper KN, Gibbons LW. 1989. Physical fitness and all-cause mortality: A prospective study of healthy men and women. *J Am Med Assoc* 262:2395–2401.

Duncan JJ, Gordan NF, Scott CB. 1991. Women walking for health and fitness: How much is enough? *J Am Med Assoc* 266:3295–3299.

HHS (U.S. Department of Health and Human Services). 1996. *Physical Activity and Health: A Report of the Surgeon General*. Atlanta, GA: U.S. Department of Health and Human Services, Centers for Disease Control and Prevention, National Center for Chronic Disease Prevention and Health Promotion.

Jakicic JM, Wing RR, Butler BA, Roberson RI. 1995. Prescribing exercise in multiple short bouts versus one continuous bout: Effects on adherence, cardiorespiratory fitness, and weight loss in overweight women. *Int J Obes Relat Metab Disord* 19:893–901.

King AC, Haskell WL, Taylor CB, Kraemer HC, DeBusk RF. 1991. Group-versus home-based exercise training in healthy older men and women: A community-based clinical trial. *J Am Med Assoc* 266:1535–1542.

King AC, Haskell WL, Young DR, Oka R, Stefanick ML. 1995. Long-term effects of varying intensities and formats of physical activity on participation rates, fitness, and lipoproteins in men and women aged 50 to 65 years. *Circulation* 91:2596–2604.

Kushi LH, Fee RM, Folsom AT, Mink PI, Anderson Ke, Sellers TA. 1997. Physical activity and mortality in postmenopausal women. *J Am Med Assoc* 277:1287–1292.

Manson JE, Colditz GA, Stampfer MJ, Willett WC, Rosner B, Nonson RR, Speizer FE, Hennekens CH. 1990. A prospective study of obesity and risk of coronary heart disease in women. *N Engl J Med* 322:882–889.

Manson JE, Hu FB, Rich-Edwards JW, Colditz GA, Stampger MJ, Willett WC, Speizer FE, Hennekens CH. 1999. A prospective study of walking as compared with vigorous exercise in the prevention of coronary heart disease in women. *N Engl J Med* 341:650–658.

McCarron DA, Oparil S, Chait A, Haynes RB, Kris-Etherton P, Stern JS, Resnick LM, Clark S, Morris CD, Hatton DC, Metz JA, McMahon M, Holcomb S, Snyder GW, Pi-Sunyer FX. 1997. Nutritional management of cardiovascular risk factors: A randomized clinical trial. *Arch Intern Med* 157:169–177.

NHLBI (National Heart, Lung and Blood Institute). 1993. *Second Report of the Expert Panel on Detection, Evaluation, and Treatment of High Blood Cholesterol in Adults* (Adult treatment panel II). NIH Publication no. 93-3095. Bethesda, MD: U.S. Department of Health and Human Services, National Institutes of Health.

NHLBI. 1998. Clinical guidelines on the identification, evaluation, and treatment of overweight and obesity in adults: The evidence report. *Obesity Res* 6:51S–209S.

Perri MG, Marin AD, Leermakers EA, Sears SF, Notelovitz M. 1997. Effects of group-versus home-based exercise in the treatment of obesity. *J Consult Clin Psychol* 65:278–285.

Simkin-Silverman LR, Wing RR, Boraz MA, Meilahn EN, Kuller LH. 1998. Maintenance of cardiovascular risk factor changes among middle aged women in a lifestyle intervention trial. *Womens Health* 4:255–272.

Stefanick ML. 1999. Physical activity for preventing and treating obesity-related dyslipoproteinemias. *Med Sci Sports Exerc* 31:S609–S618.

Stefanick ML, Mackey SM, Sheehan M, Ellsworth N, Haskell WL, Wood PD. 1998. Effects of diet and exercise in men and postmenopausal women with low levels of HDL-cholesterol and high levels of LDL-cholesterol. *N Engl J Med* 339:12–20.

Svendsen OL, Hassager C, Christiansen C. 1993. Effect of an energy-restrictive diet with or without exercise on lean tissue, resting metabolic rate, cardiovascular risk factors, and bone in overweight postmenopausal women. *Am J Med* 95:131–140.

Wood PD, Stefanick ML, Williams PT, Haskell WL. 1991. The effects on plasma in plasma lipoproteins of a prudent weight-reducing diet, with or without exercise in overweight men and women. *N Engl J Med* 325:461–468.

REPRODUCTIVE HEALTH ISSUES IN FITNESS AND WEIGHT- CONTROL PROGRAMS

Anne B. Loucks, Department of Biological Sciences Ohio University, Athens

Many women who restrict their diets or who exercise for fitness or weight-control experience a loss of menstrual cycles. In such amenorrheic women, the normal monthly rhythms of estrogen and progesterone are absent, indicating a complete suppression of ovarian follicular development, ovulation, and luteal function (Loucks et al., 1989). In addition to infertility, these estrogen-deficient women suffer an irreversible skeletal demineralization (Keen and Drinkwater, 1997) leading to osteoporosis and fractures (Loyd et al., 1986; Myburgh et al., 1990; Wilson and Wolman, 1994). Among athletic women, spinal bone mineral density is negatively proportional to the number of menstrual cycles missed (Drinkwater et al., 1990).

The proximal cause of these menstrual disorders is the slowing and disorganization of the pulsatile secretion of luteinizing hormone (LH) by the pituitary gland (Loucks et al., 1989), which reflects the disorganized secretion of gonadotropin-releasing hormone (GnRH) by the hypothalamus in the brain (Veldhuis et al., 1985). The influence of behavioral and environmental factors on the regulation of GnRH has been controversial and the subject of much research in recent years.

Early reports of amenorrhea in physically active women were attributed to low body fatness (Frisch, 1984), but many observational studies have accumulated evidence to disprove this hypothesis (Manning and Bronson, 1991; Sinning and Little, 1987). Nevertheless, this hypothesis was rejuvenated with the discovery that the adipose tissue hormone leptin is suppressed in amenorrheic women and that neurons with leptin receptors in the arcuate nucleus influence GnRH secretion via pro-opiomelanocortin and neuropeptide Y pathways (Cunningham et al., 1999). More recently, however, the secretion of leptin by adipose tissue has been found to be acutely and profoundly responsive to energy availability (Kolaczynski et al., 1996; Weigle et al., 1997), and even more specifically to carbohydrate availability (Boden et al., 1996; Grinspoon et al., 1997).

Most current research into the mechanism of menstrual disorders in exercising women is focused on two competing hypotheses. The energy availability hypothesis holds that the reproductive system is disrupted by an as yet undetermined mechanism when physically active women fail to consume enough dietary energy each day to match their daily energy expenditure (Wade and Schneider, 1992). A recent variant of this hypothesis holds that reproductive function depends specifically on glucose availability, since the brain relies on glucose for energy (Foster and Nagatani, 1999; Wade et al., 1996). The competing stress hypothesis holds that exercise activates the hypothalamic-pituitary adrenal (HPA) axis and that the hormones secreted by this axis disrupt the reproductive system.

Because the HPA axis has a glucoregulatory role, we designed experiments to measure the independent effects of energy availability and exercise stress on regularly menstruating, habitually sedentary women. Until these experiments, all investigations into the influence of exercise on reproductive function since those of Selye in the 1930s (1939) had confounded the "stress" of exercise with its impact on energy availability.

So far, these experiments appear to have taught us three lessons. First, LH pulsatility depends on energy availability, defined as dietary energy intake minus exercise energy expenditure, and not on either exercise stress or on energy intake or energy expenditure alone. In our experiments, exercise had no effect on LH pulsatility beyond the impact of its energy cost on energy availability (Loucks et al., 1998). By increasing dietary energy intake in compensation for exercise energy expenditure, we prevented the apparent disruptive effects of exercise stress on LH pulsatility.

Second, in women the disruptive effects of low energy availability appear to occur at a threshold of energy availability between 20 and 30 kcal/kglean body mass (LBM)/day. (In the women studied, 30 kcal/kgLBM/day corresponds to approximately 1,350 kcal/day.) For energy availability above 30 kcal/kgLBM/day, alterations in metabolic hormones maintain approximately normal levels of plasma glucose and ketones. Below 30 kcal/kgLBM/day, however, even larger alterations of metabolic hormones are unable to maintain normal plasma levels of these substrates, and effects on LH pulsatility begin. Below 20 kcal/kgLBM/day, the responses of certain metabolic hormones, such as insulin-like growth factor I/insulin-like growth factor-binding protein-1 and leptin, appear to have reached their limit while the responses of other metabolic hormones, such as cortisol and T_3, become exaggerated. Nevertheless, these exaggerated responses are unable to prevent further alterations in the metabolic substrates and LH pulsatility. Thus, alterations in LH pulsatility appear to be more closely associated with metabolic substrates than with metabolic hormones.

The third lesson currently emerging from these experiments is that the effects of low energy availability on LH pulsatility appear to be smaller in men than in women. Extensive observational field studies have indicated that in mammals reproductive function continues in males under conditions in which it is completely blocked in females (Aguilar et al., 1984; Widdowson et al., 1964). In our experiments at 10 kcal/kgLBM/day, effects of low energy availability on LH pulsatility appear to be blunted in men compared with women, so that we expect to find no effects in men at 20 kcal/kgLBM/day. That is, we expect to find that the threshold at which low energy availability disrupts LH pulsatility is lower in men than in women. At 10 kcal/kgLBM/day, the only metabolic parameters distinguishing men and women are leptin and absolute carbohydrate availability (i.e., dietary carbohydrate intake minus carbohydrate oxidation during exercise).

In summary, fitness and weight-control programs can damage reproductive and skeletal health. In exercising women, reproductive health appears to depend on energy availability. Damage to reproductive and skeletal health might be avoided in fitness and weight-loss programs by maintaining energy availability above 30 kcal/kgLBM/day through dietary reform alone without moderating the exercise regimen. These speculations need to be tested, though, through longer-term experiments measuring effects on ovarian function. Finally, women appear to require higher levels of energy availability than men to maintain reproductive health.

References

Aguilar E, Pinella L, Guisada R, Gonzalez D, Lopez F. 1984. Relation between body weight, growth rate, chronological age, and puberty in male and female rats. *Rev Esp Fisiol* 40:82–86.

Boden G, Chen X, Mozzoli M, Ryan I. 1996. Effect of fasting on serum leptin in normal human subjects. *J Clin Endocrinol Metab* 81:3419–3423.

Cunningham MJ, Clifton DK, Steiner RA. 1999. Leptin's actions on the reproductive axis: Perspectives and mechanisms. *Biol Reprod* 60:216–222.

Drinkwater BL, Nilson K, Chesnut CH III. 1990. Menstrual history as a determinant of current bone density in young athletes. *J Am Med Assoc* 263:545–548.

Foster DL, Nagatani S. 1999. Physiological perspectives on leptin as a regulator of reproduction: Role in timing puberty. *Biol Reprod* 60:205–215.

Frisch RE. 1984. Body fat, puberty, and fertility. *Biol Rev* 59:161–188.

Grinspoon SK, Askari H, Landt L, Nathan DM, Schoenfeld DA, Hayden DL, Laposata M, Hubbard J, Klibanski A. 1997. Effects of fasting and glucose infusion on basal and overnight leptin concentrations in normal-weight women. *Am J Clin Nutr* 66:1352–1366.

Keen AD, Drinkwater BL. 1997. Irreversible bone loss in former amenorrheic athletes. *Osteoporosis Int* 1:311–315.

Kolaczynski JW, Considine RV, Ohannesian J, Marco C, Opentanova I, Nyce MR, Myint M, Caro JF. 1996. Responses of leptin to short-term fasting and refeeding in humans: A link with ketogenesis but not ketones themselves. *Diabetes* 45:1511–1515.

Lloyd T, Triantafyllou SJ, Baker ER, Houts PS, Whiteside JA, Kalenak A, Stumpf PG. 1986. Women athletes with menstrual irregularity have increased musculoskelatal injuries. *Med Sci Sports Exerc* 18:374–379.

Loucks AB, Mortola JF, Girton L, Yen SSC. 1989. Alterations in the hypothalamicpituitary-ovarian and the hypothalamic-pituitary-adrenal axes in athletic women. *J Clin Endocrinol Metab* 68:402–411.

Loucks AB, Verdun M, Heath EM. 1998. Low energy availability, not stress of exercise, alters LH pulsatility in exercising women. *J App Physiol* 84:37–46.

Manning JM, Bronson FH. 1991. Suppression of puberty in rats by exercise: Effects on hormone levels and reversal with GnRH infusion. *Am J Physiol* 260:R717–R723.

Myburgh KH, Hutchins J, Fataar AB, Hough SF, Noakes TD. 1990. Low bone density is an etiologic factor for stress fractures in athletes. *Ann Intern Med* 113:754–759.

Selye H. 1939. The effect of adaptation to various damaging agents on the female sex organs in the rat. *Endocrinol* 25:615–624.

Sinning WE, Little KD. 1987. Body composition and menstrual function in athletes. *Sports Med* 4:34–45.

Veldhuis JD, Evans WS, Demers LM, Thorner MO, Wakat D, Rogol AD. 1985. Altered neuroendocrine regulation of gonadotropin secretion in women distance runners. *Clin Endocrinol Metab* 61:557–563.

Wade GN, Schneider JE. 1992. Metabolic fuels and reproduction in female mammals. *Neurosci Biobehav Rev* 16:235–272.

Wade GN, Schneider JE, Li HY. 1996. Control of fertility by metabolic cues. *Am J Physiol* 270:E1–E19.

Weigle DS, Duell PB, Connor WE, Steiner RA, Soules MR, Kuijper JL. 1997. Effect of fasting, refeeding, and dietary fat restriction on plasma leptin levels. *J Clin Endocrinol Metab* 82:561–565.

Widdowson EM, Mavor WO, McCance RA. 1964. The effect of undernutrition and rehabilitation on the development of the reproductive organs. *J Endocrinol* 29:119–126.

Wilson JH, Wolman RL. 1994. Osteoporosis and fracture complications in an amenorrheic athlete: Case study. *Br J Rheumatol* 33:480–481.

OBESITY: AN INFECTIOUS DISEASE?

Nikhil V. Dhurandhar, PhD

Introduction

Obesity has been called the number one public health problem in America (Bray, 1979). Although obesity is recognized as a disease of multiple etiologies, a virus infection as an etiological factor has been ignored until now. Five different viruses have been shown to cause obesity in animal models (Carter et al., 1990; Dhurandhar and Atkinson, 1996; Dhurandhar et al., 1990, 1992, 1997; Gostonyi and Ludwig, 1995; Lyons et al., 1982). Of these, we have identified two viruses, SMAM-1, an avian adenovirus, and AD-36, a human adenovirus, that produce obesity in animals. The concept that adenoviruses cause obesity and that the virus may be linked to human obesity was developed by Dr. Dhurandhar while working with SMAM-1 virus in Bombay, India, and was pursued further by Dr. Dhurandhar when he started work at the University of Wisconsin-Madison. The work led to the discovery of the obesity-promoting potential of another adenovirus, AD-36, which produced obesity in animals along with a paradoxical decrease in serum cholesterol and triglycerides levels (Dhurandhar and Atkinson, 1996). Our data described below demonstrate that a human virus produces obesity in animal models, and that a unique syndrome consisting of paradoxically low serum cholesterol and triglycerides levels, is present in about 30 percent of obese humans screened who have antibodies to this human virus. Antibodies to AD-36 were present in only 5 percent of the non-obese subjects screened to date, suggesting that infection with this syndrome carries a high probability of association (causation has not yet been proven in humans) with obesity. The possible link between a virus and obesity in humans warrants serious investigation of the obesity-promoting effect of this virus.

Adenoviruses: Background Information

Adenoviruses are naked DNA viruses with icosahedral symmetry and a diameter of 65–80 nm. The American Type Culture Collection maintains 50 types of human adenoviruses. In humans, adenoviruses are frequently associated with acute upper respiratory tract infections and may cause enteritis and conjunctivitis. Adenoviruses can easily be isolated from nasal swabs or from feces. Adenovirus infections are transmitted via respiratory, fomite, droplet, venereal, and fecal-oral routes. AD-36 was first isolated in 1978 in Germany in the feces of a 6-year-old girl with diabetes and enteritis (Wigand et al., 1980).

Review of Experiments

Experiments with SMAM-1

We demonstrated that chickens experimentally infected with SMAM-1, an avian adenovirus isolated in Bombay, India, produced excessive fat accumulation in the visceral depots and a paradoxical reduction of serum levels of cholesterol and triglycerides (Dhurandahr et al., 1990, 1992). The findings were replicated. Of 52 obese humans tested by agar gel-precipitation test, 10 had antibodies to SMAM-1 (Dhurandhar et al., 1997). These 10 individuals had a higher body weight and lower serum cholesterol and triglycerides compared with antibody-negative individuals (Dhurandhar et al., 1997).

Experiments with AD-36: Animal Studies

Chicken Experiments: Specific pathogen-free white leghorn chickens were used for three separate experiments that are summarized below. Chickens were housed under biosafety level 2 containment and were inoculated with AD-36 virus (infected group) or the tissue culture media (uninfected controls) at 3 weeks of age. Chickens were inoculated intra-nasally in experiments 1 and 2 and i.p. in experiment 3. Chickens in experiments 1, 2, and 3 were killed 3, 5, and 16 weeks post inoculation, respectively. Food intake was not different for any of the groups within any experiment. Chickens inoculated with AD-36 in experiments 1 and 2 had significantly greater visceral and total body fat and significantly lower serum cholesterol and triglycerides compared to the controls. For example, compared to the control, the AD-36 group in experiment 2 had 128 percent greater visceral fat ($p < .0005$) and 46 percent greater total body fat ($p < .0005$). These data show that AD-36 infection reliably and reproducibly induces adiposity in chickens, which is associated with a reduction in serum cholesterol and triglycerides.

The AD-36-infected group in experiment 3 had significantly greater visceral fat and the histopathological study of the brain including hypothalamic area did not show any difference in the infected versus the control groups. Unlike some other obesity promoting viruses, AD-36-induced obesity does not appear to be due to the hypothalamic damage. Virus was isolated from the oral and the rectal swabs taken from the infected chickens 1-week post inoculation, but not from the controls. Also, using capillary electrophoresis assay, AD-36 deoxyribonucleic acid (DNA) was detected in the DNA isolated from the adipose tissue and the blood of some of the infected chickens screened but not from the DNA obtained from their skeletal muscles. AD-36 DNA could not be detected in any of the control chickens screened. Absence of hypothalamic lesions and the presence of the viral DNA in the adipose tissue suggest a peripheral and not a central mechanism for the development of obesity syndrome.

Mice Experiment: The obesity promoting effect of AD-36 was tested in mice as a mammal model. Institue for Cancer Research out bred Swiss albino female mice (4 weeks old) were inoculated i.p. with AD-36 (AD-36 group), or tissue culture media (control group) and the animals were killed 22 weeks post inoculation. Food intake was not different for the two groups. Compared with the control, the AD-36 group had 9 percent greater body weight ($p < .05$), 67 percent greater visceral fat ($p < .02$) and 30 percent greater total body fat ($p < .02$). Sixty percent of the mice infected with AD-36 had total percent body-fat weights above the 85th percentile of the control group ($p < .02$). Serum cholesterol and triglycerides in the AD-36 group were significantly lower than control by 38 percent and 31 percent, respectively. This is the first report of obesity induced by a human virus in a mammal.

Monkey Experiment: This experiment was carried out to screen rhesus monkey serum for the presence of AD-36 antibodies and to ascertain any association of such antibodies to obesity and cholesterol levels. Frozen serum samples from 15 adult male rhesus monkeys were obtained from the Wisconsin Regional Primate Research Center. For each monkey, the samples were drawn every 6 months for a period of 90 months and a corresponding body weight was available for each sample drawn. Monkeys were between 8 and 14 years of age when the first sample available for this study was drawn (baseline sample) and were on an ad libitum diet. Antibodies to AD-36 in the experiment were determined with serum neutralization assay.

During the 90-month period, all 15 monkeys showed AD-36 antibodies at some point in time. Out of 15 monkeys, 7 monkeys were seropositive at the baseline and, therefore, not included in the analysis. These 7 monkeys were excluded from the analysis because a comparison for body weight and cholesterol between before and after the appearance of AD-36 antibodies was not possible. The remaining 8 monkeys were seronegative for AD-36 antibodies at baseline and became seropositive after variable periods. Body weight and serum cholesterol at 6 monthly intervals were analyzed for these 8 monkeys. Body weight and cholesterol of the 8 monkeys before turning antibody positive were compared with those after the first appearance of AD-36 antibodies. Analysis was restricted to the 90-month period for which the serum samples were obtained.

Prior to the first appearance of AD-36 antibody, body weight of the monkeys had plateaued for at least 18 months but increased by 10 percent in just 6 months after the first appearance of AD-36 antibody. The body weight was 15 percent greater after 12 months and 18 months after the first appearance of AD-36 antibody, compared with the body weight 6 months prior to the first appearance of AD-36 antibody ($p < .03$). Serum cholesterol levels increased slightly in the 18 months before the appearance of AD-36 antibodies. However, cholesterol levels decreased by 28 percent in 6 months after the first appearance of AD-36 antibody ($p < 0.03$) and remained lower for at least 18 months after the first appearance of AD-36 antibody. Thus, the increase in body weight and the reduction in cholesterol levels coincided with the first appearance of AD-36 antibody in the serum. Significant changes were observed despite the small number of monkeys. This is an indirect evidence of a possible effect of AD-36 infection on body weight and cholesterol levels. Only infecting monkeys with AD-36 can conclusively show direct effect of AD-36 on body weight and cholesterol levels.

Human Studies

Human serum samples obtained from obese (body mass index ≥ 27 kg/M^2, $N = 418$) and nonobese volunteers ($N = 93$) from three different sites (Wisconsin, Florida, and New York) were screened for the presence of AD-36 antibodies using serum neutralization test. At each of the three sites, prevalence of AD-36 antibodies was significantly greater for the obese compared with the nonobese subjects. Prevalence of AD-36 antibodies in three sites pooled together was 5 percent for the nonobese and 30 percent for the obese subjects. At each of the sites, the antibody-positive obese had significantly lower serum cholesterol compared with the antibody negative obese subjects from the respective site ($p < .002$).

Conclusion

Our data show that a human adenovirus causes adiposity in animals and is strongly associated with obesity in humans. Due to ethical reasons, humans cannot be experimentally inoculated with the virus and we have to depend on indirect evidence of the obesity-promoting effect of AD-36 in humans. Understanding the mechanism involved in promoting adiposity and reduction in serum lipid levels caused by the virus is critical. Long-term goal of this research is to develop a vaccine to prevent AD-36-induced adiposity.

References

Bray GA. 1979. *Obesity in America*. NIH Publication 79-359. Washington, D.C.: National Institutes of Health.

Carter JK, Ow CL, Smith RE. 1983. Rous-associated virus type 7 induces a syndrome in chickens characterized by stunting and obesity. *Infect Immun* 39:410–422.

Dhurandhar NV, Atkinson RL. 1996. Development of obesity in chickens after infection with a human adenovirus. *Obesity Res* 4:24S.

Dhurandhar NV, et al. 1990. Avian adenovirus leading to pathognomic obesity in chickens. *J Bombay Vet College* 2:131–132.

Dhurandhar NV, Kulkarni P, Ajinkya SM, Sherikar A. 1992. Effect of adenovirus infection on adiposity in chickens. *Vet Microbiol* 31:101–107.

Dhurandhar NV, Kulkarni PR, Ajinkya SM, Sherikar AA, Atkinson RL. 1997. Association of adenovirus infection with human obesity. *Obesity Res* 5:464–469.

Gosztonyi G, Ludwig H. 1995. Borna disease: Neuropathology and pathogenesis. *Curr Top Microbiol Immunol* 190:39–73.

Lyons MJ, Faust IM, Hemmes RB, Buskirk DR, Hirsch J, Zabriskie JB. 1982. A virally induced obesity syndrome in mice. *Science* 216:82–85.

Wigand R, Gelderblom H, Wadell G. 1980. New human adenovirus (candidate adenovirus 36), a novel member of subgroup D. *Arch Virol* 64:225–233.

FACTORS AFFECTING LONG-TERM WEIGHT LOSS/WEIGHT REGAIN

George Blackburn, MD, PhD

Introduction

Obesity has been described by the World Health Organization as an "escalating epidemic" and "one of the greatest neglected public health problems of our time with an impact on health which may well prove to be as great as smoking (Rippe et al., 1998)." An estimated 97 million adults in the United States are overweight or obese, a condition that substantially raises their risk of morbidity from hypertension, dyslipidemia, type 2 diabetes, coronary heart disease, stroke, gallbladder disease, osteoarthritis, sleep apnea, and cancer (NHLBI, 1998). The obesity epidemic is costing our country billions. The cost attributable to obesity amounted to $99.2 billion in 1995, of this total, $51.6 billion were direct medical costs associated with diseases attributable to obesity (NHLBI, 1998). Overweight and obesity prevalence has been rising at a steady pace between 1960–1994. This increase has occurred across all ages, genders and racial/ethnic groups. A recent survey reported that 59.4 percent of men and 50.7 percent of women in the United States are overweight or obese (NHLBI, 1998). Estimates show that at any one time, approximately 25 percent of men and 45 percent of women are trying to lose weight (Williamson et al., 1992). Of the participants who enter a behavioral weight-loss program, it is estimated that they will lose approximately 10 percent of their body weight over the course of 20–24 weeks (Shick et al., 1998). Unfortunately, it has also been shown that these participants also regain an average of 33 percent of their weight loss and typically return to their baseline weight within 5 years (Shick et al., 1998).

Brief Review of Factors Affecting Long-Term Weight Loss/Weight Regain

Why is America gaining weight? Consider the change in our environment over the past century. There are a greater variety of foods available. Simply consider the potato chip choices alone. There are currently a plethora of brands, varieties, and flavors available to the consumer everyday and often 24 hours a day. Compare this with the turn of the century where it was common to walk to the market and purchase a 25-pound bag of potatoes to use in cooking. Food has also become more palatable. Improved manufacturing and technology have improved colors and flavors to make food appear and taste richer and more satisfying than ever before. Food has also become increasingly convenient to obtain. Gone are the days of being forced to borrow from the neighbors because the supermarkets are closed. Many supermarkets and convenience store are open 24 hours a day, ready to sell consumers the foods that contribute to weight gain.

The fast-food market has increasingly become a staple of American food culture over the years. Effective marketing strategies coupled with broader, inexpensive choices have made this industry a prime culprit in the American obesity epidemic. Unfortunately, with the increase in variety, palatability, convenience, and availability of food, there has also been a decline in the amount of exercise performed by the average American. Sedentary desk jobs, computers, fewer safe places for exercise, and more elevators and drive-through restaurants are only a few of the contributors to this escalating problem.

With the changing environment and the discouraging rates of weight regain, it is imperative that we take a closer look at long-term weight maintenance and the various methods successful maintainers utilize to prevent weight gain. To get a better perspective in this area, it is appropriate to review a portion of the long-term data provided by the National Weight Control Registry (NWCR). The NWCR is a registry of individuals who have been followed in a prospective manner having been successful at maintaining significant weight losses. Participants in the NWCR have lost, on average, more than 65 pounds and maintained their weight losses for 5.7 years (McGuire et al., 1999b). Long-term studies of weight loss in individuals participating in the NWCR indicate that those who regain weight typically show a demonstrated decline in self-monitoring. This includes techniques such as frequent self-weighing as well as keeping food and exercise diaries. These individuals showed a marked decrease in physical activity of more than 800 calories per week, coupled with increases in the percentage of calories taken in from fat. The study also showed the re-gainers to have a higher lifetime level of intentional weight cycling (McGuire et al., 1999b). Those who regained weight were more likely to have sought assistance for weight loss rather than utilizing self-directed weight loss methods, and were more likely to have used a liquid formula diets for their initial weight loss. In comparison, it has been shown that 72 percent of successful weight losers lost weight on their own, 20 percent used commercial weight-loss programs, and 5 percent utilized a university-based program (McGuire et al., 1998). Those who gained weight also were shown to have been heavier at their maximum weight, initially lost a greater percentage of their maximum weight (> 30 percent) and had maintained their weight loss for fewer years than maintainers (McGuire et al., 1999b).

What predicts successful weight maintenance? Research has shown the five most common links appear to be (1) physical activity, (2) self-monitoring, (3) problem solving, (4) continued contact, and (5) stress management (Foreyt, 1999).

Physical Activity

Longitudinal studies with 2–10 years of follow-up results have observed that physical activity is related to less weight gain over time (NHLBI, 1998). It is a well-known fact that physical activity is a good predictor of weight maintenance (Foreyt, 1999). A review of successful weight maintainers reveals that they engaged in more strenuous activities such as running, weight lifting and aerobics than regainers, and participated in more activities that made them sweat (McGuire et al., 1999a). Specifically, 52 percent of maintainers reported engaging in three or more episodes that made them sweat in a typical 7-day week compared with 32–36 percent of the regainers and controls (McGuire et al., 1999a). Although, it is important to note it has been demonstrated that both gainers and maintainers reported decreases in total calories expended thorough physical activity. However, maintainers reported a decrease of only 500 calories per week where gainers reported a decrease of almost 1,000 calories per week at 1-year follow-up (McGuire et al., 1999b).

Self-Monitoring

Self-monitoring is the cornerstone of behavioral treatment (Foreyt, 1999). One of the common findings observed in individuals who are successful at long-term weight loss is that maintainers report extensive use of behavioral strategies for reduction in dietary fat intake, self weighing, and physical activity (McGuire et al., 1999a). Taking a closer look at self weighing as a form of self-monitoring, it has been shown that 55 percent of maintainers reported weighing themselves at least once each week, where only 35 percent of the regainers reported weighing themselves frequently (McGuire et al., 1999a). Other forms of self-monitoring, such as keeping a food or exercise record, functions to assist the patient in assessing overall intake of various foods in relation to the amount of exercise performed. Despite the fact that caloric intake may be underestimated, the records sensitize patients to the eating and exercise portion of their lifestyle (Blackburn and Kanders, 1994).

Problem Solving

Generally, it has been shown that those individuals who confront life's stressors with a positive problem-solving attitude are more likely to have greater success in any endeavor (Foreyt, 1999). All aspects of effective obesity treatment involve improved problem solving and confrontational skills. A survey of weight maintainers showed that 95 percent of them utilized problem solving or confrontational technique. In comparison, only 10 percent of those who relapsed used problem solving skills and instead, tended to use escape-avoidance ways of coping with stress, such as eating, smoking, or taking tranquilizers (Blackburn and Kanders, 1994). These findings support the theory that once an individual makes a behavioral change, relapse occurs in the face of insufficient coping skills (Blackburn and Kanders, 1994).

Continued Contact

Frequent patient-provider contact is associated with the best maintenance of weight loss (Anderson and Wadden, 1999). This contact does not have to be given solely by the physician, but by a registered dietitian, nurse, or office staff. Contact can be made to patients, via phone, fax, or email. These continued visits have been shown to enhance motivation, troubleshooting, and teach patients a new set of skills. Overall, the longer patients remain in behavioral treatment the longer they are expected to maintain their weight loss (Anderson and Wadden, 1999).

Stress Management

Literature has shown that stress has a facilitating effect on the eating behavior of individuals most likely to be patients in a weight-loss program (Blackburn and Kanders, 1994). This excessive stress appears to predict early drop out from organized weight-loss programs (Foreyt, 1999). It is essential to help patients identify a strategy when confronted with stressful events to allow them to gain quick composure in order to use other behavioral techniques (Blackburn and Kanders, 1994). Working with patients to help address and alleviate the stress-eating relationship in weight-loss treatment and maintenance is of key importance (Foreyt, 1999). Four basic stress management procedures used in weight maintenance include self-monitoring, environmental control, relaxation training, and contingent relaxation (Blackburn and Kanders, 1994).

Conclusion

Regardless of the weight-loss option selected, patients should strive to develop the skills that have been reported by successful weight-loss maintainers. These techniques include exercising regularly, monitoring weight frequently, eating a low-fat diet, recording food intake, and developing effective problem solving skills (Anderson and Wadden, 1999). In addition, believing in yourself (Fletcher, 1994) and not relying on willpower can help your patients achieve success in their weight-maintenance endeavors.

References

Anderson DA, Wadden TA. 1999. Treating the obese patient. Suggestions for primary care practice. *Arch Family Med* 8:156–167.

Blackburn GL, Kanders BS. 1994. *Obesity: Pathophysiology, Psychology and Treatment*. New York: Chapman and Hall.

Fletcher AM. 1994. *Thin for Life. 10 Keys to Success from People Who have Lost Weight and Kept it Off.* Shelburne, VT: Chapters Publishing.

Foreyt JP. 1999 (July). *Strategies for Maintenance and Relapse Prevention*. Abstract and slides presented at the Harvard Obesity Conference.

McGuire MT, Wing RR, Klem ML, Hill JO. 1999a. Behavioral strategies of individuals who have maintained long-term weight losses. *Obes Res* 7:334–341.

McGuire MT, Wing RR, Klem ML, Lang W, Hill JO. 1999b.What predicts weight regain in a group of successful weight losers? *J Consult Clin Psychol* 67:177–185.

McGuire MT, Wing RR, Klem ML, Seagle HM, Hill JO. 1998. Long-term maintenance of weight loss: Do people who lose weight through various weight loss methods use different behaviors to maintain their weight? *Int J Obes* 22:572–577.

NHLBI (National Heart, Lung and Blood Institute). 1998. Clinical guidelines on the identification, evaluation, and treatment of overweight and obesity in adults: The evidence report. *Obes Res* 6:51S–209S.

Rippe JM, Crossley S, Ringer R. 1998. Obesity as a chronic disease: Modern medical and lifestyle management. *J Am Diet Assoc* 98:S9–S15.

Shick SM, Wing RR, Klem ML, McGuire MT, Hill JO, Seagle H. 1998. Persons successful at long term weight loss and maintenance continue to consume a low energy, low fat diet. *J Am Diet Assoc* 98:408–413.

Williamson DF, Derdula MK, Serdula MK, Anda RF, Levy A, Byers T. 1992. Weight loss attempts in adults: Goal, duration and rate of weight loss. *Am J Public Health* 82:1251–1257.

FACTORS AFFECTING LONG-TERM MAINTENANCE OF WEIGHT LOSS AND WEIGHT REGAIN

John M. Jakicic, PhD, Assistant Professor, Brown University School of Medicine, Miriam Hospital Weight Control and Diabetes Research Center

Obesity is a significant health problem in the United States, and it is estimated that in excess of 50 percent of adults are considered overweight (BMI > 25 kg/m^2). Despite documented short-term success in weight-loss programs, it has been shown that typically, one-third of weight lost will be regained within 1–3 years, with total regain occurring within 3–5 years. Therefore, it is important to examine the most effective implementation of strategies that have been shown to maximize long-term weight loss and prevent weight regain.

Despite the belief that most individuals are unsuccessful at long-term weight loss, the National Weight Control Registry (NWCR) has identified a large number of individuals that have successfully maintained at least a 30-lb weight loss for a minimum of 1 year (Klem et al., 1997). Close examination of this data set shows that there are individuals that have maintained a weight loss of approximately 60 lb and have maintained this for 5.6 ± 6.8 years. Therefore, results from this study should be examined closely to determine if there are unique strategies that can be used to enhance long-term weight loss in overweight adults.

Exercise

An interesting finding in the NWCR is that individuals continue to participate in strategies to maintain both healthful eating and exercise behaviors. However, a unique finding in these data is that these individuals are maintaining extremely high levels of exercise, with leisure-time activity being 2,000 to 2,500 kcal/week for both men and women (Klem et al., 1997). This value is much greater than the current public health recommendation for physical activity to improve health (HHS, 1996; Pate et al., 1998). However, this level is similar to the amount of activity shown by Schoeller and colleagues (1997) to minimize weight regain in overweight women, and this amount of activity was verified using doubly labeled water. Jakicic and colleagues (1999) have shown that when combined with dietary modification, weight regain in the 12 months following was minimized when exercise exceeded 150 minutes per week. However, of interest is that there was no weight regain in women exercising greater than 200 minutes per week throughout the entire 18 months of treatment. Thus, overall, these results appear to verify the conclusion of Pronk and Wing (1994) based on a review of the literature, that physical activity is one of the best predictors of long-term weight maintenance.

Despite the evidence presented above, debate remains regarding the optimal intensity of the activity that will enhance long-term weight loss and minimize weight regain. In a 20-week study of overweight women, Duncan and colleagues (1991) showed that total energy expenditure rather than exercise intensity is the key factor for regulating body weight. However, data from the NWCR suggests that individuals successful at long-term weight loss participate in a high level of vigorous intensity activity (Klem et al., 1997). Despite these findings, the results of this study are cross-sectional and have not been confirmed by a randomized clinical trial. Currently, Jakicic and colleagues are conducting a randomized clinical trial to examine the dose-response of exercise (intensity and energy expenditure) on weight loss across a 24-month period of time.

Despite the debate over the optimal amount of activity that is necessary to maximize long-term weight loss, little debate exists as to the importance of physical activity for overweight adults. Data from the Center for Aerobics Research at the Cooper Institute have shown that physical fitness can have a significant impact on mortality rates independent of body weight. Lee and colleagues (1998) have shown that there is a significant reduction in mortality rates in overweight adults that also have higher levels of physical fitness, and this mortality rate is similar to leaner unfit adults. These results suggest that interventions that improve physical fitness in overweight adults can have significant health benefits independent of changes in body weight. Therefore, it is important to develop and implement strategies to increase exercise participation in overweight adults.

Recently, Dunn and colleagues (1999) have shown that a home-based lifestyle activity intervention can be as effective over 18–24 months as a structured clinic-based exercise intervention. In addition, in studies of overweight women, Jakicic and colleagues (1995, 1999) have shown that multiple short bouts of exercise can be effective in previously sedentary individuals. Therefore these strategies should be considered when implementing interventions to address body-weight regulation within the military.

Changes in the Micro and Macro Environments

It has been suggested that we live in a "toxic environment" relative to factors that affect body weight. There are a number of factors, such as accessibility of high fat/calorie foods and labor saving devices that affect our eating and exercise behaviors. However, it has been shown that the environment can be manipulated to have a positive impact on eating and exercise behaviors. For example, French and colleagues (1997) showed that lowering prices in vending machines for low-fat snacks increased the amount of low-fat snacks that were purchased. In addition, Andersen and colleagues (1998) have reported that posting signs to encourage the use of stairs in a shopping mall can have a positive impact on activity patterns.

It may also be important to increase access to healthier foods and provide opportunities for physical activity, and this can be done to both the macro and micro environments. For example, Sallis and colleagues (1990) showed that individuals living in close proximity to exercise facilities were more active than those living further away from these facilities. Jakicic and colleagues (1997) showed that there was a significant correlation between physical activity and having home-exercise equipment. More recently, Jakicic and colleagues (1999) reported that providing overweight adults with home treadmills increased exercise participation. Therefore, these findings suggests that modifications to the environment may have a positive impact on health behaviors related to body-weight regulation.

Long-Term Changes in Dietary Intake

Despite the fact that exercise appears to be one of the best predictors of long-term weight loss, the impact of eating behaviors on this process should not be overlooked. It has been shown in short-term studies that exercise alone has little impact on body weight when compared with diet or the combination of diet plus exercise (Wing et al., 1998). Moreover, the effectiveness of exercise in long-term weight loss may be partially explained by its link to healthful eating behaviors. For example, Klem and colleagues (1997) reported that individuals successful at long-term weight loss maintained healthful eating behaviors along with high levels of exercise. Unpublished data from a study conducted in our laboratory has shown that individuals that have maintained high levels of exercise also report maintaining more healthful eating behaviors than those not maintaining their exercise over a period of 18 months. Thus, these results appear to suggest that both dietary and exercise behaviors should be targeted to enhance long-term weight loss and to prevent weight regain.

Continued Contact

It has been suggested that obesity is a chronic disease and should be treated with a chronic disease intervention. Perri and colleagues (1987) have shown that maintaining contact with a weight-loss program long-term enhances weight loss. However, from a clinical perspective, it becomes difficult to keep individuals in treatment programs for long periods of time. Thus, the typical model of providing group sessions during the maintenance phase of treatment may not be appealing to individuals participating in these programs. Therefore, maintaining contact through other means may prove to be more effective in long-term intervention programs. Some of the strategies that have been shown to be successful are telephone contacts and mailings. In addition, interventions using social support strategies and computers are currently ongoing. Therefore, these intervention strategies may be appealing to the military when attempting to deliver interventions to soldiers that may be deployed throughout the world.

Targeting High Risk Periods for Weight Gain

There is some evidence that there are specific periods when individuals may be at risk for weight gain, and this may be an important factor for the military to consider. One period of time is during early adulthood, and weight gain is typically accompanied by a trend for decreases in physical activity. For example, unpublished data from our laboratory has shown that college-aged men and women participating in regular exercise gained less weight during their college years than those not regularly participating in exercise.

Weight gain may also occur in individuals that are already moderately overweight. We have shown that moderately overweight adult men left untreated will gain a significant amount of weight over a period of 16 weeks, whereas participation in a program to modify exercise behaviors and minimize fat intake appears to have a beneficial effect on body weight in these individuals (Leermakers et al., 1998). Therefore, it may be important for the military to identify individuals that are moderately overweight and encourage changes in exercise and eating behaviors to prevent further weight gain.

The postpartum period may be an extremely important time for women with regard to body-weight regulation, and interventions targeting this period may be extremely important. For example, in a study of women following pregnancy, women left untreated lost 4.9 kg with 11.5 percent returning to prepregnancy weight, whereas those participating in a correspondence-based treatment program lost 7.8 kg and 33 percent returned to prepregnancy weight (Leermakers et al., 1998). Therefore, it may be important for the military to consider offering postpartum interventions to minimize the retention of body weight in women during this period.

Application to Weight-Regulation Initiatives in the Military

There may be some debate in the various branches of the military regarding acceptable body-weight values and methods of measuring these parameters. However, regardless of the absolute value that is determined to be acceptable, it should be recognized that there are soldiers in the military that are at risk for weight gain. Therefore, the military should consider implementing strategies that may minimize weight gain in these individuals, and these could include changes in the environment and providing access to programs related to eating and exercise behaviors.

In addition, the military should consider implementing interventions early on (i.e., basic training) that will permit soldiers to transfer their activity and eating behavior outside of a controlled environment setting. For example, when an individual enters the military, it is commonly believed that they are in an environment in which they have little control over their eating and exercise behaviors, and these factors are controlled by the military. However, soon after that period of time, soldiers have more freedom of choice, and this is a period when they could potentially relapse into typical behavioral patterns. Thus, providing opportunities for soldiers to maintain their newly developed exercise and eating behaviors may minimize body weight-regulation concerns in this population. Moreover, one factor that should be considered is the history of the soldier prior to entering the military. It is likely in some cases that an individual lost weight just prior to entering the military in order to conform to the military standards and to be accepted into the military. However, the period following this initial weight loss is a high-risk time for weight regain. Identifying individuals that meet these criteria, and targeting interventions at this group of individuals may prove to be beneficial in preventing relapse while in the military.

References

Andersen RE, Franckowiak SC, Snyder J, Bartlett SJ, Fontaine KR. 1998. Can inexpensive signs encourage the use of stairs? Results from a community intervention. *Ann Intern Med* 129:363–369.

Duncan JJ, Gordon NF, Scott CB. 1991. Women walking for health and fitness: How much is enough? *J Am Med Assoc* 266:3295–3299.

Dunn AL, Marcus BH, Kampert JB, Garcia ME, Kohl III HW, Blair SN. 1999. Comparison of lifestyle and structured interventions to increase physical activity and cardiorespiratory fitness. *J Am Med Assoc* 281:327–334.

French SA, Jeffery RW, Story M, Hannan P, Snyder MP. 1997. A pricing strategy to promote low-fat snack choices through vending machines. *Am J Public Health* 87:849–851.

HHS (U.S. Department of Health and Human Services). 1996. *Physical Activity and Health: A Report of the Surgeon General.* Atlanta, GA: Centers for Disease Control and Prevention and National Center for Chronic Disease Prevention and Health Promotion.

Jakicic JM, Wing RR, Butler BA, Jeffery RW. 1997. The relationship between the presence of exercise equipment and participation in physical activity. *Am J Health Promot* 11:363–365.

Jakicic JM, Wing RR, Butler BA, Robertson RJ. 1995. Prescribing exercise in multiple short bouts versus one continuous bout: Effects on adherence, cardiorespiratory fitness, and weight loss in overweight women. *Int J Obes* 19: 893–901.

Jakicic JM, Winters C, Lang W, Wing RR. 1999. Effects of intermittent exercise and use of home exercise equipment on adherence, weight loss, and fitness in overweight women. *J Am Med Assoc* 282:1554–1560.

Klem ML, Wing RR, McGuire MT, Seagle HM, Hill JO. 1997. A descriptive study of individuals successful at long-term maintenance of substantial weight loss. *Am J Clin Nutr* 66:239–246.

Lee CD, Jackson AS, Blair SN. 1998. U.S. weight guidelines: Is it also important to consider cardiorespiratory fitness? *Int J Obes Relat Metab Disord* 22:S2–S7.

Leermakers EA, Anglin K, Wing RR. 1998. Reducing postpartum weight retention through a correspondence intervention. *Int J Obes Relat Metab Disord* 22:1103–1109.

Leermakers EA, Jakicic JM, Viteri J, Wing RR. 1998. Clinic-based vs. home-based interventions for preventing weight gain in men. *Obes Res* 6:346–352.

Pate RR, Pratt M, Blair SN, Haskell WL, Macera CA, Bouchard C, Buchner D, Ettinger W, Heath GW, King AC, Kriska A, Leon AS, Marcus BH, Morris J, Paffenbarger RS, Patrick K, Pollock ML, Rippe JM, Sallis J, Wilmore JH. 1998. Physical activity and public health: A recommendation from the Centers for Disease Control and Prevention and the American College of Sports Medicine. *J Am Med Assoc* 273:402–407.

Perri MG, McAdoo WG, McAllister DA, Lauer JB, Jordan RC, Yancey DZ, Nezu AM. 1987. Effects of peer support and therapist contact on long-term weight loss. *J Consult Clin Psychol* 55:615–617.

Pronk NP, Wing RR. 1994. Physical activity and long-term maintenance of weight loss. *Obes Res* 2:587–599.

Sallis JF, Hovell MF, Hofstetter CR, Elder JP, Hackley M, Caspersen CJ, Powell KE. 1990. Distance between homes and exercise facilities related to frequency of exercise among San Diego residents. *Public Health Rep* 105:179–185.

Schoeller DA, Shay K, Kushner RF. 1997. How much physical activity is needed to minimize weight gain in previously obese women? *Am J Clin Nutr* 66:551–556.

Wing RR, Venditti E, Jakicic JM, Polley BA, Lang W. 1998. Lifestyle intervention in overweight individuals with a family history of diabetes. *Diabetes Care* 21:350–359.

B

Biographical Sketches of the Workshop Speakers

GEORGE L. BLACKBURN serves as an associate professor of surgery and nutrition, associate director of the Division of Nutrition, and is the first incumbent of the S. Daniel Abraham Chair in Nutrition Medicine at Harvard Medical School. He is the director of the Nutrition Support Service, chief of the Nutritional/Metabolism Laboratory, director of the Center for the Study of Nutrition and Medicine, and program director for Surgical Treatment of Severe Obesity, all of which are affiliated with the Beth Israel Deaconess Medical Center in Boston, Massachusetts. He received his M.D. from the University of Kansas and completed his internship and residency at Boston City Hospital, Harvard Medical School. He obtained his Ph.D. in nutritional biochemistry from Massachusetts Institute of Technology. Dr. Blackburn has trained over 100 fellows in applied and clinical nutrition and has over 390 publications on various aspects of nutrition, medicine, and metabolism. He is on the editorial board of and reviewer for several journals and received the Grace Goldsmith Award from the American College of Nutrition and the Joseph Goldberger award in clinical nutrition from the American Medical Association. He is president of the North American Association for the Study of Obesity and immediate past president of the American Board of Nutrition. He also serves as the chair of the Scientific Advisory Committee of the C. Everett Koop Foundation Shape Up America Campaign. He remains on the Board of Advisors for the American Society of Parenteral and Enteral Nutrition of which he served as president, he was also president of the American Society for Clinical Nutrition, and is a member of numerous other medical societies. Dr. Blackburn is a principal investigator or coprincipal investigator on several National Institutes of Health-funded grants.

MAJ STEPHN V. BOWLES was the U.S. Army Recruiting Command Director of Command Psychological Operations and was located at the U.S. Army Soldier Support Institute in Columbia, South Carolina. He also serves as an assistant clinical professor in psychiatry and health behavior at the Medical College of Georgia in Augusta. Dr. Bowles has previously held positions as director of the LIFE Wellness Program, chief of Behavioral Medicine and chief of Organizational Health Psychology at Eisenhower Army Southeast Regional Medical Center in Augusta. He held a staff position at Tripler Army Medical Center and was the director of the Aeromedical Psychology Course and chief of Human Factors at the U.S. Army School of Aviation Medicine. He has an M.S.W. from Washington University in St. Louis and a Ph.D. in clinical psychology from the California School of Professional Psychology at Berkeley. He completed his internship at William Beaumont Army Medical Center in El Paso, Texas and his health psychology fellowship at Tripler Army Medical Center in Honolulu, Hawaii. His current research interests are in ASD and PTSD, aviation psychology, fitness/weight reduction, pregnancy loss, and recruiting and selection.

ANTHONY G. COMUZZIE is an associate scientist for the Southwest Foundation for Biomedical Research in San Antonio, Texas. The focus of his research is the genetic and environmental components of obesity. Dr. Comuzzie received his B.S. in biology and M.A. in biological anthropology from Texas A&M University in College Station. He received his Ph.D. in population genetics from The University of Kansas in Lawrence.

NIKHIL V. DHURANDHAR is currently an assistant professor and William Hardy Chair of Obesity Research in the Department of Nutrition and Food Science, Wayne State University, Detroit. Before moving to Wayne State, Dr. Dhurandhar was an assistant scientist and associate director of the Beers-Murphy Clinical Nutrition Center in the Clinical Nutrition Section of the Department of Medicine, University of Wisconsin School of Medicine. He received his M.S. in nutrition from North Dakota State University and his Ph.D. from the University of Bombay, India. Dr. Dhurandhar was also a medical practitioner in India, where he treated about 8,000 cases of obesity over an 8-year period. His research interests focus on the use of pharmacological aids in the treatment of obesity and, more recently, on virus-induced obesity.

GARY D. FOSTER is an assistant professor of psychology and clinical director of the Weight and Eating Disorders Program at the University of Pennsylvania School of Medicine. He received his B.S. from Duquesne University, his M.S. from the University of Pennsylvania, and his Ph.D. in clinical psychology from Temple University. He has published over 50 scientific studies, reviews, and book chapters on the causes and treatments of obesity. He also has considerable experience in the clinical aspects of obesity management, having treated obese patients in individual and group settings over the last 15 years.

FRANK GREENWAY is medical director and a professor at the Pennington Biomedical Research Center, a research campus of Louisiana State University.

He graduated from Stanford University and obtained an M.D. from the University of California at Los Angeles. He did his internship and residency in internal medicine and fellowship in endocrinology and metabolism at Harbor-UCLA Medical Center. Dr. Greenway practiced internal medicine, endocrinology and metabolism in Marina del Rey, California, from 1975 to 1995. During those years, he taught on the clinical faculty of UCLA and did obesity research, primarily through clinical trials of pharmacological agents. He moved to the Pennington Biomedical Research Center in 1995, where he has continued to do clinical research on the pharmacological treatment of obesity and its related diseases: diabetes, hypertension, and hyperlipidemia.

JOHN M. JAKICIC is currently an assistant professor at Brown University School of Medicine, with primary responsibilities in the Weight Control and Diabetes Research Center. Prior to his current position, Dr. Jakicic was an assistant professor at the University of Kansas and the University of Pittsburgh. While at the University of Pittsburgh, Dr. Jakicic was the scientific administrator of the Obesity/Nutrition Research Center. He received his Ph.D. from the University of Pittsburgh. Dr. Jakicic's primary research area is behavioral approaches for enhancing long-term weight loss. Currently, Dr. Jakicic is the principal investigator for three grants from the National Institutes of Health that focus on long-term weight loss and exercise adoption in overweight adults. He has published extensively in this area.

ANNE LOUCKS received her Ph.D. in physiology from the University of California at Santa Barbara. She did post-doctoral training and research in reproductive endocrinology at the University of California at San Diego School of Medicine. She is currently a professor and interim chair in the Department of Biological Sciences at Ohio University. Dr. Loucks' research in San Diego focused on characterizing the neuroendocrine profile of cyclic and amenorrheic athletes. At Ohio University, she has conducted short-term, prospective experiments to distinguish the independent effects of energy availability and exercise stress on LH pulsatility and metabolic substrates and hormones. Her current research is funded by the U.S. Army's Defense Women's Health Research Program. Dr. Loucks is a coauthor of the position stand of the American College of Sports Medicine on the Female Athlete Triad and a frequent participator in national and international meetings on the menstrual cycle.

PATRICK MAHLEN O'NEIL is a professor of psychiatry and behavioral sciences at the Medical University of South Carolina, where he is director of the Weight Management Center. He received his B.S. in economics from Louisiana State University and his M.S. and Ph.D. in clinical psychology from the University of Georgia. Dr. O'Neil has been professionally involved in obesity since 1977 in numerous clinical, teaching, research, and public education roles. He directs a long-standing, multidisciplinary weight-management center that offers services for people of all degrees overweight. His teaching activities include supervision of psychology interns on clinical rotations in the Center, lectures to medical and other student groups, and invited continuing education lectures to physician and other practitioner audiences. He is or has been principal investigator for a number of externally funded clinical trials of weight-loss agents and is the author of more than 100 professional publications, chapters, and presentations, primarily concerning psychological, behavioral, and other clinical aspects of obesity and its management. From 1987 to 1996, he authored *Weighing the Choices*, a weekly column on weight control in the Charleston, SC, *Sunday Post and Courier*. Dr. O'Neil has served on the Education Committee of the North American Association for the Study of Obesity (NAASO) since 1994 and is a member of the NAASO Ad Hoc Committee for Development of the Practical Guidelines. He is also immediate past president of the South Carolina Academy of Professional Psychologists, former member and chair of the South Carolina Board of Examiners in Psychology, and former chair of the Obesity and Eating Disorders Special Interest Group of the Association for the Advancement of Behavior Therapy.

LT COL LEON PAPPA was head, Training Programs Branch, Training and Education Division, Marine Corps Combat Development Command, Quantico, Virginia. An infantry officer commissioned in December 1979, he has held numerous operational assignments, both in CONUS and overseas. He reported to his current assignment in August 1995 from HQ Marine Forces Europe, Stuttgart, Germany. As head of training programs, he has oversight of a myriad of training-related programs, ranging from aviation training pipeline, recruit training, special operations, U.S. Navy field medical and religious programs, close combat, combat water survival training, physical fitness/weight control, and the Marine Corps ROTC program. Key assignments for Lt Col Pappa have included tours in the United Kingdom, Germany, recruit depot, Parris Island, Officer Candidate School, and operational tours with the 2nd battalion 8th Marines and 3rd battalion 3rd Marines, deploying to the Mediterranean, Lebanon, Okinawa, Thailand, and Southwest Asia.

LT COL JOANNE M. SPAHN was the Health Promotion Flight Commander at Elmendorf AFB, Alaska. She attended the College of St. Elizabeth in Morristown, New Jersey, where she received a B.S. in foods and nutrition. She was selected for the Air Force Dietetic Internship Program in 1982 and started her Air Force career at Malcolm Grow Medical Center, Andrews Air Force Base, Maryland. She served as chief of Medical Food Service at Tinker AFB, Oklahoma, from July 1983 to February 1986. During this time she also completed Squadron Officer's School and earned a M.S. in consumer studies from Oklahoma State University. In 1986 she transferred to Davis Monthan AFB, Arizona, as chief, Nutritional Medicine Service. In 1991 she started on an Air Force Institute of Technology assignment at the University of Arizona where she received a M.S. in human nutrition and was transferred back to Andrews AFB as chief, Clinical Dietetics, 89th Medical Group. In 1994, she became director of the USAF Dietetic Internship program and served in that capacity until July 1996. Lt Col Spahn completed Air Command and Staff College in 1996 and served as Nutritional Medicine Flight Commander at the 3rd Medical Group, Elmendorf AFB, Alaska, from 1996 to 1999. She has served as consultant dietitian, Pacific Air Forces, since 1996.

MARCIA STEFANICK received her B.S. in biology from the University of Pennsylvania in 1974 and her Ph.D. in physiology from Stanford University in 1982, focusing on reproductive physiology and neuroendocrinology. Subsequently, she did fellowship training in cardiovascular disease prevention at the Stanford Center for Research in Disease Prevention. In 1997, Dr. Stefanick was appointed an associate professor of medicine (with a courtesy appointment in gynecology and obstetrics) at Stanford University School of Medicine. Dr. Stefanick's research interests focus on the role of diet, exercise, and weight control in chronic disease prevention for both men and women, and in hormone replacement interventions for overall health issues of postmenopausal women. Dr. Stefanick is principal investigator of the Women's Health Initiative, which has a diet study focused on prevention of both breast and colon cancer and heart disease, a hormone study focused on cardiovascular disease prevention, and a calcium trial directed toward osteoporosis and prevention of hip and other bone fractures. Dr. Stefanick is also principal investigator of the Women's Healthy Eating and Living Trial, a diet study of women previously diagnosed with breast cancer. In addition, she is the research director of the Lipoprotein and Biochemistry Laboratory of the Stanford Center for Research in Disease Prevention.

JUNE STEVENS is an associate professor in the Departments of Nutrition and Epidemiology at the University of North Carolina-Chapel Hill. A graduate of the human nutrition program at Cornell University, her research career had its beginning in bench top studies of adipocytes from genetically obese rats. Her dissertation research was a clinical study of the effect of dietary fiber on food intake, gastrointestinal transit, and vitamin absorption in women. She pursued post-doctoral training in epidemiology and has since focused her career on population-based studies of obesity. Her current research examines the causes, consequences, and prevention of obesity with a focus on obesity-prone minority populations. She is principal investigator of the coordinating center for the Pathways study, a multicenter trial designed to develop and test a school-based intervention to prevent obesity in American Indian children. She also investigates the effects of obesity and fat patterning on chronic disease and mortality in African Americans. She has received attention from the popular press for her studies on the impact of age on the relationship between body weight and mortality. Dr. Stevens is an expert in epidemiological studies of obesity.

LOUIS F. TOMASI is a research physiologist for the U. S. Army Physical Fitness School (APFS). His primary responsibilities include independent research, writing army physical fitness doctrine, and teaching human performance and health-related classes for the master fitness trainer and exercise leader courses. Other fitness related projects associated with Dr. Tomasi are the civilian fitness program, physical training for pregnant soldiers, physical training for the retired officer association, and various local fitness agencies including the YMCA, American Heart Association, United States Swimming Association, regional swim teams, and many other fitness-related programs. His last project involved designing, administering, and analyzing the current army physical fitness test update study. Recently, he completed the fitness training unit exit and entrance requirement study for initial entry training. Dr. Tomasi's current project involves reviewing the hand position on the sit-up event on the APFT and developing standards for the alternate aerobic event. He is the liaison between the APFS and the American College of Sports Medicine and DSCPER process action team for fitness and health. In March 1992, Dr. Tomasi earned the Fort Benjamin Harrison Instructor of the Year and was nominated for TRADOC instructor of the year. Prior to his tenure at USAPFS, Dr. Tomasi served 13 years at the U. S. Military Academy, West Point, as an associate professor and head athletic trainer in the department of physical education. There, he was involved in community projects throughout the Hudson Valley. His earned degrees include a B.S. in physical education and biology from the University of Vermont; an M.S. from East Stroudsburg University, Pennsylvania, and a Ph.D. in education in biomechanics and physiology from New York University. Dr. Tomasi is a member of the American College of Sports Medicine, the National Athletic Trainers' Association, and other professional organizations.

CAPT TRISHA VORACHEK was a graduate student in the University of Minnesota School of Public Health. She will receive her degree this December and move to Maxwell AFB, Montgomery, Alabama, to be the Base Health Promotion Manager. Her previous assignment was at McConnel AFB, Wichita, Kansas, where she was one of four Air Force dietitians to conduct the Air Force Surgeon General's Super-Clinic Dietitian Study. The purpose of the study was to demonstrate the cost-effectiveness and need for dietitians in smaller Air Force communities, where traditionally, dietitians were not assigned. The study at McConnell AFB was highly successful, and currently a dietitian continues to be assigned there. McConnell AFB is where the Lifestyles, Exercise, Attitudes, and Nutrition (LEAN) program was developed.

LT DEBORAH WHITE was a research physiologist for the U.S. Navy, working in the Department of Operational Medicine, Naval Submarine Medical Research Laboratory, Groton, Connecticut. She received a B.S. from California

Polytechnic State University at San Luis Obispo (1988), California, and a Ph.D. in cardiovascular physiology from Colorado State University at Ft. Collins (1994). Her publications include papers on cardiovascular responses to central hypovolemia and lower body negative pressure, with emphasis on the effects of gender and fitness level on these responses. Before entering the Navy, LT White worked for a manufacturing company in the United Kingdom, working on the design, development, and testing of safety and survival equipment for fighter pilots and other military applications. Currently, she works as a program coordinator, overseeing the design, development, and testing of safety and survival equipment for submariners. LT White successfully completed Basic Enlisted Submarine School in October 1997 and is an active member of the Naval Submarine League and the Aerospace Medical Association.

C

Biographical Sketches of the Subcommittee on Military Weight Management

RICHARD ATKINSON (*Chair*) is director of the Obesity Institute of the MedStar Research Institute in Washington, D.C. Formerly, he was professor of medicine and nutritional sciences and director of the Beers-Murphy Clinical Nutrition Center at the University of Wisconsin-Madison. Previously he was a professor of internal medicine and chief, Division of Clinical Nutrition at the Eastern Virginia Medical School, and chief of staff for research and development, and chief, Medical Research Service at the VA Medical Center in Hampton, Virginia. Dr. Atkinson also served in the military as division surgeon for the 101st Airborne Division, and chief of the Department of Medicine at the U.S. Army Hospital, Fort Campbell, Kentucky following a 2-year tour as endocrine fellow at the Walter Reed Army Hospital. Dr. Atkinson's research has focused on a variety of interventions (surgical, behavioral, and pharmacological) for the treatment and prevention of obesity. He is a former member of the Committee on Military Nutrition Research.

JOHN E. VANDERVEEN (*Vice-Chair*) is a former director of the Food and Drug Administration's (FDA) Office of Plant and Dairy Foods and Beverages in Washington, D.C. His previous position at FDA was director of the Division of Nutrition at the Center for Food Safety and Applied Nutrition. He also served in various capacities at the U.S. Air Force (USAF) School of Aerospace Medicine at Brooks Air Force Base, Texas. He has received accolades for service from FDA and USAF. Dr. Vanderveen is a member of the American Society for Clinical Nutrition, American Institute of Nutrition, Aerospace Medical Association, American Dairy Science Association, Institute of Food Technologists, and American Chemical Society. In the past, he was the treasurer of the American Society of Clinical Nutrition and a member of the Institute of Food Technology, National Academy of Sciences Advisory Committee. Dr. Vanderveen holds a B.S. in agriculture from Rutgers University in New Jersey and a Ph.D. in chemistry from the University of New Hampshire.

WILLIAM DIETZ is the director of the Division of Nutrition and Physical Activity in the National Center for Chronic Disease Prevention and Health Promotion at the Centers for Disease Control and Prevention (CDC). Prior to his appointment at CDC, he was a professor of pediatrics at the Tufts University School of Medicine and director of clinical nutrition at the Floating Hospital of New England Medical Center Hospitals. He received his B.A. from Wesleyan University in 1966 and his M.D. from the University of Pennsylvania in 1970. Following an internship at Children's Hospital of Philadelphia, he spent 3 years in the Middle America Research Unit of the National Institute of Allergy and Infectious Diseases in Panama studying insect-borne viruses. After the completion of his residency at Upstate Medical Center, he received a Ph.D. in nutritional biochemistry from Massachusetts Institute of Technology (MIT). Dr. Dietz was a principal research scientist at the MIT/Harvard Division of Health Science and Technology, associate director of the Clinical Research Center at MIT, and director of the Boston Obesity/Nutrition Research Center. He served on the counsel of the American Society for Clinical Nutrition and is a past president of the North American Association for the Study of Obesity. In 1995, he received the John Stalker Award from the American School Food Service Association for his efforts to improve school lunches. Dr. Dietz served on the 1995 Dietary Guidelines Advisory Committee and is a past member of the National Institute of Diabetes and Digestive and Kidney Diseases Task Force on Obesity and president-elect of the American Society for Clinical Nutrition. In 1998, Dr. Dietz was elected to the Institute of Medicine of the National Academies. In 2000, he received the William G. Anderson Award from the American Alliance for Health, Physical Education, Recreation, and Dance. In 2002, he received the Holroyd-Sherry award for his outstanding contributions to the field of children, adolescents, and the media.

JOHN D. FERNSTROM is a professor of psychiatry, pharmacology, and neuroscience at the University of Pittsburgh School of Medicine and research director of the UPMC Health System Weight Management Center. He received his B.S. in biology and his Ph.D. in nutritional biochemistry from the Massachusetts Institute of Technology (MIT). He was a postdoctoral fellow in neuroendocrinology at the Roche Institute for Molecular Biology in Nutley, New Jersey. Before coming to the University of Pittsburgh, Dr. Fernstrom was an assistant and then associate professor in the Department of Nutrition and Food Science at MIT. He served on numerous governmental advisory committees and is a member of several professional societies, including the American Society for Nutritional Sciences, the American Society for Clinical Nutrition, The North American Society for the Study of Obesity, the American Physiological Society, the American Society for Pharmacology and Experimental Therapeutics, the American Society for Neurochemistry, the Society for Neuroscience, and the Endocrine Society. Among other awards, Dr.

Fernstrom received the Mead-Johnson Award of the American Society for Nutritional Sciences, a Research Scientist Award from the National Institute of Mental Health, a Wellcome Visiting Professorship in the Basic Medical Sciences, and an Alfred P. Sloan Fellowship in Neurochemistry. His current research interests include the influence of the diet and drugs (particularly appetite suppressants) on neurotransmitters in the central and peripheral nervous systems.

ARTHUR FRANK, an internist, is the medical director of the George Washington University Weight Management Program in Washington, D.C. He received his B.S. in chemistry from the Massachusetts Institute of Technology, his M.S. in biochemistry from the University of Pennsylvania, and his M.D. from New York University. His residency was completed at the Stanford Medical Center. He was a U.S. Public Health Service post-doctoral fellow in endocrinology and metabolism at Stanford and a post-doctoral fellow at the National Heart Institute. Subsequently, he directed the food and nutrition programs at the Office of Economic Opportunity and served as an adviser to the Assistant Secretary for Health at the Department of Health and Human Services. He has been responsible for the provision and management of medical care of overweight and obese patients since 1977. He has been the principle investigator in a number of clinical research trials involving the pharmacotherapy of obesity. His research interests also involve the development of systems for the organization and evaluation of weight-management services (he was on the National Academies committee that wrote the book *Weighing the Options*) and the evaluation and measurement of the maintenance of weight loss. Dr. Frank has been the chairman of the Clinical Committee of the North American Association for the Study of Obesity (NAASO). In this position he was responsible for facilitating NAASO's increasing involvement in the scientific aspects of clinical activities. He has been a member of the Board of Directors and treasurer of the American Obesity Association since its inception and has actively participated in litigation related to the protection of the rights of obese patients who were subjected to discrimination.

BARBARA C. HANSEN is the director of the Obesity and Diabetes Research Center at the University of Maryland School of Medicine and a professor of physiology. She received her B.S. and M.S. from the University of California, Los Angeles. She completed a Ph.D. in physiology and psychology at the University of Washington, Seattle. Dr. Hansen is a past president of the North American Association for the Study of Obesity and served as the first president of the International Association for the Study of Obesity for four years. She was president of the American Society for Clinical Nutrition from 1995 to 1996. She is a member of the Institute of Medicine and has served on its program committee and in other consulting roles. Dr. Hansen has also served as a member of several organizations, including the Advisory Committee to the Director of the National Institutes of Health, the U.S.-Japan Nutrition and Metabolism Panel, and the Armed Forces Epidemiological Board of the Department of Defense. She has published extensively in biomedical journals and lectures widely in the field of obesity and diabetes. Dr. Hansen is an associate editor of the *Journal of Obesity Research* and coeditor of *Diabetes/Metabolism Research and Reviews* and has served as associate editor/editorial board roles for *Diabetes Care*, *International Journal of Obesity*, *International Journal of Primatology*, and *Journal of Parental and Enteral Nutrition*. Dr. Hansen's laboratory is involved in the study and evaluation of new compounds for the treatment of diabetes, obesity, and dyslipidemia.

STEVEN B. HEYMSFIELD is a professor of medicine at Columbia University, College of Physicians and Surgeons in New York. He also serves as deputy director of the New York Obesity Research Center and is director of the Human Body Composition Laboratory. Dr. Heymsfield is immediate past president of the American Society of Parenteral and Enteral Nutrition and is an active member of the American Society of Clinical Nutrition and the North American Society for the Study of Obesity. He was recently made an honorary member of the American Dietetic Association. He received his B.A. in chemistry from Hunter College of the City University of New York and his M.D. from Mt. Sinai School of Medicine. Dr. Heymsfield has done extensive research and has clinical experience in the areas of body composition, weight cycling, nutrition, and obesity, especially as they relate to women.

ROBIN B. KANAREK is dean of the Graduate School of Arts and Sciences and professor of psychology and nutrition at Tufts University in Medford, Massachusetts. Her prior experience includes research fellow, Division of Endocrinology, University of California, Los Angeles School of Medicine and research fellow in nutrition at Harvard University. In addition to reviewing for several journals, including *Science*, *Brain Research Bulletin*, *Journal of Nutrition*, *American Journal of Clinical Nutrition*, and *Annals of Internal Medicine*, she is a member of the editorial boards of *Physiology and Behavior* and the *Tufts Diet and Nutrition Newsletter* and is a past editor-in-chief of *Nutrition and Behavior*. Dr. Kanarek has served on ad hoc review committees for the National Science Foundation, National Institutes of Health, and U.S. Department of Agriculture nutrition research, as well as the Member Program Committee of the Eastern Psychological Association. She is a fellow of the American College of Nutrition, and her other professional memberships include the American Society for Nutritional Sciences, New York Academy of Sciences, Society for the Study of Ingestive Behavior, and Society for Neurosciences. Dr. Kanarek received a B.A. in biology from Antioch College in Yellow Springs,

Ohio, and an M.S. and a Ph.D. in psychology from Rutgers University in New Brunswick, New Jersey.

BARBARA J. MOORE is president and chief executive officer of Shape Up America!, a national initiative to promote healthy weight and increased physical activity in the United States. Committed to providing achievable science-based messages, Shape Up America! was founded by C. Everett Koop in 1994. Dr. Moore joined in June 1995 and serves as key liaison with the scientific, professional, and corporate communities. Dr. Moore earned a B.S. from Skidmore College and an M.S. and Ph.D. in nutrition from Columbia University. She has several years of postdoctoral training at the University of California at Davis. Dr. Moore was appointed a Henry Rutgers Fellow at Rutgers University, where she held a tenure track position in the Department of Nutritional Sciences. After leaving academia, Dr. Moore served as general manager of program development and primary technical policy advisor for Weight Watchers International. Dr. Moore joined the Executive Office of the President in 1993 as acting assistant for social and behavioral science in the Office of Science and Technology Policy. She was involved in the process of policy formation and budgetary support of fundamental scientific research policy. Prior to joining Shape Up America!, Dr. Moore worked at the National Institutes of Health, Division of Nutrition Research Coordination, where she was responsible for providing guidance on nutrition policy and dietary guidance materials promulgated by the federal government. In this position, Dr. Moore focused on the development of the 1994 Progress Report to the Assistant Secretary of Health on the nutrition objectives of Healthy People 2000. She maintains active membership in the American Society for Nutritional Sciences, American Society for Clinical Nutrition, North American Association for the Study of Obesity, Society for the Study of Ingestive Behavior, and Sigma Xi.

MARY I. POOS (*FNB Staff, Study Director*) is project director for the Committee on Military Nutrition Research. She joined the Food and Nutrition Board (FNB) of the Institute of Medicine in November 1997. She has been a project director for the National Academies since 1990. Prior to officially joining the FNB staff, she served as a project director for the National Research Council's Board on Agriculture for more than seven years, two of which were spent on loan to FNB. Her work with FNB includes senior staff officer for the IOM report *The Program of Research for Military Nursing* and study director for the reports *A Review of the Department of Defense's Program for Breast Cancer Research* and *Vitamin C Fortification of Food Aid Commodities.* Currently, she also serves as study director to the Subcommittee on Interpretation and Uses of Dietary Reference Intakes. While working with the Board on Agriculture, Dr. Poos was responsible for the Committee on Animal Nutrition and directed the production of seven reports in the *Nutrient Requirements of Domestic Animals* series, including a letter report to the commissioner of the Food and Drug Administration concerning the importance of selenium in animal nutrition. Prior to joining the National Academies, she was consultant/owner of Nutrition Consulting Services of Greenfield, Massachusetts; assistant professor in the Department of Veterinary and Animal Sciences at the University of Massachusetts, Amherst; and adjunct assistant professor in the Department of Animal Sciences, University of Vermont. She received her B.S. in biology from Virginia Polytechnic Institute and State University and a Ph.D. in animal sciences (nutrition/biochemistry) from the University of Kentucky. She completed a postdoctoral fellowship in the Department of Animal Sciences Area of Excellence Program at the University of Nebraska.

D

Acronyms

AA	Asian American
AD	Active duty
AFB	Air Force base
AI	American Indian
AN	Alaska Native
APFS	Army physical fitness school
APFS	Army physical fitness test
AR	Army regulation
AWCP	Army weight control program
BCT	Basic combat training
BF	Body fat
BMI	Body mass index
BOTS	Basic Officer Training School
BUMED	Bureau of Medicine and Surgery
CDPCP	Command-directed physical conditioning program
CEA	Cost effectiveness analysis
CFL	Command fitness leader
CHD	Coronary heart disease
CHO	Carbohydrate
CLA	Conjugated linoleic acid
CMNR	Committee on Military Nutrition Research
CNS	Central nervous system
CONUS	Continential United States
CVD	Cardiovascular disease
DEA	U.S. Drug Enforcement Agency
DHEA	Dehydroepiandrosterone

DMED	Defense medical epidemiology database
DOD	U.S. Department of Defense
DNA	Deoxyribonucleic acid
DRG	Diagnosis related group
FDA	U.S. Food and Drug Administration
FEP	Fitness Enhancement Program
FFM	Fat-free mass
FNB	Food and Nutrition Board
GnRH	Gonadotropin-releasing hormone
GW	Gastric wrapping
HAWC	Health and Wellness Center
HCA	Hydroxycitrate
HDL	High-density lipoprotein
HMB	Beta-hydroxy-beta-methylbutyrate
HPA	Hypothalamic-pituitary adrenal
HPM	Health promotion manager
HRT	Hormone replacement therapy
IC	Immediate Commander
IDC	Independent Duty Corpsman
LBM	Lean body mass
LDL	Low-density lipoprotein
LH	Luteinizing hormone
LEAN	Lifestyle, exercise, attitude, and nutrition
MAJCOM	Major Command
MAW	Maximum allowable weight
MD	Medical doctor
MFT	Master fitness trainer
MO	Medical officer
MOS	Military operational specialities
MRE	Meals ready to eat
MTF	Medical treatment facilities
MWR	Morale, welfare, and recreation
NE	Norepinephrine
NHANES	National Health and Nutrition Examination Survey
NIH	National Institutes of Health

NOS	Not otherwise specified
NP	Nurse practioner
NWCR	National weight control registry
OA	Overeaters anonyomous
OTC	Over-the-counter
PA	Physicians assistant
PCS	Permanent change of station
PFA	Physical Fitness Assessment
PI	Pacific Islander
PME	Professional military education
PRT	Physical Readiness Test
PT	Physical training
QTL	Quantitative trait loci
RCMAS	Retrospective case mix analysis system
RD	Registered dietitian
REE	Resting energy expenditure
RER	Respiratory exchange rate
RMR	Resting metabolic rate
RPCP	Remedial Physical Conditioning Program
SBWC	Shipboard weight-control program
SES	Socioeconomic status
SS	Shipshape
SSRI	Selective serotonin reuptake inhibitors
T_3	triiodothyronine
TDY	Temporary duty away
TMD	Temporary medical deferral
UC	Unit commander
UCP	Uncoupling protein
USAMRMC	U.S. Army Medical Research and Materiel Command
USDA	U.S. Department of Agriculture
VBG	Vertical banded gastroplasty
VLCD	Very-low-calorie diets
VO_{2max}	Maximal oxygen consumption
W	Waist circumference

WBFMP	Weight and Body Fat Management Program
WMP	Weight management program